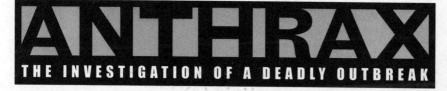

ANTHRAX
THE INVESTIGATION OF A DEADLY OUTBREAK

JEANNE GUILLEMIN

UNIVERSITY OF
CALIFORNIA
PRESS

berkeley | los angeles | london

The quotation in Chap. 1 from Homer, *Iliad,*
trans. R. Fitzgerald, is reprinted by permission of
Doubleday, a division of Bantam Doubleday Dell
Publishing Group, Inc. The quotation in Chap. 1
from Virgil, *Georgics,* is from the Loeb Classical
Library, *Virgil,* Vol. 1, trans. H. Rushton Fair-
clough, Cambridge, Mass.: Harvard University
Press, 1916, rev. 1935. The quotation in Chap. 9
from Osip Mandelstam is reprinted with the
permission of Scribner, a Division of Simon &
Schuster, Inc., from *Osip Mandelstam: Selected
Poems*, trans. Clarence Brown and W. S. Merwin.
Copyright © 1979 Clarence Brown and W. S.
Merwin. The quotation in Chap. 26 from Pushkin,
Feast in Time of Plague, trans. E. M. Kayden, is
reprinted by permission of the University of
Colorado Foundation, Inc.

University of California Press
Berkeley and Los Angeles, California

University of California Press, Ltd.
London, England

First Paperback Printing 2001

Library of Congress Cataloging-in-Publication Data

Guillemin, Jeanne, 1943–.
    Anthrax : the investigation of a deadly
outbreak / Jeanne Guillemin.
      p.   cm.
    Includes bibliographical references and index.
    ISBN 0-520-22917-7 (pbk. : alk. paper)
    1. Anthrax—Russia—Ekaterinburg—
Epidemiology.   2. Biological weapons—
Russia—Ekaterinburg.   I. Title.

RA644.A6G85   1999
614.5'61'094743—dc21   99-32927
                        CIP

Printed in the United States of America

10 09 08 07 06 05 04 03 02 01
10 9 8 7 6 5 4 3 2

The paper used in this publication meets
the minimum requirements of ANSI/NISO
Z39.48-1992 (R 1997) (Permanence of Paper). ∞

ANTHRAX

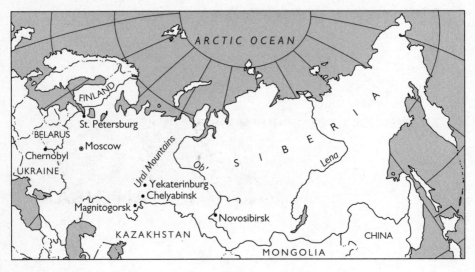

Russia

Contents

Illustrations follow pages 142 and 238.

Maps 1–3 appear at the end of the second illustration section.

List of Figures

Preface

The tragic event described in this book is unique, and I hope it will remain so. Twenty years ago, in April 1979, the Soviet city of Sverdlovsk was suddenly struck by an epidemic of anthrax, a disease rare in humans and, in its worst forms, highly lethal. Reportedly, sixty-four people died, although U.S. intelligence sources claimed the toll might have reached a thousand. *Bacillus anthracis* is found naturally in soil and can infect grazing livestock, whose tainted meat or hides can pass it on to humans. The disease has long been familiar in Russia and still persists in many rural parts of the world. Yet in the last sixty years anthrax has also been developed as a biological weapon—by Japan, Britain, Canada, the United States, and the Soviet Union. Had the USSR in 1979 been developing anthrax as part of its Cold War arsenal, even though it was party to the Biological Weapons Convention, which forbids such activity? Or was the Sverdlovsk outbreak the result of contaminated meat being sold in the city, a breakdown in public health and sanitation?

On one level, this book is a detective story that aims to determine an unknown cause of death in all its detail. But it is also an account of a scientific investigation, within which the facts about the epidemic—not suppositions or guesses—were the only goal. From the first, political ideology, hearsay, and media distortions threatened to bury not only the facts but the real human tragedy of the Sverdlovsk outbreak. Only the end of the Cold War and the creation of a new Russia permitted a working team to make inquiries in the city in 1992 and, with the help of Russian colleagues, to subsequently piece together what information time and political censorship had not destroyed.

Ludwig Fleck in *The Genesis and Development of a Scientific Fact* maintains that the scientist should remain modestly in the background. The reader is advised that, far from staying in the shadows, I present this investigation very much in the first person, exposing its process of fact-finding as both an emotional and an intellectual experience. The insights of a wide range of writers on gender and science, from Londa Schiebinger to Evelyn Fox Keller, have made it much easier for me to appreciate the integration of the subjective and the objective in the process of research. Every scientific quest has its high and low moments, its times of confusion and doubt. At the same time there is nothing like the satisfaction of having tracked the evidence, checked it against multiple sources, and solved a mystery.

For me there has been an additional benefit to this quest. My previous field research took me to the British West Indies, to Canadian Indian reserves, and to elite American and European hospitals to study the culture of medicine. Yet, raised in a conservative Catholic family in the 1950s, I had more qualms about venturing to the Soviet Union than about immersing myself in those other societies. My childhood (like that of many others in my generation) was regularly punctuated with drills to prepare us for a nuclear bomb attack from the USSR; at the same time, in my grade school, we prayed for the salvation of atheist Russians. I was well out of college before I learned that my family is related to John Reed, author of *Ten Days That Shook the World* and the only American buried as a hero in the Kremlin Wall in Moscow. The connection was, given the tenor of the times, something of an embarrassment. So on my first visit to the Soviet Union in 1988, to interview physicians about the health care system, I went with great trepidation. If the political climate then was not exactly reassuring, two later visits to Moscow, during the heady days when democracy was in ascendance, were extremely gratifying. Embarking for Russia once again in 1992, I had the sense, later confirmed, that the moment was perfect for the open communication that is vital to science—and that it might not last. We had but a short time to retrieve precious information from different quarters.

The troubles that beset the Soviet Union are part of the present Russian dilemma: decaying bureaucracies, political cronyism, pervasive cynicism about law and authority, to name a few. Yet, and this was the surprise for me, Russians are still Europeans, even in the outlying cities of the Urals, and therefore not so terribly foreign or exotic. I found myself enjoying them and was eager to understand them better. Not fluent in the language, I nonetheless took pleasure improving my command of it, and drew on some of the literature Russia has given the world—Chekhov, Pasternak, Akhmatova, Mandelstam, and Tsvetaeva—as windows to this compelling culture. Had there been a substantial social science literature, I would gladly have relied on that as well, but the Soviet Union was harshest in subverting that kind of knowledge. Throughout the Cold War, American journalists have also provided a window on Russian life and politics. Another whole book should be written about that contribution which, though never disinterested and at times distorted, can be a powerful lens for understanding current events. The work of David Remnick, Eleanor Randolph, and David Hoffman, among others, sets the current standard. Whatever criticism one might levy against contemporary Russia, one cannot ignore its problems, though they seem as vast as its geography and its enormous resources in people, industry, and nature.

The driving force in this investigation has been Matthew Meselson, Thomas Dudley Cabot Professor of the Natural Sciences at Harvard University, and also my husband. We met by chance in 1981 at the Aspen Institute in Colorado at a conference on health care, ethics, and science. The participants' presentations alternated widely, even wildly, between the social organization of medicine and stunning revelations about the new biotechnologies. Matthew and I were married in 1986.

In that same year, Matthew had become involved in investigating U.S. allegations that the Soviet Union aided Laotians in attacking Hmong tribes with dangerous trichothecene mycotoxins—known as Yellow Rain. I immediately joined in that inquiry and interviewed Hmong refugees in Rhode Island and Minnesota, as well as officials from the United Nations and the U.S. and other governments who played a part in the controversy. (Particularly memorable was the meeting with an ex-CIA agent at a McDonald's in Arlington, Virginia. A Joseph Conrad figure who had spent years in Southeast Asia, he claimed to have killed several men with his big, bare hands.) The inquiry eventually revealed that harmless bee feces, not mycotoxins, were misinterpreted by the U.S. government as evidence of Yellow Rain attacks. Through the Freedom of Information Act, I was able to obtain U.S. army cable traffic showing that the initial Yellow Rain reports were probably based on rumor, though no one could deny the Hmong were brutally mistreated by the Laotian government, in some measure because of their alliance with the United States during the Vietnam War.

The Yellow Rain investigation was good practice for the Sverdlovsk project. Both were fundamentally private academic inquiries into arms control controversies that the governments concerned seemed unable to resolve. In both studies, if there was the likelihood of being rebuffed or seen as a threat by one or more government agencies or individuals, there was also the freedom to keep up the scientific investigation until the mystery was solved.

The work of Matthew Meselson and his colleague in the Harvard-Sussex Program, Julian Perry Robinson, has been a consistent, unique force against biological and chemical weapons for more than thirty years. Before the ebbing of the Cold War drew heightened attention to biological and chemical weapons, these two advocates for disarmament promoted the 1972 Biological Weapons Convention and its strengthening and laid the groundwork for the 1993 Chemical Weapons Convention. With passionate diligence and scientific expertise they have kept the world informed of the risks of arms proliferation. It has been a privilege to work with them both, and a special bonus to be included on the team that went to Russia to investigate the 1979 anthrax outbreak. Matthew and I have had our share of disagreements about the results of this research, the ambiguities of which preoccupied us throughout the 1990s. He is an exacting scientist, not easily drawn to conclusions. In this venture to the Urals, I believe I convinced him that the social science perspective can bring a needed balance to medical and scientific facts. Without his extraordinary persistence in tracking the source of the 1979 outbreak, irrefutable evidence of the cause of the nearly seventy deaths in Sverdlovsk would probably never have been revealed and certainly this chronicle would not exist. Of late, the attitude of some who followed accounts of the Sverdlovsk anthrax outbreak has been that they knew the source of the outbreak all along. In truth, until this project reached completion no one had more than suspicions. In matters of death, suspicions are simply not enough.

Many people played a part in the ultimate success of our investigation. Faina Abramova, Irina Belaeva, Sergei Borisov, Lev Grinberg, Margarita Ilyenko, Larissa Mishustina, Ilona Popova, Vladimir Shepetkin, Paragoriy Suetin, Alexey Yablokov, and Olga Yampolskaya all helped keep the 1979 Sverdlovsk victims from being forgotten. My thanks go also to the Ural State University, the public officials in Yekaterinburg (as Sverdlovsk is once again called) who gave us their time, and the staff at the Military Museum there; to the John T. and Catherine D. MacArthur Foundation for field research support; to Boston College for research grants; and to the O'Neill Library staff and the Harvard University libraries as well. I also thank the colleagues and friends who criticized the manuscript in its various phases, especially Paul Doty, my brother J. B. Garrigan, Zvi and Diane Griliches, Hugh Gusterson, Peter Pringle, Julian Robinson, and Betsy Seifter. Important document translation came from Irina Arkipova, Cynthia Simmons, Alexis Shelokov, Stephan Turek, and Svetlana Tutorskaya, and organizational genius from Barbara Ring. Special mention must be made of the U.S. Foreign Broadcast Information Service, an invaluable means for translating Soviet and now Russian media. The photographs of Sophia Bliumova, Anna Komina, Mukhametalin Mukhametshin, and Alexey Syskov are courtesy of Martin Hugh-Jones; all other photos are my own or are from the Sverdlovsk project files of Matthew Meselson. Howard Boyer, my editor at the University of California Press, lived up to his excellent reputation for responsible commitment to the manuscript in all its phases; Jan Spauschus Johnson skillfully guided this book to completion; and Ellen F. Smith's copy-editing was superb. My special appreciation goes to Ivanna Bergese, a peerless research and editorial assistant, to Erik Dowling for computer graphics, and to Matthew Meselson for production of Maps 1–3. With all this help, I nonetheless remain responsible for any flaws in this book.

I have made a special effort to include as much about deceased victims of the epidemic as possible, especially their names. The last names of survivors of the 1979 outbreak, as well as various neighbors and friends, are indicated by a first letter only. The names of victims who died are complete, as a way of memorializing them. For readers unfamiliar with Russian, many of the victims' names, as well as those of other Russians who figure in this story, will seem difficult to remember and to distinguish. I have attempted consistency in spelling these names, although there are a few variations where individuals themselves indicated a preference (for example, Sergei instead of Sergey). A list of the victims' names is included at the back of the book, as Appendix A, and a guide to names of principal participants described in this account follows the table of contents.

This book is dedicated to Matthew Meselson and Julian Perry Robinson; to the 1979 anthrax victims and their families and friends in Yekaterinburg; and to the next generation, that it may inherit sufficient controls over biological weapons, and all weapons of mass destruction, to live in freedom, peace, and dignity.

Principal Participants

The following list gives names and background information for the important figures in the investigation of the 1979 anthrax outbreak in Sverdlovsk, including the other American members of the team and the many Russians who contributed significantly to our efforts. A list of those who died in 1979 can be found in Appendix A. For simplicity's sake, throughout the text, I generally use only Russian first and last names, without the traditional patronymic. Also, in stories that combine the personal and the professional, as this one does, it is always a question how to refer to those who are more than colleagues. I have chosen to use first names for those with whom I have close personal relationships.

Dr. Faina Abramova, chief pathologist at Hospital 40 in Sverdlovsk during the 1979 anthrax outbreak.

Dr. Viktor Arenskiy, epidemiologist during the 1979 epidemic and, in 1992, chief of the Sverdlovsk Medical Institute.

Dr. Nikolay Babich, in 1979 head of the Sverdlovsk Oblast Sanitary Epidemiological Station (SES).

Professor Irina Belaeva of the Ural State University, interpreter and colleague in 1993 and 1998 trips to Yekaterinburg.

Dr. Ivan Bezdenezhnikh, chief epidemiologist for the Russian Republic, who was in Sverdlovsk in the last two weeks of April 1979.

Professor Sergei Borisov, physicist at the Ural State University who organized meetings for the American team during the 1992 study visit.

Dr. Pyotr Burgasov, Soviet Deputy Minister of Health in charge of the official USSR medical and public health response to the 1979 outbreak and chief spokesman in 1988 for the official explanation of its cause.

Dr. Tamara Chernich, head of the health clinic at the ceramics factory in 1979 and still head in 1993.

Dr. Lev Grinberg, pathologist who was Dr. Abramova's assistant in 1979 and later the head of the Tuberculosis and Pulmonary Diseases Unit, Yekaterinburg.

Professor Vladimir Gubanov, physicist at the Ural State University who assisted the 1992 team in having the university serve as its host in Yekaterinburg.

Yuriy Gusev, director of the ceramics factory in 1979 and still director in 1993.

Dr. Martin Hugh-Jones, professor of veterinary medicine, Louisiana State University, Baton Rouge, consultant to the World Health Organization on anthrax, and member of the 1992 study team.

Dr. Margarita Ilyenko, head of Hospital 24 in 1979 and 1992.

General A. T. Kharechko, in 1992 and subsequently the head of Military Compound 19.

Dr. Yakov Klipnitzer, head of Hospital 20 in Chkalovskiy rayon during the 1979 epidemic.

Dr. Vladimir Krasnoperov, in 1993 the chief veterinarian of the Yekaterinburg Sanitary Epidemiological Station (SES).

Dr. Alexander Langmuir, retired Chief Epidemiologist at the Centers for Disease Control, Atlanta, and project mentor.

Professor Anatoliy Marenkov, sociologist of education at the Ural State University who introduced his colleague Professor Ilona Nikonova (Popova) to the 1992–93 study.

Matthew Meselson, Thomas Dudley Cabot Professor of the Natural Sciences, Harvard University, and the organizer and leader of the 1992 team.

Larissa Mishustina, a journalist and Peoples Deputy who in 1991 successfully petitioned President Boris Yeltsin for pensions to compensate the families of victims of the 1979 epidemic.

Dr. Vladimir I. Nikiforov, chief of infectious diseases at Botkin hospital in Moscow and head clinician in Sverdlovsk during the 1979 outbreak.

Dr. Vladimir V. Nikiforov, son of the above Dr. Nikiforov and also a specialist in infectious diseases at the Botkin Hospital.

Professor Ilona Nikonova (later Popova) of the Ural State University, project interpreter and researcher in 1992 and 1993.

Dr. D. N. Ponomaryev, chief epidemiologist for the Sverdlovsk oblast in 1979.

Dr. Viktor Romanenko, public health epidemiologist in 1979 and in 1992 Assistant Chief Inspector of the Sverdlovsk Oblast Sanitary Epidemiological Station (SES).

Dr. Yuriy Semyonov, in 1992 the director of the Sverdlovsk Oblast Sanitary Epidemiological Station (SES).

Dr. Vladimir Sergiev, in 1979 secretary to Dr. Burgasov; accompanied Drs. Burgasov and V. N. Nikiforov on their 1988 trip to the United States and was later director of the Institute of Medical Parisitology and Tropical Medicine, Moscow.

Dr. Alexis Shelokov, public health and vaccine expert from the Salk Institute who also served as an interpreter for the American team.

Rector Parigoriy Suetin, physicist and in 1992 head of the Ural State University, the team's host institution in 1992.

Dr. Yevgeniy Sverdlov, head of the Institute of Molecular Genetics, our Moscow base for the 1992 study trip.

Dr. David Walker, head of the Pathology Department at the University of Texas Medical Branch, Galveston, and 1992 team member.

Dr. Alexey Yablokov, in 1992 Russian Counselor of the Environment and Public Health and later advisor to the government on environmental affairs, who successfully promoted the national law criminalizing chemical and biological weapons development, production, and use.

Dr. Olga Yampolskaya, specialist in infectious diseases at Botkin Hospital, Moscow, and Dr. V. N. Nikiforov's assistant, who treated victims of the 1979 anthrax outbreak and was also a member of the 1992 study team.

Boris Yeltsin, Communist Party boss of Sverdlovsk oblast in 1979 and first democratically elected president of Russia.

General Valentin Yevstigneyev, in 1992 and subsequently Russian Federation Chief of Directorate for Protection Against Biological Weapons and in the 1980s science director at Military Compound 19, Sverdlovsk.

Anthrax

ACCURSED FIRE
AND BIOLOGICAL WEAPON

Tuesday, June 2, 1992. After a long transatlantic flight from New York, our research team arrives in the new post-Soviet Russia, a nation that six months before did not exist. We are in the first stage of a trip to investigate the cause of the worst anthrax epidemic recorded in a modern industrial nation. The outbreak occurred in April and May 1979 in Sverdlovsk, an industrial city in the Ural Mountains, nine hundred miles east of Moscow. According to Soviet reports, by the time it was over, at least sixty-four people had died from this rare disease.

Leading the team is Matthew Meselson, a Harvard University biologist. I am the expedition's anthropologist, from Boston College, a Jesuit university that has unblinkingly supported my research for nearly twenty years. Matthew and I are also husband and wife. Doing research with a spouse can be problematic, especially when both are strong-minded individuals. Working on a politically charged issue in a foreign country can compound the difficulties, particularly when that country is the former Soviet Union, where censorship and political repression were the norm. But we have researched and written together before, on the "Yellow Rain" controversy. That investigation, during the 1980s, involved clarifying whether or not a dangerous mycotoxin had, with Soviet assistance, been used by Laos against its Hmong minority.[1] By 1991, when Matthew began recruiting the Sverdlovsk team, I was well immersed in the details of this new problem and had made several trips to the Soviet Union, although none with the purpose and potential of this foray.

Matthew's commitment to discovering the Sverdlovsk epidemic's cause goes back to 1980, when he was consulted by the CIA after news of the event leaked to the West. In the years that followed, the world learned little about the outbreak, though speculations and suspicions abounded. Claims by a few Soviet dissidents that an explosion in a secret biological weapons laboratory caused thousands of deaths were countered by the Soviet government's contention that a much smaller number of people died from eating anthrax-infected meat sold on the black market. For years, Matthew, who has long been an advocate for the prohibition of chemical and biological weapons, has requested permission from the USSR for impartial experts to investigate the outbreak firsthand, but these requests have been denied.[2] After the dissolution of the Soviet Union, however, the political doors have opened for our travel to Sverdlovsk, which has reclaimed its prerevolutionary name, Yekaterinburg. We have allowed ourselves only two weeks to attempt to discover conclusive evidence about the source of the 1979 anthrax deaths.

My part of the assignment is to interview the victims' families, if I can find them. We have no record of names or addresses. Yekaterinburg, an industrial city with a population of 1.2 million, as yet has no public telephone directory. Nonetheless, I optimistically carry in my suitcase a hundred copies of a brief questionnaire that I have prepared and tested in translation. Our team brings other expertise to the expedition. The congenial Dr. Alexis Shelokov, who speaks fluent Russian, is a vaccine expert from the Salk Institute with a long career in public health. The more reserved Dr. David Walker is chief of pathology at the University of Texas Medical Branch in Galveston. We are hoping that reports in the Russian press will prove true, that autopsy samples have been preserved by two pathologists who worked during the 1979 outbreak.

The fifth member of our team is veterinarian Martin Hugh-Jones from Louisiana State University, a member of the World Health Organization's Anthrax Research and Control Working Group, and an avid world traveler. The veterinary perspective is essential. Anthrax is a zoonosis, a disease that can travel from animals to humans. It is almost always associated with grazing animals, especially sheep, cows, goats, and horses, that pick it up from contaminated soil, by either eating or inhaling the tough spores that are the dormant form of its deadly bacteria.

Anthrax is as old as pastoralism and the origins of civilization. It might be the Sixth Plague, the sooty "morain," in the Book of Exodus that kills livestock and affects people with black spots. It is probably Apollo's "burning wind of plague" that begins Homer's *Iliad*.

Pack animals were his target first, and dogs
but soldiers, too, soon felt transfixing pain from
his hard shots, and pyres burned night and day.[3]

In ancient Roman times, Virgil's *Georgics* lamented the shortage of animals caused by what again was most likely anthrax.

Ghastly Tisphone rages, and . . . drives before her Disease and Dread. . . . The rivers and thirsty banks and sloping hills echo to the bleating of flocks and incessant lowing of kine. And now in droves she deals out death, and in the very stalls piles up the bodies, rotting with putrid foulness, till men learn to cover them in earth and bury them in pits.

Virgil also noted the other hazard of anthrax, that it spreads to humans, not by human-to-human contact, but by human contact with infected animals:

For neither might the hides be used, nor could one cleanse the flesh by water or master it by fire. They could not even sheer the fleeces, eaten up with sores and filth, nor touch the rotten web. Nay, if any man donned the loathsome garb, feverish blisters and foul sweat would run along his fetid limbs, and not long had he to wait ere the accursed fire was feeding on his stricken limbs.[4]

Veterinarians can often tell an animal has died from anthrax by its sudden death and by the blood and bloody fluid that have oozed from its orifices. Anthrax bacteria in the decaying carcass are likely to be killed off by the bacteria of putrefaction; anaerobes (bacteria that can multiply without free oxygen) from the intestines do the clean-up work.[5] The greater danger of anthrax lies in the blood that spills from the animal and drains into the soil, where the bacteria can then assume a protective spore form. (In a real sense, then, anthrax needs its host to die so that the disease may continue.) Relative temperature, along with varying blood and soil conditions, determines whether spores actually will form.[6] Once formed, though, they can be devilishly hard to eliminate.

Burying dead animals in pits, as Virgil suggested, never really disposed of anthrax. In spore form, its bacteria have been known to persist in soil for as long as seventy years, well after the memory of the site is lost. When an old site is disturbed—as new fields are plowed, new gravel pits dug, or new roads laid—or when a spring flood brings spores to the surface, animal outbreaks can flare as if from nowhere. Animal and human anthrax ravaged Europe and Asia throughout history, with major outbreaks in Germany in the fourteenth century and in central Europe and Russia in the seventeenth century, and these epidemics most likely originated from old reservoirs where diseased animals had been buried.

Attacking anthrax contamination has its problems, especially when attempted on a large scale. It takes three hours at 140 degrees centigrade to sterilize a five-ton load of bones in an industrial digester.[7] Four decades after the World War II testing of anthrax weapons at Gruinard Island off the coast of Scotland, the British used formaldehyde to the depth of six inches to ensure the soil was rid of spores.[8]

In humans, an anthrax infection can begin in one of three ways. Infection through the skin (cutaneous anthrax) is what Virgil described and is the most common and obvious form. It begins with a tiny pimple. In a few hours this eruption becomes a reddish-brown irritation and swelling that turns into an ulcer, the "feverish blister" that splits the skin. The black scablike crust that the lesion develops gives the disease its name, *anthracis*, the Latin transliteration of the Greek word for coal. In Russian, anthrax is also called "Siberian ulcer" (*Siberskaya yazva*), because of the prevalence of the disease in that region. Indeed, czarist Russia and the former Soviet Union, with their huge rural area, had among the world's highest levels of recorded anthrax outbreaks.[9] Without treatment, the fatality rate for cutaneous anthrax can be 20 percent. In this century, sulfamides, penicillin, tetracycline, and other relatively accessible drugs have reduced fatality to 5 percent and less.

As noted, there are two other ways of contracting anthrax in humans: Over the years, a distinction has been drawn between gastrointestinal anthrax, acquired by eating tainted meat, and inhalation anthrax, acquired by breathing in the deadly spores. This distinction immediately raises the issue of "portal of entry," of whether the spores enter the body through the mouth and digestive system or through the respiratory system, an issue central to the Sverdlovsk outbreak.

Outbreaks of gastrointestinal anthrax, rare and dangerous, usually afflict villages in developing countries, where animal vaccination and meat inspection programs are not in place or simply fail. They can occur when undercooked infected meat from local livestock or from wild animals makes it to the table. Depending on the outbreak, 25 to 100 percent of gastrointestinal anthrax victims are likely to die. Medical research (autopsy and tissue analysis) on the process of infection in authentic gastrointestinal anthrax is almost nonexistent.

Inhalation anthrax results from inhaling microscopic anthrax spores (one to five microns in diameter) deep into the lungs. Untreated inhalation anthrax is almost always fatal, but even in textile factory settings, where it has been best documented, it has proved exceptionally rare. For example, in one report of 117 cases of "woolsorter's disease" (as anthrax has been called since early industrial times), strung out over more than two decades, from 1933 to 1955, there was only one (fatal) case of inhalation anthrax; the rest were cutaneous.[10] Other scattered fatal cases of inhalation anthrax were reported in the United States during this same time period: a football player who may have contracted the disease from playing-field soil, a San Francisco woman who beat bongo drums made of infected skin, a construction worker who handled contaminated felt, and several gardeners whose infection was traced to contaminated bone meal fertilizer. In the best-researched incident, in Manchester, New Hampshire, in 1957, inhalation anthrax killed four woolen-mill workers.[11] In the same year, a man and woman living near a Philadelphia tannery also died of inhalation anthrax.[12]

The terms gastrointestinal and inhalation, as noted, refer to the portal of entry, how the pathogen entered the body, not necessarily to specific clinical manifestations. According to the few published reports of cases, fatal gastrointestinal anthrax and inhalation anthrax are characterized by similar initial symptoms. At first the patient may experience the aches, chills, mild fever, and nausea characteristic of influenza. In many cases, there is a brief respite from the symptoms, a "false recovery." Then, as the infection progresses, there may be high fever, severe pain in either the abdomen or chest or both, congested breathing, dizziness, bloody vomiting, and diarrhea.[13]

Regardless of the portal of entry, if the anthrax infection is internal, not merely cutaneous, it is termed systemic, and its treatment is highly problematic. Antibiotics are the first line of defense and can kill the anthrax bacteria or halt its growth. But because the bacteria produce a toxin that rapidly floods the blood and lymph system, sending the patient into shock, no remedy may be possible once serious symptoms begin. An unchecked anthrax infection sweeps rapidly through the body, causing massive toxic shock and internal ulceration and bleeding. During this process, a secondary pneumonia infection can develop, possibly in both patients who have eaten infected meat and patients who have inhaled anthrax spores.

Until World War II scientific interest in human anthrax cases was relatively minor compared to the focus on animal disease. *Bacillus anthracis* was discovered in 1850 by the French parasitologist Casimir-Joseph Davaine, who examined the blood of infected sheep under the microscope. Subsequent work, especially by Robert Koch, the famous German biologist, and the legendary Louis Pasteur in France, proved beyond doubt that this bacterium caused anthrax. It was with anthrax, in fact, that the germ theory of disease was firmly established. In 1876, Koch employed his pure culture techniques to discover the life cycle of anthrax (from the bacterium, with its bamboo-like rods, to its hardy spore form and back to bacterium again). At the time, though, he was much less concerned with the victims of "ragpicker's disease" (the colloquial German term for anthrax) than with the hundreds of thousands of grazing animals his native country was losing each year to anthrax. These repeated epizootics, common also in France and other European countries, damaged the food, textile, and leather industries dependent on animal products.[14] In 1881 Pasteur followed up his successful development of a vaccine against chicken cholera with one for animal anthrax. In May of that year, he was pressured into an early public demonstration of the vaccine at a farm in Pouilly-le-Fort, forty kilometers outside Paris. The risk paid off. On June 2, with twenty-five vaccinated sheep alive and twenty-five unvaccinated ones dead, Pasteur was proclaimed a hero in the press and by his scientific colleagues.[15]

Since World War II, the potential of anthrax as a biological weapon has focused national and international attention on its lethality for humans. Anthrax spores, tough enough to withstand bomb detonation and small enough to aerosolize, have been a preferred agent for every nation that has sought to develop and produce biological weapons. But the primary attribute of biological weapons, including anthrax, is that they have been experimented with but almost never deployed. Some restraints are a matter of international norms. Born of a repugnance for chemical weapons used in World War I, the Geneva Protocol of 1925, for example, prohibits the use in war of both chemical and biological weapons. Although several nations, including the United States and the USSR, formally reserved the right to use such weapons in reprisal if first used against them—and thus implicitly maintained the right to develop and stockpile them—only very rarely do the norms against using biological or chemical weapons break down. In modern times, the only significant use of biological weapons, including anthrax and plague, was in the late 1930s and early 1940s, when the Japanese Imperial Army undertook covert experiments on humans (which included vivisection) and deployed biological weapons against Chinese troops and civilians in Manchuria. The details of this historical anomaly have only recently been revealed.[16]

During World War II, American, British, and Canadian laboratories moved far along in developing and producing biological weapons, especially anthrax, which had the code name "N."[17] By 1944, thousands of anthrax bombs were ready for use by Allied Forces, but intelligence sources could find no indication that Nazi Germany had any investment in biological weapons (BW) capability. Indeed, directives from Hitler forbade BW offensive research. Late in the war some subordinates, notably Reich Marshall Hermann Göring, supported research at a small, secret facility outside the city of Posen (Poznan) in Poland,[18] where anthrax was the most seriously considered BW agent against both humans and animals. The war ended before the effort produced any results.

After the war, the United States and Britain continued BW research and testing, with the U. S. program (centered at Fort Detrick, Maryland) at times having more money than it could spend. In 1969, after reviewing the extensive U.S. investment in offensive BW, President Richard Nixon categorically renounced biological weapons. "Mankind already carries in its own hands too many of the seeds of its own destruction" was his public statement. Nixon limited U.S. BW activities to strictly defined defensive purposes: "techniques of immunization, safety measures, and the control and prevention of the spread of disease."[19] All U.S. programs were then dismantled or converted to protective or other peaceful defensive uses.

At the same time, President Nixon declared U.S. support for a British proposal for an international treaty banning biological weapons. With the concurrence of the United States, Great Britain, and the Soviet Union, the Biological Weapons Convention (BWC) was completed in 1972, and some 140 states are now party to it. The BWC forbids development, production, stockpiling, or otherwise retaining biological agents or toxins "of types or in quantities that have no justification for prophylactic, protective or other peaceful purposes." It also forbids "weapons, equipment or means of delivery designed to use such agents or toxins for hostile purposes or in armed conflict." Lacking investigatory or punitive powers, the convention eventually came to rely on "confidence-building measures," such as good-faith revelations by those states party to it of past offensive and current defensive BW activities and review sessions every five years, starting in 1980. It also allows one state party to lodge a complaint against another with the United Nations Security Council, in order to begin a formal investigation that all states party to the convention would support.

The BWC has remained largely a good-faith pact among nations, but it is because of it that our research team has become involved with investigating the 1979 anthrax outbreak in Sverdlovsk. In March 1980, during the first review session of the BWC in Geneva, the U.S. State Department raised its initial concern that the Sverdlovsk outbreak signaled a Soviet violation of the convention. Soviet invasion of Afghanistan the previous December had already ruptured relations between the two superpowers and precipitated a long list of U.S. economic and political sanctions against the Soviets. U.S. suspicions about Sverdlovsk were based on satellite photographs of the city's military Compound 19, on covert intelligence reports, and on an anonymous article published in January 1980 in West Germany, in the Russian dissident broadside *Posev (Sowing)*. This account of the outbreak was translated by the CIA and made available to American reporters just in time to rock the BWC review session. The article's author described hearing about a tremendous "explosion" of anthrax in Sverdlovsk and laid the blame on the military. "During a month or so an average of 30–40 people died each day," the author wrote. "The total number of deaths can be estimated at about 1000." The report described the removal of contaminated topsoil and the paving of streets in a nearby village to cover the contaminated earth. "One would imagine this is the only asphalted village in the Urals," the anonymous author commented. The article also added that no animal cases occurred, although within the city stray dogs were reportedly destroyed to control the spread of the disease.[20]

Taken by surprise, the Soviet Foreign Ministry in Moscow at first denied the outbreak. Then it followed up with a statement that an anthrax epidemic in the Urals had occurred but had been caused by "improper handling of meat products." On March 21, the last day of the BWC review meetings, Viktor Israelyan, the head of the Soviet delegation, stood and delivered a final response to the U.S. suspicions of forbidden work in biological weapons and a leak of deadly anthrax:

> In March–April 1979 in the area of Sverdlovsk there did in fact occur an ordinary outbreak of anthrax among animals, which arose from natural causes, and there were cases where people contracted an intestinal form of this infection as a result of eating meat from cattle which was sold against the regulations established by the veterinary inspectorate. In this connection an appropriate warning appeared in the press. However, this incident has no bearing on the question of compliance by the USSR with the Convention on the Prohibition of Bacteriological and Toxin Weapons. In this connection there are no grounds whatsoever for the question which was raised by the U.S. delegation.

U.S. intelligence analysts believed otherwise. Rumors of hundreds, even thousands of people killed in the 1979 outbreak continued to come in from Moscow, from emigrés in Western Europe, and from Soviet Jews newly settled in Israel, although no firsthand witnesses ever emerged. Calculations of the anthrax dose by some U.S. intelligence experts further inflamed the issue. A single gram of anthrax contains around a trillion potentially lethal spores. In a briefing on Sverdlovsk for President Jimmy Carter by Central Intelligence Director Stansfield Turner, the amount of anthrax released in the outbreak was estimated at seventy kilograms, an amount that could seriously infect tens of thousands of square miles. Matthew Meselson and U. S. government BW experts at the army's Dugway Proving Ground, who better understood the basic aerodynamics involved in such estimates, reckoned that as little as a gram of aerosolized anthrax, with its trillion spores, could have caused the Sverdlovsk outbreak. The figure settled on in Defense Intelligence Agency reports was ten kilograms.

The Soviet response to these suspicions was to adamantly stand by its tainted-meat explanation. In the spring of 1980 the U.S. government formed a working group on the Sverdlovsk outbreak, consisting of representatives from the Joint Chiefs of Staff, the National Security Council, the State Department, the CIA, and other agencies, to consider the incident. The group called on several outside experts: Philip Brachman from the Centers for Disease Control, Nobel Laureate microbiologist Joshua Lederberg at Rockefeller University in New York, Paul Doty, professor of biochemistry at Harvard, and Matthew Meselson. After some months, the majority judgment of the group was that an accidental explosion at the Sverdlovsk military factory caused an aerosol emission of virulent anthrax spores and that this emission resulted in many deaths from inhalation anthrax. The group also surmised that the emission caused an epizootic that brought infected meat to the black market. This inclusion of infected meat in the scenario (meat that could have been stored and eaten over a period of weeks) would account for the epidemic's reported long duration into early May, with people still falling ill and dying long after the initial explosion.[21]

During the 1980s, as Cold War tensions heightened, the U.S. investment in weapons systems (including renewed production of chemical weapons) quadrupled, and American press reports about alleged Soviet treaty violations, in Sverdlovsk and elsewhere, filled the news.[22] Yet during this time no formal complaint about the 1979 epidemic was lodged against the Soviet Union at the United Nations Security Council by the United States or any other nation. Meanwhile, throughout these years, Matthew kept pressing for a full on-site investigation of the Sverdlovsk incident and sent numerous missives to Soviet officials and fellow scientists, asking for research cooperation. In August 1986, after Mikhail Gorbachev began to liberalize contact with the West, Matthew was invited to Moscow for a private meeting with the three principal public health physicians who had been sent from Moscow to Sverdlovsk in the 1979 epidemic and who now offered their evidence for the Soviet infected-meat explanation of the outbreak. Later, in October of that year, a delegation to Moscow from the U.S. National Academy of Sciences, chaired by Joshua Lederberg, heard the physicians' case, in both a formal presentation and informal discussion. Following that, in 1988, with Matthew handling the arrangements, two of those Soviet physicians came to the United States to present and defend their government's explanation of the 1979 anthrax outbreak. They spoke to professional audiences at the National Academy of Sciences in Washington, the Johns Hopkins School of Public Health in Baltimore, and the American Academy of Arts and Sciences in Cambridge.[23] Their detailed presentation of the infected-meat scenario was judged plausible, even persuasive, although it lacked substantive clinical and epidemiological evidence.

Following that 1988 visit, Matthew persisted in expressing the need for a scientific investigation of the outbreak—in Congressional testimony, in print, and on the radio.[24] In 1990, he wrote, "On the Soviet side there needs to be a political decision to allow qualified US officials freely to examine what remains of the relevant evidence and to meet with surviving patients and local medical, public health, and veterinary personnel in Sverdlovsk. In addition, US experts should be invited to visit, on a suitable reciprocal basis, the facility described in the allegations."[25]

As the Cold War came to an end, the question remained whether all trust in the Soviet Union's adherence to the BWC had been misplaced. More to the point now perhaps was whether the new Russia was capable of fully revealing any violations at Soviet facilities. And if not, could the world trust this new government? In 1992, as we begin our investigation, the two explanations for the cause of the 1979 anthrax outbreak—a meat-borne infection or an aerosol biological weapons leak—continue to rest on conflicting assertions, neither as yet proven by facts. But now the doors to Russia are open so wide that even an unofficial group like ours can walk in and start asking questions. Will they be answered?

Moscow

FRAGMENTS OF EVIDENCE

Wednesday, June 3. In Moscow, the atmosphere of excited anticipation I remember from my last visit, in 1990, has turned edgy.[1] Only last December the Soviet Union dissolved, and a democratic Russia has begun its attempt to undo seventy years of central state control. In the capital, signs of disruption and change are visible. The streets are full of potholes, of speeding Mercedes sedans, of refuse from the new McDonald's near the Foreign Ministry. Palatial hotels have sprung up in the center city. On a street corner near the Bolshoi Theater, decent-looking people desperate for money are selling their own furniture and clothes. Kiosks on every corner vend Pepsi and Snickers bars, German herbal tea, and Italian spring water, but few products from Russia's industries, which were already faltering before the breakup of the USSR. Outside the Oktyabrskaya subway station near our hotel, a dignified gray-haired woman in a woolen suit holds out wilted flowers for sale for fifty rubles. When I offer a dollar, she takes it, thrusts the flowers at me, and bolts. The dollar is worth six hundred inflated rubles, a day's wages, maybe more. Across the street, rock music is blaring from an arcade market where customers are mulling over the purchase of fresh flowers, bread, meat, fruits, and vegetables, a bounty not everyone can afford, but, in contrast to the Soviet era, now they can see and desire it. Meanwhile, up from the Metro percolates the heady, authentic sound of Klezmer musicians playing with abandon.

Our hotel, the Academicheskaya, is no palace. It once provided modest accommodations for members of the scientific and scholarly academy. According to the desk clerk, it is now owned by its employees. Its rates have gone up, but its ambiance has changed for the worse. The leather-jacketed men in the lobby look like the mobsters who used to hang around the Ukraina Hotel, the grandiose and grim Stalinist edifice where I stayed in 1988 on my first trip to Russia, when Matthew participated in an arms control conference and I interviewed physicians at Moscow's largest maternity hospital. In the rooms we have booked for the team at the Academicheskaya, pale brown cockroaches skitter over the walls in broad daylight. But our stay is just for two nights, not worth the effort of finding another hotel, and the adjacent restaurant has decent food.

There is a sixth member of our team, Dr. Olga Yampolskaya, a specialist in infectious diseases at Moscow's Botkin Hospital, who joins us for dinner. In April 1979, with a brand new degree in infectious diseases, she spent three weeks in Sverdlovsk treating the victims of the outbreak. That experience, she recounts, was a desperate, round-the-clock struggle to save lives. She has not returned since 1979, but she remembers the city, now called Yekaterinburg, and the hospital where the anthrax patients were treated—in her recollection, by the dozens, not by the hundreds or thousands. Fair-haired, with flawless skin, Yampolskaya still looks fresh out of medical training, but she has a married daughter who is expecting her first child. She doesn't smile easily or often. Being a physician at Moscow's best hospital hardly guarantees a large, secure salary or a luxurious life. Doctors' salaries are small and, with economic change, becoming erratic. In addition, Yampolskaya, who also has a nine-year-old son, works the double shift of jobs and housework that Soviet women normally shouldered. Still, like the perestroika-influenced women described in Francine du Plessix Gray's *Soviet Women*, she is increasingly aware of Western culture and would like to travel outside Russia, though she doubts she will have the chance. For now, Yampolskaya is willing to join our expedition and renew contacts with medical colleagues from 1979. As a bonus, her English is excellent, and she will help me interview any relatives of the 1979 victims we can locate. We take time after dinner to review the questionnaire I have prepared for the victims' families.

The task before the team is a basic inquiry into a "point epidemic," that is, a large but temporary excess in disease frequency, usually lasting days or weeks rather than months. Understanding the dimensions of a point epidemic requires assessing the response of a group to an infection source to which each member was exposed at nearly the same time.[2]

The purpose of my interviews is to reconstruct what each anthrax victim was doing in 1979, in the days prior to falling ill: the place where each was, what each ate, what unusual or routine circumstances involved each in the collective disaster.

Before flying to Yekaterinburg, our group has business to take care of in Moscow. This morning, June 3, the six of us go to the Institute of Molecular Genetics, our Moscow host organization, where we have two separate appointments, each with someone who has promised to bring us important evidence about the 1979 outbreak. We are met by our host at the Institute, Dr. Yevgeniy Sverdlov (no relation to the Bolshevik Sverdlov for whom Yekaterinburg was previously named), the institute's director and an internationally known molecular geneticist. In the institute's conference room waits the former Deputy Minister of Health, Dr. Pyotr Burgasov, the lone survivor of the three key Soviet physicians who developed evidence that the Sverdlovsk epidemic was gastrointestinal. In 1979 Burgasov was the senior official sent from Moscow to handle the outbreak. Together he, Dr. Ivan Bezdenezhnikh, and Dr. Vladimir Nikiforov created and sustained the official Soviet explanation of the incident. It was these three physicians that Matthew met with in Moscow in 1986. Later, in 1988, Burgasov was the principal spokesman for the Soviet government when he and Nikiforov made a two-week visit to the United States to discuss the epidemic, as described in Chapter 1.

Dr. Ivan Bezdenezhnikh (whose last name means "without a penny" in Russian) was the Russian Federation chief epidemiologist in 1979. Although he died in September 1986, the infected-meat explanation based on evidence he compiled lives on. In 1986, when Matthew visited Moscow, Dr. Bezdenezhnikh gave him a graph he had made illustrating the course of hospital admissions in April 1979, a crucial representation of how people fell ill over a three-week period. An expanded version of this graph was included in a summary document by the three physicians, which was given to the U.S. State Department after Burgasov and Nikiforov's 1988 visit (see Figure 1). The information in these graphs clearly showed the temporal contour, not of a cataclysmic explosion, but a seven-week epidemic that peaked in its second week, around mid-April. By that time two-thirds of the total of sixty-four recorded fatalities had occurred. Then the epidemic trailed off over another four-plus weeks, ending May 18. This duration has been described (but not explained) in Soviet dissident accounts and is accepted by the U.S. government.

In 1986, as evidence of the public health response, Matthew also received a folder of printed material that supported the animal outbreak explanation. It included a copy of a leaflet dated April 19, 1979, that was reportedly distributed in Sverdlovsk. The leaflet described all three means of transmitting anthrax ("through damaged skin while caring for an animal," "through the upper respiratory pathways," and "through the gastrointestinal tract" from tainted meat or food). It added a fourth vector, insect bites, a caution based on Soviet evidence for anthrax transmission by horseflies.[3] Yet the leaflet warned citizens about only two clinical forms of the disease, cutaneous and "septic," that is, either a skin infection or a general systemic infection (sepsis, which would cover both inhalation and gastrointestinal forms). For the latter, the leaflet described symptoms ranging from general malaise, fever, chills, headaches, and back pains to bloody coughing, chest pains, stomach pains, bloody vomiting, and bloody diarrhea. Instructions were clear: in case of symptoms, call a physician, isolate the patient, do not allow the patient's excretions to get into the sewer system. Then, after the patient is hospitalized, relations should disinfect the rooms and any utensils or objects used and put personal belongings and clothes "through a disinfection chamber" at the hospital. Then caretakers "must undergo daily medical examination" to make sure they are not infected. These prescribed "measures of social prevention" were based entirely on veterinary control over sick farm animals, at animal feed processing plants, and on the vaccination of "individuals who care for animals and process animal products," and not at all on possible airborne factors.

Another item in the folder was a broadsheet dated April 18, 1979, that was distributed to the local community in the southern part of the city where infected meat was allegedly distributed. This listed the initial symptoms of anthrax as headache, fever, head cold, and cough, after which "intestinal disorders develop [and] pains in the abdomen appear," with a fever of 39–40 degrees centigrade (102–4 degrees Fahrenheit). The publication declared that to prevent anthrax, "it is necessary to strictly observe the rules of personal hygiene when caring for animals" and that "under no circumstances should unstamped meat, fur, or uncured pelts be purchased on the open market or from private individuals. . . . It is also forbidden to slaughter animals and butcher the carcasses without veterinary permission." Presumably people who ignored these warnings and ate from cooked or frozen stores of infected meat were those who died in the late days of the epidemic.

In 1979 Dr. Vladimir Nikiforov was Director of the Infectious Diseases Department at Moscow's Central Postgraduate Institute at the Botkin Hospital. He arrived in Sverdlovsk at the peak of the epidemic, on April 12, and took over clinical treatment of the dying victims. In May 1980 he and Dr. Bezdenezhnikh published an article about the epidemiology and clinical aspects of the outbreak.[4] In 1988, it was Nikiforov and Burgasov who traveled to the United States to present the Soviet explanation of the anthrax outbreak. Together, at the three presentations (in Washington, Baltimore, and Cambridge), they fielded questions about the epidemic from invited experts from the CIA, Defense Intelligence Agency (DIA), and other government offices and from academic centers. Having accompanied the Soviet delegation during this trip, I remember Dr. Nikiforov as a fragile man with a gentle, aristocratic manner, and a refined St. Petersburg accent. Olga Yampolskaya, who for twelve years worked for him at the Botkin Hospital, still refers to him as a "saint." In August 1990, Nikiforov suddenly collapsed and died of a heart attack in his country garden.

Dr. Burgasov, the only survivor of the three key figures, is now retired from his post as Deputy Minister of Health and lives at his dacha on the Moscow River. He has come to Moscow today to argue once again the case for anthrax-infected meat as the source of the epidemic, and he has brought documents to support his case. I have not seen him since his 1988 visit to the United States. That he is visibly older and thinner reminds me of how each year diminishes the cast of players from 1979. Still, at over six feet tall, with thick white hair, a heavy brow with protruding platinum eyebrows, and a barrel chest, Burgasov remains a commanding, almost operatic presence, like a character in *Boris Godunov*. With vigorous hand gestures, in booming phrases, he complains about the rough treatment he has received in the newly liberated Russian press. He describes one interview in which the journalist implied he was close to the KGB.[5] Much has also been made of Burgasov's handling of the 1979 epidemic, particularly the washing of buildings and repaving of roads, which the media have interpreted as a giveaway that he must have known the outbreak was airborne and from the laboratory in Military Compound 19. In 1988, in the United States, he denied giving any such orders and attributed the cleanup to local authorities getting the city in shape for the traditional Soviet celebrations on May 1. One recent Russian newspaper account, he tells us, portrays him in a helicopter flying over the city while the cleanup goes on. "What would I be doing in a helicopter?" he protests. We assure him that while we are familiar with some, though not all, of the newspaper articles on the Sverdlovsk epidemic, we are here on a scientific mission, not a search for anecdotes.

Dr. Burgasov is even more agitated about a missing manuscript on the

Sverdlovsk epidemic, which he says he was writing with Dr. Nikiforov just before the clinician's death. In late 1988, the Soviet Foreign Ministry presented to the U.S. government the official version of the outbreak (with Bezdenezhnikh, Burgasov, and Nikiforov listed as authors, in that order). It included a detailed description of gastrointestinal anthrax infection, apparently summarized from Nikiforov's records, along with epidemiological data from Dr. Bezdenezhnikh. The report also pointed out that the Sverdlovsk oblast (the regional political division in which the city of Sverdlovsk/Yekaterinburg lies), which is about the size of France, has 371 separate sites where anthrax has occurred in modern times, and forty-eight of them had caused repeated outbreaks. But Burgasov is referring to yet another manuscript about the epidemic, which he says contains even more authoritative data. He asserts it is being wrongfully withheld by Dr. Nikiforov's son, who is also named Vladimir and is also a Moscow physician, a toxicologist who co-authored a text on botulism with his father. The former deputy minister has reason to feel proprietary. Anthrax was one of his specialties long before the 1979 outbreak. He was lead author of a 1970 book on the disease's history, causes, symptomology, treatment, and prevention; it is one of the few comprehensive sources of information on both human and animal anthrax in any language.[6] He is also co-author of a 1984 monograph on anthrax infections. Although he has documentation for us, the missing manuscript would, he insists, clinch his case.

In fact our second appointment this morning is with the young Dr. Nikiforov, who is bringing photographic slides of autopsy material from the 1979 outbreak, which were among his father's office records. Olga Yampolskaya has warned us that the two men might come to blows if they meet. Our scheduling of appointments is admittedly not brilliant, but we have arranged for Nikiforov to be shown to an office securely distant, we hope, from the conference room. Yampolskaya and David Walker are waiting for him there, ready to review whatever the photographs reveal. Leaving Matthew, Alexis Shelokov, and our veterinarian, Martin Hugh-Jones, to begin discussion with Burgasov, I cross the hall and traverse several connecting rooms to check that our second visitor has safely reached his destination.

Dr. Vladimir Nikiforov has arrived with his father's cache of photographic slides. Slightly built, in his forties, the young Nikiforov strongly resembles his father, except his manner is hardly hesitant. Immediately and forcefully, he asserts that his father was coerced by Soviet authorities into supporting the infected-meat hypothesis. A slide projector and screen have been set up. With Yampolskaya interpreting, Nikiforov begins to show us the color slides taken, he says, by his father during the autopsies of the epidemic's victims. The slides are of internal organs glistening with lesions and of microscopic tissue samples shot through with signature minute rods of *B. anthracis*. Interspersed among these slides are full body pictures of autopsies in progress.

Most prominent in this display are the photographs of infected lymph nodes, which are crucial for understanding how the body contends with anthrax or any other kind of infection. The human body has mighty resources to protect itself against harmful microbes. The inflammatory response to an invading microorganism produces increased antibodies and phagocytes (the policing "cell-eaters"). In addition, the body is endowed with a dynamic system that continually filters foreign material and debris: the constantly circulating lymph, a clear liquid derived from blood serum, flows out of capillaries and washes through tissues on a surveillance mission for harmful invaders. It eventually delivers its "cargo" to the lymph nodes for filtration, after which it returns to the blood stream via the great veins of the thorax or abdomen. Beset by bacteria like those of anthrax, the lymph accelerates its already fast flow, moving policing cells and bacteria alike toward the nearest lymph nodes, where antimicrobial forces (the node's own macrophages and other reinforcements the immune system calls into play) should destroy the harmful invader. Major nodes serve the lungs (thoracic nodes) and the intestines (mesentery nodes), as well as other areas of the body. When the lymph nodes fail to overcome an infection, bacteria can multiply, and in the process the node itself becomes inflamed and bleeds. In bubonic plague, as one example, the affected node becomes a pocket of pus, "a battlefield containing dead and living microorganisms, host cells and inflammatory exudate."[7] Still-active bacteria, carried along by the flow of the lymph, can escape the node, enter the bloodstream, and cause a general infection. This secondary onslaught can beset other lymph nodes than the one nearest the initial site of infection and turn them into battlefields as well.

In anthrax, the bacteria themselves are not the killers. Rather, once spores germinate, the bacteria produce a toxin that causes the edema and hemorrhaging that the younger Dr. Nikiforov is showing us in slide after photographic slide, not just in lymph nodes but throughout the organs of the body. Although he seems certain of his case for inhalation anthrax, Nikiforov keeps looking to Walker as if expecting confirmation. But Walker, busily taking notes, is keeping his own counsel.

As one slide after another lights up the screen, the elder Nikiforov's prior testimony in favor of gastrointestinal anthrax preoccupies me. The question in my mind is whether an old-school clinician not trained as a pathologist could in fact look at autopsy materials and distinguish between gastrointestinal and inhalation anthrax. There is no question that he knew about anthrax, but how much? In 1973 he wrote a monograph (*Cutaneous Anthrax in Humans*) on cutaneous anthrax, after having monitored an outbreak in Albania, where he was stationed for three years. Certainly in 1979, he was familiar with patients' clinical symptoms. But what did he see in the autopsy materials?

In 1986 in Moscow, Nikiforov showed Matthew fourteen photographic slides of both lungs and intestines (some perhaps the same we are now reviewing) to illustrate the official belief that gastrointestinal anthrax had killed the Sverdlovsk victims. He said then: "Nodes throughout the body cavity, including around the lungs and intestines, were black and necrotic. In all cases, however, the lungs were undamaged and free of hemorrhage."[8] Shortly after, he told the U.S. National Academy of Sciences delegation that he had seen cases of inhalation anthrax in Albania, with hemorrhagic edema as their main, most telling characteristic. He also claimed to have witnessed more than one hundred cases of intestinal anthrax in his career, all of them fatal, except for fifteen Sverdlovsk victims he was able to save with antibiotics. Nikiforov also showed the delegation a range of autopsy slides, including some of infected lungs, which he saw as the result of systemic anthrax. Ostensibly, he believed in the description in the 1970 Burgasov book, according to which inhalation anthrax is accompanied by extensive damage within the lungs: "With the pulmonary form of anthrax, numerous pneumonic lesions are found in the lungs, which take up a significant part of the stricken organ. There are hemorrhages, bloody infarcts, and gangrenous lesions in different parts of the lungs." Yet even in that text, the importance of the lymph nodes is cited, albeit without discussion:

> The experimental data of a number of authors indicate that inhaled anthracic spores do not proliferate into the lungs, but after being captured by the macrophages they are carried with the flow of the lymph into the tracheobronchial lymph nodes. There they develop within the phagocytes that captured them, then enter the blood stream and cause general infection.[9]

If to Nikiforov (as to Yampolskaya, who witnessed some dozen autopsies), the lungs looked less damaged than the intestinal organs, he might have concluded that the anthrax infection had spread from the intestines via the blood stream to the lungs and not vice versa, from the lungs to the rest of the body.[10]

Knowing what Dr. Nikiforov perceived or believed is by now impossible, and in fairness, the diagnosis remains problematic. In 1979, even an American clinician would probably have had difficulty distinguishing the two rare forms of anthrax from one another, especially if the systemic infection in the victim's body had become massive. An American, though, would have had access to case descriptions as far back as the 1940s, one of a 1942 Pennsylvania textile worker, which offers a rare description of human lungs infected with anthrax by inhalation, and another of a rug salesman who died of inhalation anthrax, also presented in detail.[11] In both, the thoracic lymph nodes, rather than the lungs, are where infection is most evident. In 1970, an American clinician of Dr. Nikiforov's rank, faced with handling a massive outbreak, could also have consulted with government experts Wilhelm Albrink or Philip Brachman or one of the U.S. or British researchers who worked on inhalation anthrax. In the postwar decades, while the United States and Britain were heavily invested in biological weapons development, major animal experiments, many on nonhuman primates, were conducted, both in closed chambers and in open-air settings in the Caribbean and the Pacific. Government experts could have discussed with him what to look for in the thoracic lymph nodes and in the interior of the lung.

Even so, no Western expert at that time could have laid out infallible criteria for distinguishing inhalation from intestinal anthrax. From 1939 on, the framework for investigating the disease was weapons, which meant no research was done on gastrointestinal anthrax, just on the inhalatory form. Even today, a lack of published studies on authentic gastrointestinal anthrax in humans leaves us wondering exactly how it infects the body. It is plausible that heavy mesentery (intestinal) lymph node infection, without major impact on thoracic lymph nodes, would characterize it, but direct proof is lacking. An autopsy might allow a comparison of the degree of infection in the mesentery and thoracic lymph nodes, enough to estimate which was the primary portal of entry. Or the quality and severity of lesions in the intestinal walls could be compared with the progress of damage in the lungs. An inquisitive clinician in Nikiforov's position would have followed the pathologist to the autopsy table to find out more about the thoracic lymph nodes and the interior condition of each lung, as well as about the mesentery nodes and the degree of damage to the intestines, great and small, and to the stomach. According to Yampolskaya, Nikiforov did attend autopsies. Perhaps he was satisfied that, by his criteria, the portal of entry was not the lungs. Or maybe he was simply more preoccupied at the time with how he might save his critically ill patients. Or maybe, as his son believes, he was co-erced into supporting the infected-meat hypothesis.

The slides (there are more than eighty in the tray) follow one another haphazardly. Walker, sitting ramrod straight, is completely focused on the pictures; he continues to take notes without much comment or ques-tion. Yampolskaya, who seems tense, is taking her cue from him. For all I know, all these photos could be from just a few victims, from any epi-demic. One of the slides, though, has a certain fame. It shows a severely infected large intestine covered with dark hemorrhagic spots. Dr. Niki-forov brought it with him to the United States in 1988 and was roundly criticized for having picked only this kind of representation of autopsy results, unbalanced by photos of lungs and thoracic lymph nodes. As I remember, the trip was not a happy one for him, as it was for Dr. Bur-gasov, who, like many high-level officials in public health, enjoyed his international contacts and travel. And because in 1979 Burgasov had di-rected the organizational response to the outbreak and was far removed from the clinical care of patients and the autopsy room, the considerable demands from the American audiences for scientific evidence fell on Niki-forov's shoulders. He was not prepared.

As this morning's slide show continues, I suddenly recognize one of the photographs. It shows a naked man, his skin blue and his trunk cut open, his penis relaxed against his thigh, his face obscured. In 1986, when Nikiforov offered to give Matthew his choice of slides, he picked this one, depicting an early autopsy. Soon after, I happened upon a copy of this slide that Matthew had unintentionally left at home. Despite all the research I'd done in hospital settings, I was taken aback—and I am again. It isn't simply that the man is dead or that he is naked; it is that he is both, doubly vulnerable, and then triply so, with his insides on exhibi-tion, as if for scientific scrutiny. But the science of this display is eluding me. I decide to leave David Walker to his job and go back to hear what Dr. Burgasov has to say.

In the conference room, the former deputy minister is still complain-ing that the young Nikiforov has heisted the only copy of the missing anthrax manuscript. In it, Burgasov tells us, the elder Nikiforov wrote a descriptive section with two of the Sverdlovsk pathologists (Faina Abra-mova and Lev Grinberg) who performed autopsies of victims in 1979. Then there was a section of Burgasov's own on the survivors of the epi-demic. Just before his death, Nikiforov was editing the final version. Now the son is apparently holding up publication. "And," Burgasov adds, "the autopsy slides he has belonged to my son."

The tragedy of Dr. Burgasov's only son, Dimitriy, is intertwined with that of the 1979 epidemic. A doctoral candidate at Moscow University, he traveled with his father to Sverdlovsk, to study the epidemic as a thesis project. Not long after returning to Moscow, we understand, he died of pancreatitis. Rumors persist that Burgasov's son alone knew the real story of the outbreak and that only his untimely death prevented the true facts from emerging. Our attempts to find his thesis, supposedly filed at Moscow University, have yielded nothing.

So today two survivors of two different generations, Dr. Burgasov and the younger Dr. Nikiforov, are squabbling over the scientific legacy of their dead relatives. The younger Nikiforov clearly has the advantage: his father's papers and files (as well as his Moscow apartment) are in his possession. There is also a subtext of class conflict in this dispute. The Nikiforovs are from the educated elite of the old system, which persisted under Stalin and subsequent Soviet leaders. Burgasov was born a peasant and became a physician by accident, as he tells the story. In his youth, he went to a large hall in Moscow where welders were being recruited. He stood in the wrong line and was drafted into medical school instead. That was in the early 1930s, when Soviet professional education was thrown open to the proletariat. By 1936, the educational system had reverted to its former elitism; peasant youth like Burgasov were routinely sent to technical schools, and the children of the privileged regained their university places. Equipped with his medical degree, Burgasov rose as high in the Soviet public health ranks as a physician could, achieving the rank of Army General and becoming a member of the Academy of Medical Science. He did not need the KGB for privileges. But, unlike the elder Nikiforov, he now has no male heir to the privileges he might have passed along.

Our vaccine expert Alexis Shelokov knows Burgasov from the Soviet physicians' 1988 visit to the United States. At the presentation at the National Academy in Washington, it was Shelokov who stood up in the audience and corrected a serious mistake the interpreter, unfamiliar with biological terms, had made, a confusion of pneumonia with influenza. Shelokov, with his gray hair and mustache, is from the same generation as Burgasov (both men are in their seventies), but Shelokov, from a White Russian family that lived in Manchuria, immigrated to California in 1938 and went to medical school at Stanford University. After the war, when the Soviet army drove the Japanese out of Manchuria, Shelokov's father was arrested and most likely executed or died in a gulag. Despite this history, Shelokov has traveled many times to the Soviet Union on professional trips. Now he converses affably with the former Deputy Minister and also interprets for us.

Martin Hugh-Jones, our veterinarian, has not met Burgasov before. In his pronounced British accent (of Welsh descent, he was born in the U.K.), he takes the lead in asking questions about the alleged animal outbreak, the dates of which are crucial for understanding the cause of the epidemic. Burgasov has come prepared. Out of a folder, he takes eight veterinary documents, which he says are originals. Each pertains to cases of animal anthrax in the spring of 1979. Four are laboratory reports from the Sverdlovsk Oblast Veterinary Bacteriological Laboratory. One documents that on April 6, the remains of three sheep from a village near Sverdlovsk tested positive for anthrax. One details positive results from meat confiscated April 22, 1979, "from an unknown citizen" attempting to sell it in the central market. The other documents refer to seven infected sheep and a cow that died between April 5 and 10 in Abramova village, south of Sverdlovsk. Still other reports cite the slaughter of sick sheep in Rudniy village, also south of the city, on March 28 and April 7 and 8, and a subsequent legal case against a local family for distributing the infected meat.

"This animal outbreak began before the epidemic," Burgasov emphasizes. For him, there is no doubt that the consumption of anthrax-infected meat caused the 1979 outbreak in Sverdlovsk. He pushes the documents across the table. "Here is the proof!"

Moscow

CONFLICTING VISIONS

The precedent that Pyotr Burgasov leans on for explaining the Sverdlovsk deaths is the 1927 anthrax epidemic in Yaroslavl, 250 kilometers northeast of Moscow, which is known to have been caused by infected meat. In that outbreak, twenty-two of the twenty-seven victims were men who worked at and lived near the railroad station, just south of the town. They were bachelors, mobile and without families, probably much like the roughneck railroad laborers Chekhov described in one of his stories, men who "drank, ate, and used bad language, and pursued with shrill whistles every woman of light behavior who passed by."[1] The epidemic lasted from July 6 to 17, with most deaths occurring in the first week. At first it was thought to be influenza or mild gastroenteritis, because the victims' symptoms were diverse and such infections were common in the summer. But as the deadly infection ran its course, the victim's temperature usually declined sharply and there was "unexpected cardiac collapse accompanied by sudden chilling of the limbs, cyanosis, and a fast and thready pulse."[2] The diagnosis changed to anthrax, but from where?

The speculation was that sausages sold by private venders were the source of contamination. Yet local physicians, unschooled in the appropriate laboratory techniques, found no proof of food contamination. Nor did tests done on blood and tissue samples from victims prove conclusive. To be on the safe side, the local public health officials banned all consumption of sausage and fish products and called for help from Moscow. By the time three physicians arrived in Yaroslavl from Moscow's State

Microbiological Institute, it was the end of the epidemic, and the very last patient was dying. Using better laboratory techniques, they proved anthrax was the source of the outbreak, by injecting materials from the last autopsied corpse and a blood culture from the dying patient into white mice and guinea pigs. All the animals died within two days of anthrax septicemia. The last patient (as they noted in their report) died before they could explain his suffering to him.

The Moscow physicians who wrote the account of the Yaroslavl epidemic faulted the victims' lifestyles:

> Individual analysis of the victims showed that the overwhelming majority consisted of working bachelors having no possibility of proper and regular nutrition; these persons irregularly consumed whatever food happened to be available, with cooked sausage occupying a prominent place. In contrast to the situation of these working bachelors, not a single case of illness was observed among working family members who enjoyed normal home cooking.[3]

The homely moral of the physicians' account is that an unsettled life can be fatal.

Historically, explanations of epidemics almost always include some blame for misbehavior.[4] In Burgasov's scenario one moral is that is that honest citizens should never eat black-market meat when the legitimate source was state stores selling inspected meat, or they might suffer for it. Yet, since in the 1970s (and probably still today), the "second economy" accounted for as much as 20 percent of national output, many Russian people acquired food, especially farm products, from nonofficial sources.[5] Perhaps the citizens of Sverdlovsk should not have bought black-market meat, but it was hardly unusual to do so.

And what about those who sold on the black market, the venders of the contaminated meat? An article in a Soviet law journal in September 1980 reported a Sverdlovsk court case in which two people from a village just outside the city were found guilty of selling bad meat in April 1979.[6] Each had butchered his own sick livestock, given some meat to relatives, and marketed the rest. One culprit was fined and the other given a year's suspended sentence. The court's judgment was that their "not taking into consideration the dangerous consequences to people grossly violated the regulations of the veterinary directorate." But, "taking into consideration the personalities of the guilty persons [and] their repentance," the court let them off easily. And again, what they had done, many others were doing—vending their own domestic products.

The more fundamental source of the outbreak, as Burgasov argues (and

as is described in the Soviet explanation given to the U.S. State Department in 1988), lies in the food industry. To begin, in March 1979,
a failure to properly sterilize anthrax-infected waste products at a meat-
processing plant resulted in contaminated bone meal. This bone meal
was mixed with grain and other slaughterhouse products to make combined feed, as is used worldwide for cattle. Reaching again into his folder,
Burgasov takes out a signed statement by the manager of a grain products factory located in the village of Aramil, a few kilometers south of
Sverdlovsk. The document states that 2,121 tons of combined feed for
cattle were produced in March 1979. According to the official Soviet explanation, this shipment was delivered to local farms, both private and
state, just one or two days before the anthrax outbreak among animals
began. At the one state farm (*sovkohz*) where a small load of this feed had
been received, a breeding bull (apparently not effectively vaccinated) became ill and died, and the feed was confiscated. The meat processing plant
officials were reprimanded for being "in violation of technical protocol."

> Grinding of raw materials, heat treatment, sifting and filling of bags with the
> final product all were done in the same building. The shop had no records of
> the starting and final temperatures during treatment of the raw materials.
> Manometers were found at the height of 4 meters above the boilers, making
> it impossible to read the dials. The uncrushed bone fragments left after the
> sifting of the dried product were loaded back into the boilers. There were two
> wheelbarrows in the shop used to transport bathed raw materials and the
> meat-bone meal. The meat-bone meal was not tested for vegetative and spore-
> forming microflora, as is required.[7]

Once livestock became sick, private parties presumably slaughtered
their animals and sold them illegally, either as raw or as processed meat
(cutlets and mincemeat are mentioned in the 1988 report). In addition,
by mistake, fifteen infected carcasses from a state farm were reportedly
trucked in from the countryside and sold at the Sverdlovsk ceramics factory to workers and local residents. This sale point (ostensibly legal)
would explain why a disproportionate number of the victims in 1979,
perhaps as many as a third, were ceramics workers. Those who purchased
this contaminated meat took it to their homes for consumption, homes
both near the factory and scattered randomly throughout the city. In sum,
multiple errors in the complex procedure of getting meat to market caused
the 1979 anthrax epidemic. Misbehavior was endemic.

Nothing is terribly amiss with Burgasov's argument, but a few aspects
of it are puzzling. First of all, from the point of view of evidence, the
statement from the Aramil factory director tells us nothing about an-

thrax contamination. The combined feed was simply mixed there. Why give us this document, rather than something about the culprits at the plant that failed to sterilize the bone meal? Not wishing to appear ungrateful for any documentation, we focus on other questions. For example, only one person per household caught anthrax, while all family members might have been expected to eat from the same pot, as it were, and share the risk of infection. It could be argued that the dose was too low to infect more than one person in a family. But Burgasov has an interpretation that explains not only the lack of family clusters, but another curious feature of the 1979 outbreak, that no children died. Most of the victims were men, Burgasov tells us, and male heads of households eat more meat because they do more physically strenuous labor. Therefore in 1979 they were more vulnerable than their wives. No children were affected (except for a six-year-old girl who had cutaneous anthrax and was cured) because, Burgasov explains, children are largely fed their main noon meal with meat at school, not at home.

Burgasov's belief that Yaroslavl is a valid model for what happened at Sverdlovsk gains some support from the profile of the epidemic included in the 1988 Soviet report, based on the work of Dr. Bezdenezhnikh. The report contained a graph charting the dates of what appear to be hospital admissions for ninety-six cases (sixty-four fatalities, the rest survivors) during the 1979 anthrax epidemic (Figure 1). The course of the Yaroslavl epidemic showed a comparable initial peak in cases, which declined after the first week.

A more professional approach on Bezdenezhnikh's part would have been to plot the distribution of times of the onset of each patient's illness, the true epidemic curve, rather than when each arrived at the hospital.[8] Every infectious disease has a characteristic incubation period, that is, the likely interval between contact or entry of a disease agent and the emergence of symptoms. For any particular disease, incubation depends the portal of entry, the dose, and the individual's susceptibility to the disease. Of any three people exposed to even a common cold virus, one person might start sneezing in eight hours, another in two days, a third not at all. To identify the source of a disease outbreak, the epidemic curve of the onset of patients' symptoms provides a vital clue, like arrows pointing back in time to when the infection took place. A good rule is to investigate the earliest cases to find out the source. That Dr. Bezdenezhnikh, Chief Epidemiologist of the Russian Federation, plotted only hospital admission dates underscores our impression that his study of the extraordinary 1979 outbreak lacked thoroughness.

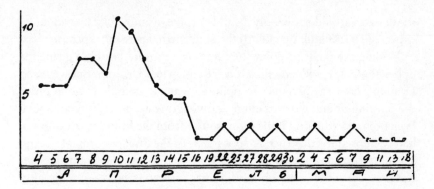

FIGURE 1. The 1988 graph of hospitalization dates for ninety-six victims of the 1979 Sverdlovsk anthrax outbreak, from the Soviet document (Bezdenezhnikh, Burgasov, and Nikiforov 1988) that was given to the U.S. State Department to explain the outbreak. The graph includes both fatalities and survivors. It begins with six patients admitted to hospital on April 4, illustrates a peak around April 10, and ends with the record of a single patient on May 18.

A key for understanding the Sverdlovsk outbreak, then, is knowing the incubation period for anthrax. The scant literature on human anthrax cases points to patients' developing the disease and succumbing rapidly, in two to seven days after exposure,[9] which again fits the Yaroslavl outbreak with its peak in fatalities six to seven days into the epidemic. It also fits the "wedding banquet" scenarios of other anthrax outbreaks, as well as common food-poisoning episodes from *E. coli* and salmonella. The modern history of anthrax contains accounts of feasts in Iran, Kazakhstan, the Philippines, Siberia, and various African countries where infected meat (not cooked enough to kill the anthrax bacteria) is shared by a large group, some of whom then fall ill. One need only learn from those affected what and where they recently ate to find the common vector, the bad meat. The Sverdlovsk epidemic, with patients dying over the course of about seven weeks, is just too prolonged for such an explanation, unless one accepts that some victims continued eating from stores of infected meat during April and May and became ill later than the majority. Burgasov's proof that this happened is conversations with local residents. Two pensioners, for example, kept eating from meat they had bought and cooked weeks before, which laboratory tests, he says, then revealed to be contaminated with anthrax. In another family, the fatty meat was recooked to obtain lard, which they ate as food. It, too, had anthrax in it. Thus, Burgasov argues, if the anthrax outbreak had been caused by a single point of exposure, such as an emission resulting from an explosion at the military laboratory, the graph of death dates would show only a sudden spike, as most victims would be expected to succumb quickly to the single lethal aerosol exposure.

Finding the point or points of common exposure has been a rule for understanding epidemics since the 1850s, when Dr. John Snow traced London's cholera epidemics to polluted water sources.[10] In addition to the plotting of an epidemic curve showing disease onset, it would have been even more helpful if the information from the Sverdlovsk outbreak had been used to construct a "spot map" of the disease outbreak. Using a map of the city, one could plot where victims lived and, through interviews, trace the common relation of those households—presumably to the tainted meat sold at the ceramics factory or marketed unofficially elsewhere. Information from each household should reveal that the consumption of that meat was the "common vehicle" for transmitting the fatal anthrax. According to the Soviet report, Dr. Bezdenezhnikh did look at the distribution of residences but concluded they bore no relation to the outbreak, except that the homes of many but not all victims were near the countryside where the epizootic took place and the infected meat originated.

An additional point for the tainted-meat explanation would be if, as Burgasov claims, 30 percent of the 1979 anthrax victims really did live scattered throughout the city, some at a distance of fifteen kilometers. Meat bought from a market and eaten at home might account for this dispersion. In contrast, an airborne dissemination of anthrax spores would follow the wind direction. The locations of victims in the path of a passing anthrax cloud, of those we would say were in the wrong place at the wrong time, would appear in some pattern, depending on the source of the anthrax and the direction of the wind. Without verifying what individuals did and where they were just before becoming ill, we cannot be certain where the lethal anthrax of 1979 originated and how it infected its victims.

As I listen to Dr. Burgasov, I have one thought in my head: I have no facts. I have neither the home addresses to confirm that the victims were dispersed throughout the city nor the interview information for estimating what common circumstances the victims might have shared outside their homes. Epidemiology is key, but Bezdenezhnikh, the penniless one, has left us wanting.

"Do you think Bezdenezhnikh kept records?" Matthew asks. "Might we be able to find them?"

"I have no idea," Dr. Burgasov replies with a grimace. "When a man dies, who knows what happens to his things!" He is obviously thinking of his quarrel with Nikiforov's son. And he is generally pessimistic about our prospects for successful research of the epidemic. "Hospital and legal records are not kept long," he says. "After a few years, they're destroyed."

"How do you think I should try to reach the families of victims?" I ask.

"Beware of money-seekers," he warns and makes an offhand remark about pensions that I write down without understanding, and we quickly move on to other questions.

As a creator and defender of the official Soviet position, Burgasov might well wish we would simply accept his word and book our return flight to the States. But he has been aware since 1986 that Matthew was nevertheless intent on an on-site investigation of the 1979 epidemic. The surprise for Burgasov is probably less that we have shown up than that people in his own world, the world of Moscow opinion makers, politicians, and journalists, would doubt a deputy minister's authority.

In response to our other questions, Burgasov recounts that in 1979 there were no cases of anthrax at Compound 19, the Sverdlovsk military base with a biological facility, although two cases of visitors there were indirectly associated with it. "Compound 19 has a polyclinic, but no one there died of anthrax," he insists. About the low death toll during the outbreak, he shows some pride. He reiterates the official numbers: sixty-four people died of intestinal anthrax, but fifteen survived. In addition, six of the seventeen cases of cutaneous anthrax became systemic, but all these lived. These are survival rates to be proud of, he insists.

Other items in Burgasov's folder are letters he has written to the newspaper *Izvestia*, complaining about his interview with journalist Aleksandr Pashkov, parts of which are going to be televised. He resents being portrayed as affiliated with the KGB.[11] His letters have been ignored. "So," he asks us, "if our democracy is so widespread, why is nothing I write ever published?"

That is not the only news in the press about Burgasov. Apparently he had spent quite a bit of time in Sverdlovsk before the 1979 epidemic. Press reports claim that in the 1950s he worked in the laboratory at Compound 19, a fact that never came up during his 1988 visit to America.[12]

"Is it true?" Matthew asks.

"Yes," Burgasov replies, unabashed. "In 1957 and 1958 I was working at Compound 19 on antidotes for botulinal toxin. But that had nothing to do with my role in containing the 1979 epidemic." His assertion has some weight. Not only Burgasov's rank as Deputy Minister of Health, but his experience with and prior publications on epidemics made him the logical person to handle the 1979 crisis. Moreover, in the final chapter he wrote for the 1970 book *Anthrax* (on "Possible Use of *B. anthracis* for Bacteriological Warfare"), he sharply criticizes the United States' biological weapons activities on universal grounds:

> The greatest discoveries of our times, which made it possible to produce large amounts of bacterial mass (deep-layer method of cultivation), to use various cellular systems to accumulate viruses, to alter the genetic code of viruses and bacteria are now subordinated to the goals of developing and producing bacteriological weapons in the world's largest capitalistic country, the United States. This research . . . is a negation of everything that has already been achieved by physicians, a negation of medicine itself.[13]

The former deputy minister is also a man with a long and impressive track record in fighting major epidemics. After Burgasov's 1988 presentation at the National Academy, polio vaccine pioneer Albert Sabin, his hair as white as Burgasov's, came forward to embrace him. They had worked together in the Soviet Union's successful antipolio campaign in 1960–61, when seventy-eight million people, nearly one-third of the population of the USSR, were inoculated with the vaccine Sabin developed. Burgasov's reception from Dr. Donald A. Henderson, dean of the Johns Hopkins University School of Public Health, was also welcoming. Burgasov had worked with Henderson on the World Health Organization campaign to eradicate smallpox.

Burgasov still denies knowing of any military involvement in the outbreak or if the Soviet scientists at Compound 19 were engaged in producing anthrax weapons. He staked out his position in 1979, repeated it in the United States in 1988, and stands by it now. I am reminded of his angry response in Washington in 1988 to repeated questions from the audience about the Soviet army's culpability: "Go ask them!"

At the conclusion of the interview, Dr. Burgasov invites us to visit him at his dacha once we have finished our work in Yekaterinburg. Then, when Matthew asks his permission to photocopy the 1979 veterinarian documents, Burgasov not only agrees but says that we can have the originals, to help in our research on the animal outbreak. After Matthew has escorted Burgasov out, Hugh-Jones, who heartily shook hands with the old man, exclaims, "He's telling the truth!"

The words are hardly out of his mouth when Walker (who has left the young Dr. Nikiforov across the hall) enters the conference room to announce authoritatively that he is certain he has seen two, possibly three, instances of inhalation anthrax in the slides. But he has to admit that the slides suggesting infection of the lymph nodes in the lung area are mixed with others that look like gastrointestinal anthrax or what might have been general systemic infection. He will need to see more and better material to make a judgment.

Young Dr. Nikiforov joins us for lunch at the Presidium of the Russian Academy of Sciences. The Presidium is a massive futuristic edifice with wide, echoing corridors. The main restaurant, with a ceiling as high as an airplane hangar, is nearly empty. Soviet science, like so much of the Soviet economy, was deeply involved with the military. With the Cold War over, one hears stories of entire laboratories shut down for want of equipment, materials, electricity, or salaries to pay their employees. Scientists have emigrated or perhaps haven't the means to eat here any more.

"I believe the anthrax was inhalatory," Dr. Nikiforov tells us. Then he adds, "Though I never discussed this with Papa." When asked by Walker why his father went to the States in 1988 without a full range of slides, Nikiforov answers, "Because he was forced to!"

This lunch sets the unfortunate precedent of discussing at mealtime the destructive effects of anthrax infection on the body. Hugh-Jones and Nikiforov converse in detail about the damage to oral mucous membranes and the gut in animals as possible analogues to paths of infection in humans. Walker joins in with the specifics of throat tissue degeneration in experimentally infected pigs. All the while, we are being served *pelimeni*, little dumplings stuffed with pork, and platters of sliced sausage, some gray, some pink.

In addition to the autopsy slides he is willing to share, Nikiforov says he also has at home copies of hospital records for some of the survivors of the 1979 epidemic, which he might allow us to peruse. Like Burgasov, he is proud that twenty-one people survived systemic anthrax infection, but he credits his father alone for this victory. Because of time pressures, we delay taking up the offer to see these hospital records until we return to Moscow from Yekaterinburg. My expectation is that hospital records still exist in Yekaterinburg and that we have only to nose around to find them.

That evening, the team convenes for the first of the nightly discussions we plan to have throughout this research. It is my idea that each evening we should sort out our intake of information and that I will use my tape recorder to keep us straight on what happened when. Matthew and I have already begun to take notes during and after interviews and at quiet moments, day and night. This last evening in Moscow, our group meets in one of the hotel lounges. We have a lot of questions. Primary among them is the familiar puzzle of whether the elder Dr. Nikiforov would have recognized inhalatory anthrax if he had seen it. In the twelve years since the 1979 epidemic, and in part because of it, Western science has moved ahead on anthrax research. Much of this work builds on the discovery in the 1950s by British biochemist Harry Smith of the three components of anthrax that combine to make it deadly: protective antigen, lethal factor, and edema factor. Between 1980 and 1989, while little was heard from Soviet scientists, no less than twenty-six American and British articles documented the efforts of researchers to apply molecular and cellular biology to explore the disease's lethal properties in laboratory animals and to improve vaccines for soldiers.[14] But, again, how sophisticated is anyone in interpreting human pathoanatomical evidence, the actual infection in the body? How sophisticated was anyone in 1979?

"The evidence I saw today," Walker asserts, referring to the Nikiforov slides, "was intestinal *and* inhalatory. We must find the autopsy materials." He bets he can settle the question with twenty tissue slides per case. I am more interested in what we can discover from families about the victims' clinical symptoms, from the onset of the disease to death. I have organized my questionnaire for family members with that in mind, and hospital records would be helpful, too.

The next morning we go to Domodevedo Airport to fly to Yekaterinburg. The Aeroflot plane we board looks run-down, nothing like the new Finnair plane that brought us to Moscow. The seats creak, the upholstery is ragged, and the interior walls are scarred with scrapes and gouges. The plane's one advantage is that it has open access to the baggage area down a flight of stairs. Hugh-Jones has lugged along a global positioning device that relies on satellites to determine locations. He wants to test it in Yekaterinburg, to check existing maps. We have each brought cameras, and Matthew and I packed tape recorders as well. Our suitcases are in full view, and we can check on them any time to be sure they are safe.

To get to our flight early, we left before the hotel canteen opened at seven, and the airport offers nothing to eat or drink. Not a good traveler under the best of circumstances, I also feel physically wretched from jet lag, and my mind is bothered by the problem of whom and what to believe. Strapped in my seat and nervous with anticipation, I take out my notebook and write:

Why would Burgasov agree to come to the States if he felt his case was in the least shaky? He could have just said no, unless some higher-up gave him marching orders, i.e., the military. But would they do that if the case were at any point open to refutation? Was this a cocky venture in 1988? Or did Burgasov really believe his explanation? How should we interpret Nikiforov's neglecting to bring lung-photo slides?

A little while later, aching for breakfast, I add:

10:18. It looks as if the plane is ready to take off, nearly on time. A cart has been wheeled by with candy bars, chewing gum, and magazines on it. I hear the rattle of bottles in the back of the plane. But no hope. "Ou vas yest chai?" I asked. (Do you have tea?) And got a sulky "nyet" from the stewardess.

In less than three hours we pass over the Ural Mountains, which despite the spread of industrial pollution are still impressive. As Boris Pasternak, who was always fascinated by these mountains, wrote in one of his poems, "Arrayed in majesty, the firs arose / In ranks of glory."[15] The Russian passengers cram the windows to gaze down on the great north-to-south stretch of rocky peaks and taiga, the green conifer forest.

I feel less romantic about nature. Civilizations dominate it any way they can, with brutality or with affection.[16] Nature always fights back, with floods, storms, earthquakes, fires, volcanic eruptions—and disease. The emphatic gray concrete and asphalt of Moscow has kept me from thinking about Russia's long history with anthrax outbreaks. In czarist times, the Russian incidence of anthrax reportedly hovered around 50,000 animal deaths per year, 11,500 human skin infections, and 3,500 human deaths. In 1649, after a terrible anthrax epidemic, Czar Aleksey decreed that no more animal carcasses could be dumped in Moscow streets. The general situation led one contemporary to pronounce, "Anthrax exists permanently in Russia. This is our self-styled national disease."[17]

But ultimately it was one of Russia's own who helped control the disease. In 1888 the great biologist Ilya Metchnikoff worked in Louis Pasteur's laboratory on anthrax. Through him the czars soon had their own animal vaccine, and by the end of the nineteenth century, all rates of anthrax were dropping. By the 1930s, Soviet morbidity and mortality rates from anthrax were halved, but so, too, were the numbers of livestock. The disastrous policies of collectivization prompted peasants to kill animals they thought would be taken from them in the name of the state. At that time, before World War II, human anthrax rates in the remote Soviet republics such as Azerbaijan, Bessarabia, and Kazakhstan still recalled the czarist era, with animal and human cases in the thousands. By the 1950s, animal anthrax cases in the Soviet Union were reduced to several thousand per year, human infections to some twelve hundred, and human fatalities were in the low hundreds. This improvement resulted not only from better vaccines but also from the stupendously large Soviet programs to get those vaccines to animals and people. By the 1960s, more than ten million animals and two million people per year were being vaccinated against anthrax. Unlike the West, the Soviets developed and used live spore vaccine on humans; produced in Tblisi, Georgia, and known as STI vaccine, its side effects restrict its use to healthy adults.[18]

Globally, according to World Health Organization reports, modern outbreaks of anthrax, animal and human, have occurred mainly in contaminated environments in rural enclaves of Asia, Asia Minor, and Africa, where vaccination programs are lacking or erratic. Yet anthrax can emerge even in industrial countries with long histories of enforced public health laws.[19] In 1976, in Texas and Louisiana, large herds of horses and cattle came down with anthrax. Industrialized nations with small dispersed private farms, such as the United Kingdom and Italy, still remain relatively susceptible to anthrax. And yet, among all industrialized countries, by 1990 the USSR averaged the most anthrax outbreaks, nearly three hundred animal outbreaks per year over the last two decades and around twenty human cases, with one or two fatalities among them. Unvaccinated privately owned cattle have been one source of infection; in 1975 infected goat hair from Iran caused an outbreak in a mill near Moscow.[20]

The 1979 outbreak (if the Soviet number of ninety-six cases, including the cutaneous ones, and sixty-four fatalities, is correct) tripled the USSR's yearly average morbidity from anthrax and pushed its death rate off the chart. And yet the invasion of infected meat into a populous urban area might do that much damage. All it would take is a breakdown in the veterinary service and public health surveillance, leading to the scenario we have been given, of contaminated feed and meat. If the other scenario is true, however, if the breakdown was an accident at the Soviet military facility, the full explanation for the disaster lies hidden within that organization. Either way, there was much to hide. Why then should the responsible civic or military personnel wax confessional for us? They would have to be willing to repudiate the Soviet Union's public health sector or its army. If they had been principal actors in the disaster, they might be implicating themselves. But the government is letting us in; we have been told that a good number of officials in Yekaterinburg are willing to speak to us. Is it possible that some basic honesty, a need for truth-telling, has emerged as part of the glasnost spirit? On the last pages of Gogol's novel *Dead Souls*, the Russian prince exhorts his officials to put aside dishonesty by appealing to "those who still have a Russian heart and who have still some understanding of the word 'honour.'"[21] That is lofty rhetoric; reality may let us down. These thoughts, not the romantic beauty of the Urals, preoccupy me as we fly across the mountains and begin our descent into Asia.

4

In the Urals

THE QUEST BEGINS

Thursday, June 4. We arrive in Yekaterinburg just before 3 P.M. Tell a friend you are going to Siberia and the conversation will turn to tigers and massive forests, or to the gulags. The Urals region is far less exotic and harsh, its history and tragedies of another order. It was to the eastern side of the mountain range that Stalin transferred major military industries during the 1930s and 1940s, to protect them from Nazi aggression. But hundreds of years before that the natural riches of the region, especially iron ore, had fostered Yekaterinburg's intimate connection to weapons manufacture. At the end of the seventeenth century, Czar Peter I commissioned the blacksmith Nikita Demidov to forge cannons to fight the Swedes in Russia's successful battle for control of the Baltic. The city of Neviansk became Demidov's empire, and around it sprang up a constellation of factory towns, including Yekaterinburg, which eventually came to dominate the region.

Technically in Asia—the Urals mark the division between Europe and Asia—and some two hundred kilometers west of the Siberian border, Yekaterinburg sits on a north-central break in the mountains. It was established in 1723 and named for the saint (not the great Empress Catherine, who had yet to make her appearance in history). The old maps show the first nub of settlement on a widening of the Iset River, in what is now the northern part of the city. By 1727 the area had enlarged into a grid of streets, like a Roman encampment. In 1831 the emerald boom began, with crates of the gems supposedly shipped monthly to the czars. By 1856 the town had tripled in size, its grid spreading in orderly fashion north, south, and east. By 1891 the completion of the Trans-Siberian railroad made it a major way station between Russia and Asia. By 1923, Yekaterinburg, doubled in size again, was a complete city, with postrevolutionary factories sprouting up on its eastern and southern edges.

Yekaterinburg was and is more than a military-industrial enclave. Over the years, it attracted mining barons and merchants who profited from the deposits of coal and bauxite and nonferrous metals (copper, titanium, manganese, vanadium, nickel, chromium) and precious gems—the enduring emeralds and diamonds, and semiprecious stones like malachite, the symbol of the Urals, which still is used to decorate tourist pins and mementos. The city also has the benefit of a rich agricultural hinterland, stretching south toward Chelyabinsk and east toward Novosibirsk, two other major industrial cities. As early as 1763, the territory for thousands of kilometers east of Yekaterinburg and the Urals was within the Russian empire. The Trans-Siberian Railroad further increased national reliance on the Urals' natural and industrial resources, and incorporated the city even more securely within the Russian empire. From the perspective of St. Petersburg and Moscow, the city was provincial. In 1890, Anton Chekhov, on his pilgrimage to the Far East to visit the Sakhalin Island prison, stopped in Yekaterinburg for three days. He wrote home to his sister about the city's velvet-toned church bells. But he was more impressed by how the iron-works industry dominated the center city with its noise and smoke. He described the local people, including one of his mother's relatives, as having "prominent cheekbones, big brows, broad shoulders, tiny eyes, and huge fists." He added, "They are born in the local cast-iron foundries and are brought into the world not by a midwife but by a machinist."[1]

On Yekaterinburg's highest bluff, overlooking the Iset River, the wealthiest merchants built ornate mansions. In 1918, one of those mansions, the house of an engineer, N. N. Ipatiev, became the prison of Czar Nicholas II and his family. Seized in their flight from Moscow to St. Petersburg, the Romanovs were eventually brought as captives to the Urals. In Yekaterinburg, they lived under house arrest on Voznesenskiy Prospekt (Ascension Avenue). In October 1918, as White forces were encroaching on Yekaterinburg, the royal family, their physician, and three servants were shot to death in the mansion's basement. Later their remains were burned and buried outside the city. The order to murder the Romanovs, only recently discovered in archives, was telegraphed from Yakov Sverdlov, Lenin's right-hand supporter and confidant. The order presumably came to him directly from Lenin, who wanted to eliminate the "living flag" around which monarchists might rally but who also cloaked his order for their violent execution in secrecy.[2] Sverdlov, not the Romanovs, would be memorialized by the city of Sverdlovsk and by the region (Sverdlovsk oblast) as well.

A Bolshevik at age seventeen, Yakov Sverdlov was twice exiled by the czarist government to Siberia. Both times he lived with fellow revolutionist Joseph Stalin, whom he described in letters as an arrogant loner and "egoist." In the fall of 1905, at age twenty, Sverdlov was dispatched to Yekaterinburg to convene an all-Urals party congress. He never forgot the names of the people he met or underestimated the importance of the rank-and-file organizers, and the workers of the Urals did not forget their "Yasha" when it came time to show party loyalty. Often elected by workers to preside over debates, Sverdlov developed a domineering style that in 1918 allowed him to quell factional opposition to Lenin. Most important, he almost single-handedly pushed through the centralization of the Communist Party's administrative and legislative systems. He "stressed the need for a centralized party with each local unit bound to the decisions of a higher one and the entirety subordinated to the Central Committee. This was pure Leninism."[3]

Sverdlov, having driven himself to exhaustion with committee work, died of influenza in 1919, when he was thirty-three. At the time he was the Soviet Republic's first president, as well as its secretary general. Lenin, despite his fears of the influenza epidemic, visited his dying comrade and found him making notes for the next Council meeting. Sverdlov was quickly made an icon of Bolshevik loyalty, a model for aspiring *pratiki* (the party organizers who left grand theory to others) who never fell from grace. Afterward, while purging the living loyalists, Stalin eulogized Sverdlov as the man who skillfully created the organizational forms of the interrelation between the Party and the Soviets, securing the leadership of the Party. Stalin had reason to be grateful to his old comrade in exile, for what Sverdlov had unwittingly created was the political foundation of the Stalinist dictatorship.

Sverdlov's mentor Lenin did not long outlive him. He suffered his first stroke in May 1922, his last in January 1924, after which he quickly succumbed. In that same year, Yekaterinburg was renamed for Sverdlov as part of the overflow from the party's posthumous mania for glorifying Lenin. This is when Petrograd, which had been St. Petersburg until 1914, became Leningrad; and when Sverdlov University in Moscow, a major center for agit-prop, was created. Yekaterinburg would stay Sverdlovsk until September 1991, when its city's soviet (council) voted to reclaim the prerevolutionary name, even before the Soviet Union officially dissolved.

Russia has long had a vigorous and confusing tradition of naming and renaming. Political figures have changed their names to denote their public roles, for which ordinary identification will not suffice. Vladimir Ulyanov was only an exiled Marxist until he invented the name Lenin and became the architect of a new empire. Josef Dzhugashvili was an undistinguished Georgian Bolshevik who became first the minor revolutionary "Koba" and then Stalin ("man of steel"). Russian places, too, have been precipitously renamed—or rather recoded—to fit political change. After the revolution many cities and towns, and the streets and places within them, lost their traditional and ecclesiastical associations and became dedicated to the dates and heroes of the new order. The repressed names of individuals and places signify a Russian tolerance for the displacement (rather than the obliteration) of former identities.[4] The effect is like a shell game, not because the identifying names do not matter, but because they matter so much.

As Sverdlovsk, Yekaterinburg became an elaborately bureaucratized party outpost. To begin, some thirty churches were destroyed and with them the velvet-toned bells that Chekhov admired. Lest anyone doubt its new identity, in 1931, in the center city, an entire building, a monument to communism, was constructed in the shape of a hammer and sickle. New factories overshadowed but did not eliminate the ornate wooden cottages on the city's outskirts. Instead, the burden of modernity in this region of the USSR was born by Magnitogorsk, the new industrial city to the south,[5] while Sverdlovsk became the capital of the Urals, with its own opera house, theaters, cinemas, parks, museums, and educational institutions dedicated to Soviet dogma.

For Stalin, Sverdlovsk ultimately bore testimony to the successful conversion of the USSR to a great military power. Although it had militarized its industries during the late 1930s, the Soviet Union was nonetheless taken unaware by Germany's June 1941 attack on its western border ("Operation Barbarossa"). By winter, the Germans had captured three million Soviet soldiers and controlled roughly two-fifths of the population and half the nation's vital resources. Yet after November, when Hitler's troops foundered in the mud and snow outside Moscow, the Soviets started to rebound. Stalin's purges of 1936–38 had depleted whole cadres of officers, but by 1943, the Soviet military leadership had grown in numbers and experience, learning from bitter failures. Soviet factory work, transported to the Urals, supported its army. Between 1940 and 1944, the USSR managed to quadruple its output of munitions.

> By the end of the war, 3,400 military planes were being produced monthly. Industry in the first four years of fighting supplied the red forces with 100,000 tanks, 130,000 aircraft and 800,000 field guns. At the peak of mobilization there were twelve million men under arms. The USSR produced double the amount of soldiers and fighting equipment that Germany produced.[6]

During the war, Sverdlovsk became a major armaments producer. The design of the T-34 tank was created here, and though the tanks, essential to the defeat of Nazi forces, were manufactured in Chelyabinsk, just south of Sverdlovsk, the trucks for carrying them to the front were made in Sverdlovsk. Artillery and munitions were also made in Sverdlovsk and shipped across the Urals. The city expanded south and east, down the slopes, with more factories. During the war, institutes of biology, chemistry, and physics were also transplanted from Moscow.

Just after World War II, between 1947 and 1949, the military base called Compound 19 was built, abutting the southern industrialized sector of the city. Later, in the 1960s, Compound 32, an army base with barracks and apartments for soldiers and their families was added to the southern edge of Compound 19. Past the western walls of Compound 32 lies farm land, with *sovkhozes* (state farms) and *kolkhozes* (collective farms) identical to those dotting the southern hinterlands, called the Sysertskiy district, where animal outbreaks of anthrax were supposed to have taken place in 1979.

During the Cold War, Sverdlovsk became a Soviet "closed city," to which travel was restricted for foreigners. The military presence, which early on included scientific laboratories, justified this designation, as did the continued production of weapons. By the 1970s, according to one source, 87 percent of Sverdlovsk's industrial production was military; only 13 percent was for public consumption. The city's educational resources, such as the Gorky Ural State University and the Ural Polytechnic Institute, from which Boris Yeltsin was graduated,[7] and other institutes for engineering and science, also set it apart.

Our host for the next ten days in Yekaterinburg is the rector at the Ural State University, Parigoriy Suetin. The arrangement was made only a month before our arrival, and not without difficulty. To get Russian visas, we needed an invitation from an appropriate person in Yekaterinburg. In January 1992 Matthew wrote to Alexey Yablokov, President

Boris Yeltsin's Counselor on Ecology and Health, to ask for assistance. He had previously met Yablokov, a zoologist, during a visit of Russian scientists to Fort Detrick, the U.S. biodefense center. On February 5, 1992, Yablokov, who was accompanying Yeltsin on his first trip to the United States, responded on Hyatt Hotel stationery that he doubted any scientific evidence could be found and, anyway, the Russian press had already covered the story. He advised us that someone in Yekaterinburg would have to organize the trip at that end. (He knows the city: during the 1991 attempted coup against Mikhail Gorbachev, he was designated a member of the shadow government Yeltsin would establish there, in case the military sided with the Central Committee and chased all reformers from Moscow.) In his letter, Yablokov also mentioned proudly that he was trying to get a criminal law against biological weapons passed in the Russian Parliament, similar to the one in the United States. But he was unenthusiastic about the Sverdlovsk study trip.

Matthew petitioned Yablokov at his Kremlin office, with a letter hand-delivered by Dr. Yevgeniy Sverdlov (our host in Moscow), who had passed through Boston on his way back to Russia after a science lecture trip. The response to this more pointed request for assistance (communicated by e-mail from Dr. Sverdlov) was that there was "no reason to disturb a skeleton in the cupboard." In a follow-up letter in March, Yablokov said that although there was no scientific evidence, "we [are] all sure it was [a] connection with some activities in Sverdlovsk[Compound]-19. It's enough!"[8] There was nothing to do now in Yekaterinburg but "catch some rumors, and visit [the] cemetery with 64 graves." In conclusion, he said he was willing to meet with the team at his Kremlin office when our work was done, but he offered no helpful leads to contacts in Yekaterinburg. With less than two months before our scheduled departure, the trip was stalled for lack of a Russian invitation.

Then Matthew remembered that in 1979 a Northwestern University physicist, Donald Ellis, had spent time as an exchange scholar in Sverdlovsk. Ellis had worked on theories of molecular structure in rare earth metals with a colleague there, Vladimir Gubanov. In a remnant of the exchange programs that had flourished during the Nixon administration, the U.S. National Academy of Sciences and the Soviet Academy of Sciences supported Ellis, his wife, and two small children for two months in Sverdlovsk. Ellis and his family arrived in the city on April 12, 1979, at the height of the epidemic, but he knew nothing about the disaster the whole time he was in the Soviet Union. In his trip report to the National Academy, he wrote, "We traveled freely about the city, and did quite a bit of exploring through the older sections of wooden houses that are gradually giving way to multistory apartments and office buildings." No security precautions, he stated, prevented him from traveling to villages outside the city. In mid-May, as the epidemic was ending, Ellis and his family departed for a month's stay in Novosibirsk, and then returned to Sverdlovsk in mid-June for a final month of research. That Ellis, who read and spoke Russian, heard nothing about the epidemic cast serious doubt on its having involved a thousand victims or more.[9] But it was also true that he lived and worked in a university institute in the center city, perhaps cut off from wider events.

On April 1, 1992, with the team's travel plans otherwise in order, Matthew telephoned Donald Ellis at Northwestern University to ask his advice about getting the proper official invitation. Ellis said he hadn't been back to Sverdlovsk since that 1979 trip.

"How can I reach that physicist you worked with?" Matthew asked.

"I'll pass the phone to him," Ellis replied. "He's here in my office."

Professor Vladimir Gubanov, who was traveling in the United States, was indeed in Ellis's office at that moment, and he agreed to ask his university to cooperate on our behalf.

On April 27, at last, the necessary letter of invitation arrived by fax from Rector Suetin, who is also a physicist. It concluded on a cheerful note: "So, welcome to Yekaterinburg and to the Ural State University. We'll be happy to see here all the participants of your research program. As a president of the university and a chairman of the Rector's Council of the city, I'll do my best to make your visit useful and fruitful." On May 21, however, an e-mail from the university strongly advised us that local officials were unwilling to cooperate in any sort of investigation without documentation from high-level Moscow officials that this study trip was permitted. Another request to Councilor Yablokov yielded a batch of letters of support that did the trick.

Now that we have arrived, we are in the hands of scientists. At the airport, Professor Sergei Borisov, another physicist from the university, and his son-in-law, Sasha Tiutiunnik, a graduate student in physical chemistry, meet us with two cars. The two men, slim and handsome, look almost like brothers. We drive immediately to the main building of the university, a neoclassical edifice that, except for its worn marble floors and chipped banisters, might be anywhere in Europe or even on a campus in the United States. The university dates back to 1920, when Lenin decreed its founding and gave it the mandate "to educate the people of the Soviet Urals."

Naming the Ural State University after the famous author Maxim Gorky came later, after his somewhat mysterious death in 1936. Gorky, who lacked a formal education and called the impoverished of Russia his "university," would have appreciated the irony of the gesture. The tribute was not so much to Gorky's genius as to his maintaining the posture of party loyalty into his old age. Stalin made him an icon by spreading his name (not his real name but the pseudonym he chose, which means "bitter") all over the Soviet Union, attaching it to streets and schools, to the old town of Nizhni-Novgorod and its university, and to Moscow's most celebrated park.

We ascend a grand staircase and go through a pair of high wooden doors into a large foyer where three secretaries work at their desks on old, gleaming typewriters. In the corner to the right is a small desk-top copying machine. Rector Suetin meets with us in his expansive office to the left of the secretarial desks. The rector is another bearish, barrel-chested Russian like Dr. Burgasov, but younger and more genial. Three other university administrators join us, including the Pro-Rector for Research, Y. E. Tretyakov. Vladimir Shepetkin, a biologist of courtly shyness who speaks little English, is also there. He and Professor Borisov will assist us during our stay.

All of us sit down around a long, heavily carved conference table, with Rector Suetin at the head. By miscalculation, I find myself seated on the same side as the solemn university administrators, facing the other members of my team. Though I dislike being isolated from them, I am at the end of the table, with a good vantage on the meeting. Sergei Borisov handles the interpreting of the pro forma greetings and salutations. Pro-Rector for Research Tretyakov will allow us to use his spacious office opposite the rector's as a base. We can also use the small copying machine in the main office. The other resources, a computer, e-mail, and fax machines, are in Sergei Borisov's office in another building a few blocks away.

Earlier, on April 30, Matthew e-mailed Professor Borisov our proposed study plan, which included meetings with public heath officials, physicians, and families of the victims. Borisov then consulted about it with the rector and the others and made telephone calls around the city. On May 4, in his first e-mail to Matthew, he remarked that some local experts who were involved in the 1979 outbreak are reluctant to come forward. A head clinician who worked under Dr. Nikiforov, for example, does not want to talk to us. (Another physician in Moscow, who served at the same time as Olga Yampolskaya, felt the same way.) Nonetheless,

Borisov is committed to involving all who are willing in our research. He now distributes evidence of his success: a detailed agenda, in English and Russian, to structure our time for the next ten days. Meanwhile, we have agreed not to release any of our findings to the press until we are sure they are conclusive, to avoid sensationalizing the epidemic.

On reading the agenda, I realize with dismay that we are in for ten days of official presentations, mainly by public health officials, at various offices around the city; no contacts have been arranged with victims' families. At 2:30 the next day is an important meeting with Dr. Faina Abramova and Dr. Lev Grinberg, the two pathologists who performed autopsies during the 1979 epidemic. Even that is designated "a presentation." On the bright side, a trip outside the city is scheduled on Wednesday, June 10, to visit the villages where the epizootics are alleged to have taken place. The only other deviation from official presentations is a trip to the Vostochniy (East) Cemetery. The cemetery is our primary and perhaps only source of the names of 1979 anthrax victims who were buried, we have been told, in a segregated sector. But the trip is planned for June 12, right before our departure. Alarmed, I begin waving to Matthew. We ask to have the cemetery visit rescheduled to Saturday June 6, in just two days. Finding the families will be difficult; no one seems to know how.

I wait for the Russians to initiate discussion of our research, but after the rector's welcome, silence reigns. I have the distinct impression that our hosts, on the whole sophisticated gentlemen, believe we have come on a fool's errand. Like several million other Russians, they are motivated to establish American contacts, to generate joint research projects, but an event that happened thirteen years before lacks the luster of a great science venture. Maybe if we were interested in titanium or space craft or cancer cures, their expressions would be less bored and their exit less swift.

On the next day, Friday, June 5, at 10 A.M. at the Oblast SES (Sanitarno-epidemiologicheskaya stanciya, the Sanitary Epidemiological Station), our group files through an anteroom packed with secretaries' desks into an office jammed with file cabinets and brightly lit by fluorescent lights and a brilliant sun shining through large windows.[10] We are scheduled to meet with the present director, Dr. Yuriy Semyonov, and then with the retired director. Dr. Nikolay Babich, who was in charge of public health measures during the 1979 epidemic. Instead of Director Semyonov, however, a young doctor named Viktor Romanenko greets us; he is the assistant chief sanitary inspector, filling in for his boss. When we are seated at the small conference table, Dr. Romanenko begins his presentation. His demeanor is solemn, with not the slightest trace of humor, which is thoroughly in keeping with the old Soviet-style norms for public address. At the same time, with his shaggy hair and crew-neck sweater, he looks very much the modern young European professional.

"We have no records from the 1979 epidemic," he begins, and then quickly assures us that all current records—on diphtheria, tuberculosis, influenza, as well as animal anthrax and other outbreaks—are computerized and in good order. The station is in charge of monitoring the health of the entire Sverdlov oblast, with a population of 5.5 million in forty-nine wards (*rayoni*), and is also responsible for investigating, with their veterinarians, any epizootics. "A record of every case presenting at the rayon level is recorded at the oblast level and can be examined by date, by diagnosis, and so forth—except for the anthrax epidemic of 1979."

Dr. Romanenko was employed at SES as a junior physician at the time of the outbreak, so he is able to give us his perspective on what had happened. But first he explains that the Sverdlov oblast is continuously monitored for anthrax because it has thirty-seven known contaminated livestock burial sites. Aside from the 1979 outbreak, no fatal human cases have occurred for more than fifty years. In Yekaterinburg, despite extensive annual surveys, only negative soil samples have ever been found. "In short," he concludes, without a trace of a smile, "no one should have to fear getting anthrax in Yekaterinburg."

Romanenko organizes his presentation according to what he calls three hypotheses for explaining the epidemic. He is willing to consider the first, that it came from mixed feed contaminated by bone meal. From reports he remembers reading, though, hundreds of tests were done and only one or two were positive—not in samples of feed, but in residues on farm machinery. He thinks the mixed-feed factory, which he believes combines fodder and bone meal from Kazakhstan, is somewhere to the south, in Sysertskiy rayon, perhaps between the towns of Aramil and Bolshoi Istok, but he has never been there. However, he does note that during the outbreak the anthrax pathogen was found in meat taken from "the refrigerators of private persons," in about ten homes in the city's southern Chkalovskiy rayon.

"Had there been an animal outbreak in March in Sysertskiy rayon?" we ask.

"Definitely," he answers. "It was sometime around International Woman's Day, maybe in the first week. I was annoyed that I had to give up my holiday to go there." As he recalls, a few early animal cases were followed by others. "Later there were many cases, with much hysteria and the wholesale slaughter of animals."

Dr. Romanenko's second hypothesis is more innovative. He speculates that wild animals might have been a source of the outbreak. A wild boar and a wild goat were captured and fed by farmers and then, around the time of the outbreak, the animals died. We happen to know that pigs and goats are not prime candidates for anthrax, but we listen attentively, straining to separate good information from bad. Tests of these animals and their feed, he admits, proved negative.

His third speculation is that an aerosol leak from Compound 19 caused the outbreak. "This is a very disturbing hypothesis," he comments somberly. "The SES investigated but could not prove it. Samples were taken from inside and outside walls of stables, roofs, and from soil in the city. From houses and from the air. All were negative."

"What did you think then was the cause?" I ask.

"Classical epidemiology taught me that human anthrax is acquired from animals. I believed this at the time. Now I do not know what to believe."

Dr. Romanenko then excuses himself and leaves the office. Immediately, Dr. Babich, the former head of SES, arrives and unceremoniously introduces himself. He is a weathered man with hunched shoulders and the unhealthy smell of tobacco emanating from his clothes. The first two fingers on his right hand are deep yellow from cigarette smoking, not what one expects from a public health official. Unlike Romanenko, Babich was a principal player in the public health response to the epidemic. Dr. Burgasov has described going with him to Compound 19 to take soil and water samples from outside its walls, which Burgasov said proved negative. I lean forward to listen.

"I speak only from memory," Babich says, "since there are no documents. Everything was taken a few months after the outbreak. All documents are in the hands of Burgasov." Then he goes on to describe the epidemic. "People died in streetcars and in the lobbies of buildings. There was no time for an ambulance. Everything happened at once. Following regulations, the clinics trying to diagnose the illness notified Moscow."

As Babich remembers, Dr. Nikiforov arrived the third or fourth day after the initial outbreak, before it was recognized as an anthrax epidemic. He thought that Nikiforov deserved great credit for saving at least some patients when a 100 percent fatality rate was expected. At first, the victims were taken to Hospitals 20 and 24, but after three to four days,

Hospital 40 was devoted to the epidemic. Anyone with a temperature above 38 degrees centigrade was sent there for screening, with special attention paid to pulmonary distress. Dr. Babich is emphatic that the outbreak was airborne and claims that "clinical, pathoanatomical, and bacteriological evidence" support this diagnosis. "There were no intestinal symptoms and no intestinal lesions," he says, in direct contradiction to the elder Dr. Nikiforov's report.

And what about an epizootic in the south preceding the human outbreak?

"There was none," Babich insists. "Maybe there was a suspected case of a wild goat in Syserts, but nothing came of it."

"Were there any unusual animal deaths in Sysertskiy rayon?"

"You should ask a veterinarian," he replies impatiently.

"Was the SES asked to investigate an epizootic on Woman's Day in 1979?" Matthew asks.

Dr. Babich's face turns deep red, whether with embarrassment or anger, we cannot tell. After a pause, he says insistently, "I believe the animal deaths occurred only after the epidemic began." He appears reluctant to elaborate.

On hearing two different stories, first that there was an epizootic before the human anthrax cases and then that there was none, we begin exchanging worried glances. Were Burgasov's documents about animal deaths valid or forgeries? Was Dr. Babich aware of Romanenko's account of epizootics? Could he tell us about any late-occurring epizootic? Alexis Shelokov refuses to translate any confrontational questions, saying that they would be insulting and might get us in trouble. More than the rest of us, he is highly conscious of the fact that we are nine thousand miles from home and completely dependent on the good will of officials, which he trusts not at all. My exhortation, "just ask him," falls on deaf ears.

Matthew moves the discussion along by passing Dr. Babich a copy of the graph of recorded deaths from the 1988 official Soviet statement.

"It's approximately correct," Babich concludes, but grudgingly, as if the graph cannot possibly matter.

"And the extended tail of the distribution, to mid-May?"

"You are assuming you know the strain," Babich retorts. "Maybe this was a different strain. We do not know its properties, do we?"

When told we want to make a map plotting both the work places and homes of victims, he dismisses the effort with the wave of his yellow-fingered hand. "Nothing will come of making such maps."

Dr. Romanenko returns and, as soon as he does, Dr. Babich seems eager to leave. We all stand, crowded between file cabinets. At that moment, Professor Borisov also appears, ready to drive us to lunch at the university. We tell him what seems to be the most important fact we have learned, that the SES has no records from the outbreak, and therefore no list of the victims' names. Borisov replies that fairly recently he saw a television news report that alluded to an official government list of names, but he remembers no details. Neither Romanenko nor Babich saw the news report or know about any government list of victims.

At this juncture, Dr. Semyonov, the current chief of SES, comes briskly into the office and joins our little crowd. He looks displeased to see his old predecessor. In haste, he announces that he understands our purposes are humane and that he will help as much as he can in introducing us to the hospital personnel under his jurisdiction. He adds that he will help arrange a meeting with the veterinarians in Sysertskiy rayon. Then he breezes out, across the anteroom to his office.

"Why see today's officials?" Dr. Babich complains, in pointed reference to Romanenko and Semyonov. "They know nothing. There were no intestinal infections."

Dr. Romanenko and he exchange glares. Then Dr. Babich shakes our hands and shambles off. After Dr. Babich leaves, Dr. Romanenko leads us to an adjoining room, where an oversized map of the Sverdlov oblast covers one wall. While he points out villages and towns to the south, I scribble in my notebook, "Who should we believe?"

On the way back to the car, we debate this question. Why did Babich suddenly blush when asked about animal deaths in March? Is he just an old man suffering memory loss? Why was Romanenko so definite about the timing of the epizootic? Is he just a young man suffering memory loss? Shelokov, who did most of the interpreting, has no explanation for the contradictions, nor does Yampolskaya. Romanenko seems serious and intelligent, Babich impassioned. But was there a serious epizootic before the epidemic or not?

"Romanenko's a liar," concludes David Walker, who has little tolerance for ambiguity. But the rest of us are unsure. And what about this list of victims alluded to on television? I ask Professor Borisov to find out more, explaining that my primary research goal is to find the families of victims. He replies rather obliquely that he will ask a friend who is in politics about it. We return to the university for lunch, to the basement cafeteria where the faculty and administrators eat. Rector Suetin joins us, but it is a strictly egalitarian arrangement, with each person selecting a plate of salad and meat and then paying for it after eating, on the honor system. I find myself sitting next to a woman who teaches literature and who was living in the city in 1979, near the university. I explain I am in Yekaterinburg to investigate the anthrax epidemic.

"Really? I know nothing about it," she says.

"Nothing at all? Sixty-four people died. It affected Chkalovskiy rayon."

"Oh, that explains it. I never go there."

Here, in a phrase, I discover the division between the center city in the north, with its broad boulevards and office buildings, educational institutions and riverside parks, and the working class Chkalovskiy district to the south.

I think of Donald Ellis, the American physicist who lived in Sverdlov in April 1979, also in the center city, and heard nothing about the epidemic. A catastrophic anthrax epidemic was raging no more than ten miles from here, and no newspaper, no radio or television station, no word-of-mouth bridged the divide. Or maybe it never happened. After all, there are no records, no names of victims, no agreement on its cause, just gory photographic slides of anthrax-infected organs that might be from any anthrax epidemic.

The literature professor is interested in Western ideas, especially postmodernism and the breakdown of rationality. The subject is popular in Russia, with some ex-Soviet writers claiming that postmodernism with its simulacra and apocalyptic visions was invented here before it ever found expression in Western philosophy.[11] What is authentic human experience amid the corporate (for the Soviet Union, read statist) packaging of pseudoevents and simulated memories that disguise a rigid hierarchy of power?[12] She asks me what I know.

"Not enough," I reply.

5

Autopsy Visions

In the afternoon, we go to the Tuberculosis and Pulmonary Diseases Unit for the city of Yekaterinburg, located just three blocks from the university dormitory where we are housed, down a quiet tree-lined street. The area is gated and the main building, dating from the 1920s, has a loading platform. Maybe the platform is only for scientific supplies, but since pathology is part of the center's work, I imagine that other, more morbid cargo is unloaded there.

Dr. Lev Grinberg's office is in a single-story wing, which we enter directly from a parking lot. Tall and hefty, with tinted glasses and a black beard, and wearing a white laboratory coat, Grinberg makes it clear from the beginning that he will dominate this meeting. In a deep bass voice, he invites us to follow him down a narrow hall past a conference room to his small office. There he sits commandingly behind his desk, while the six of us squeeze onto a small couch or sit in uncomfortable plastic chairs. Even Dr. Faina Abramova, a radiant woman in her mid-sixties with wavy white hair, is wedged on the couch next to Olga Yampolskaya. Dr. Grinberg states directly and clearly that he and Dr. Abramova are determined to publish the autopsy data from the anthrax epidemic. There is a brief pause in which the implications of this statement sink in. Then, recalling that Grinberg was only a medical student in 1979, I pointedly ask what Dr. Abramova has to say. A good deal, as it turns out.

Speaking in a low voice, she describes how, in 1982, she and Grin-

berg traveled to Moscow, expecting to give a lecture on the 1979 outbreak. Instead, they were allowed no opportunity to speak. They met
Dr. Nikiforov at his office and left with him their manuscript and eighty-
nine slides.[1] By her account, then, the slides the young Nikiforov showed
us in Moscow, or some portion of them, belong neither to him nor to
Dr. Burgasov. According to Dr. Abramova, she was in charge of the autopsies and ordered the photographs, so the slides belong to her and, by
extension, to her collaborator, Dr. Grinberg. I try to be impartial, but I
have the feeling this composed, grandmotherly figure in her pink sweater
and laced shoes was too trusting of Nikiforov.

When Matthew requests permission for Walker and Yampolskaya to
begin examining the autopsy material, Grinberg replies, "First we must
discuss protection of our property, of our intellectual property rights."

We all agree that their ownership of the data is a fair assumption. Grinberg then announces he will give a presentation of the material that will
illustrate inhalation anthrax. He leads us to the conference table, where
a slide projector and screen have been set up. Before turning on the projector, Dr. Grinberg narrates a synopsis of the 1979 outbreak, from the
pathologists' point of view. On April 10, at one of the city's smaller hospitals, Dr. Abramova and he took part in the autopsy of a young man.
Abramova noted that, along with massive thoracic and gastrointestinal
hemorrhaging, there was a distinctive pattern of bleeding in the brain.
She remembered a photograph from an old medical textbook that associated anthrax with a circular "Cardinal's cap" of red hemorrhagic tissue and immediately made her guess. Then she sent Grinberg by car to
take samples of the brain and spleen for bacteriological analysis at the
SES hazardous infection laboratory. By the end of the next day, April 11,
her guess was confirmed: the disease was anthrax. By then the outbreak
was reaching its peak. Screening, diagnosis, and treatment had already
been set up at Hospital 40, which also became a center for autopsying.
Abramova, who was now directing the autopsies, began, along with Grinberg, to investigate a series of ninety-six bodies of people who died in
April and May after being admitted to the hospital as possible anthrax
cases. Of these, forty-two were diagnosed at autopsy as having died of
anthrax; the rest, as having died of other causes. Abramova and Grinberg did all but one of the autopsies themselves. There was a barrage of
fatal cases at the peak of the epidemic, with fewer but still often multiple autopsies per day continuing over the subsequent month. It is not a
scene one wants to contemplate at length.

"And the other twenty-two autopsies?" we ask, since Grinberg has agreed with the official Soviet account that the total fatal cases of anthrax numbered sixty-four.

"The remaining twenty-two anthrax deaths must have occurred before April 10 and been autopsied elsewhere."

From the start, he continues, the medical staff was fearful about the epidemic. Was it contagious or not? Then Dr. Nikiforov arrived on April 12 and assured everyone that contagion was not a serious problem, although for the first week the staff was on antibiotics. Nikiforov demanded complete autopsies, which, out of fear and revulsion, not everyone wanted done. Ordinarily nearly all patients who died at the main hospital were autopsied, but this time the staff refused. Nikiforov, however, had his reasons and insisted. He thought it was important to determine which patients had really died of anthrax (as opposed to other infections, heart attacks, cancer, or other causes). In addition, as Abramova represents him, he had spent his whole life studying anthrax and realized how scientifically valuable autopsies might be in this case. Like Dr. Babich, Grinberg seems to respect Nikiforov, even though their explanations of the cause of the 1979 outbreak may differ. Perhaps what impressed the Sverdlovsk doctors was Nikiforov's clinical competence, which they seem to separate from his defense of the official "bad meat" explanation.

Grinberg goes on to describe how in doing the autopsies, he and Abramova used no special protection except gauze face masks. They did, however, take the precaution of closing off the floor drains, and they tried not to spill blood. Afterward, buckets of chloramine were used to disinfect the autopsy room surfaces. At the height of the epidemic, they had to move quickly from one corpse to another, without rest and sometimes without time to clean equipment between autopsies. They sent tissue samples from each autopsy for bacteriologic confirmation and have the results to show us.

Dr. Grinberg turns off the lights and his slide show begins. It is much more coherent than the one I saw in Moscow. Grinberg will argue as a pathologist who has studied the cases. He shows us twenty-five color and black-and-white slides to illustrate what he feels are the general characteristics of the impact that anthrax had on the victims. Of the forty-two cases, thirty-nine had gastrointestinal lesions; thirty-six of these had lesions in the small intestine, and thirty had small multiple gastric lesions. If correct, this puts to rest Babich's assertion that there were no gastrointestinal lesions. But Grinberg has seen infection in the mesentery lymph nodes in only nine victims. He therefore considers these signs of gastrointestinal infection to be secondary to inhalation anthrax.

In contrast, he says in his deep voice, all forty-two cases show signs of massive infection in the chest area, with hemorrhagic thoracic lymph nodes and with hemorrhaging in the mediastinum (the area between the lungs). In most cases the inside surfaces of the lungs appeared to be without serious lesions, but in eleven cases there was a hemorrhagic lesion inside the lung. Twenty-one patients had cerebral hemorrhage, including sixteen with definite Cardinal's cap.

Grinberg also notes that two or three victims had cutaneous anthrax, apparently at the sites of vaccinations. He remembers in particular one victim, a man who was vaccinated once on April 21 and died May 1. Dr. Nikiforov believed that the vaccine inoculations were given too late to offer protection to anyone. Abramova and Grinberg think the vaccinations (three successive shots were prescribed) may have intensified existing infections. In any event, the one shot of the vaccine this victim received was certainly not effective.

Grinberg's review reminds us that, while weapons experts might think of anthrax spores as uniform little bullets, they are organic entities with a definite life cycle, just as Robert Koch demonstrated more than a century ago (see Chapter 1). We see in these coherently organized slides what happens as the bacillus form of the disease develops and invades, a glimmering of the mysterious processes that direct the spread of infection and the production of toxins that flood the body and kill the host. And, not depicted here, there is the anthrax that can be rendered innocuous, when its spores and bacteria are defeated by the immune system of mammals that survive the disease.

I am struck by how far all this detail takes us from actual victims, from human beings. No symptoms matter here, no chills or fever, no tightness in the chest or how many times the victim vomited. Now it is only the indelible marks the disease left inside the body that count.[2]

After his talk ends, Grinberg lists the materials he and Abramova have for their forty-two cases. For many of the cases, they have gross organs preserved in 10 percent formalin, paraffin blocks of tissues, and glass slides of histological preparations. For all forty-two cases, there is some documentation, such as pathological description and diagnosis, brief histological (tissue analysis) descriptions, bacteriological test results, some clinical notes, and the patients' names, with the dates of onset, admission, death, and autopsy. Dr. Abramova has kept all this material under her personal protection since 1979.

Our group is impressed. Unless the autopsy materials are of poor quality or have been seriously degraded, Walker should be able to draw some basic conclusions about the portal of entry, whether pulmonary or gastrointestinal. For Grinberg to assert he has proof is one thing; for a colleague to confirm it is another. My particular interest is in the onset data, with which we could begin to construct an epidemic curve, and whether we can have access to the name of the patients and perhaps help in finding their families.

But this is no time to ask for more. Grinberg wants to hammer out the details of the intellectual property rights issue. He suggests an agreement between institutions. On their side, the Sverdlovsk oblast SES can provide an umbrella to protect their rights, including publications, future contacts, exchange of materials, and presentations at meetings. He wants us to make the request for this protection from his supervisor, Dr. Semyonov, the director of SES, who greeted us so hurriedly this morning.

No American member of our group, each employed by a different institution, rushes to offer reciprocal guarantees. Nor do we pause to discuss our commitment among ourselves. Grinberg has been so quick to answer our questions, at times interrupting Shelokov's interpreting, that we are sure he understands English. So we agree to reflect on this proposal overnight and meet again with the two pathologists the next day. An unfortunate glumness settles over us. Nothing is decided. We are not shaking hands and celebrating glasnost and international cooperation. But Grinberg, not pushing his advantage, says that Dr. Walker and Dr. Yampolskaya are welcome to come back to the center the next morning to take a closer look at the glass slides of some tissue samples.

Before we leave, I ask Grinberg if in 1979 he and Abramova had believed doing the autopsies was dangerous. I am thinking of Everett Hughes's concept of "dirty work," which distinguishes among social activities by the degree of taboo they carry.[3] Why pick an older woman (Abramova was called out of retirement to direct the 1979 autopsies) and a medical student to face first an unknown epidemic and then the threat of anthrax bacteria and spores?

Dr. Grinberg replies that, at the beginning, the medical staff speculated that the epidemic was plague. Everyone was terrified, and some physicians refused to come to work. He deliberately quarantined himself at the hospital to protect his family, as did other clinicians. In a few days, once it became clear the disease was anthrax, he was no longer afraid. And he and Abramova were not completely alone at their work. Two other pathologists worked with them, under Abramova's direction.

"My feeling then," Grinberg, standing tall, explains, "was one of tremendous commitment in the course of hard work."

Dr. Abramova, more modest, refrains from comment. Maybe she doesn't want to remember how bad it was.

Dinner tonight is instant soup and peanut butter on crackers, provisions I am glad I had the forethought to pack at home in Cambridge. We are being quartered in one of the student dormitories, which are in a somewhat isolated area, and the nearby university canteen closes early. Our suite of rooms, reserved for special visitors, is on the seventh floor. We each have rooms with showers; there is a lounge area where we can meet, and next to it a small refrigerator and hot plate. Yampolskaya makes tea, which takes the chill out of my hands and feet. The temperature outside is just above freezing, and I have come dressed for early summer. We are making do with an elevator that is almost always "temporarily out of order," no hot water, narrow beds with spent springs that touch the floor, and light bulbs that randomly explode. Strangely enough, none of this really matters to me. I am too preoccupied with my disappointment about how little solid information we have wrested from both the day's appointments. I naively expected that, in the spirit of glasnost, the SES people would somehow reach into their obviously ample files and pull out stacks of forgotten records, leftovers of bureaucratic memory penned in black ink by some unknowing but careful scribe. No such luck.

That evening our group mulls over the question of whether an animal outbreak of anthrax did occur in 1979, before the human deaths. Though Walker has a low tolerance for ambiguity, Shelokov's is considerable. With little trouble, he conjures up five or six hypothetical reasons, not only for Babich's blush, but for Burgasov's claim to Abramova's slides, and even for why our original hotel reservations fell through and landed us in a student dormitory. Most of his hypotheses predicate the heavy use of *vranyo*, the verbal presentation of non-facts as truths for which Soviet bureaucrats (among others) were well known. As journalist David Shipler once had *vranyo* explained to him, "You know that I'm lying, and I know that you know, and you know that I know that you know, but I go ahead with a straight face, and you nod seriously and take notes."[4] In *The Russian Mind* Ronald Hingley likens *vranyo* to Irish blarney and leg-pulling.[5] The analogy is apt. Verbal gaming may be no ordinary game, but the product of a repressive social system that dictates and even distorts the forms of communication.[6] Under Czarist rule and then the Soviets, the political consequences of speaking one's mind could be catastrophic. Russian words are charged with extraordinary power; poetry and death sentences have been imbued into the language.

But I am in the liberated Russia of 1992, where no purges persist and everyone can talk freely. So how does one get a straight answer to a straight question? How can we discern the facts when stories conflict? How will we find out anything, except that there is disagreement?

A little after 7 P.M., these meanderings are interrupted by a surprise telephone call. Our shy biologist from the university, Dr. Vladimir Shepetkin, has for us five names of victims, with their addresses and snippets of information on hospital admission. Apparently Sergei Borisov conveyed my anxiety to him. But what is the source of this information?

"A physician who is a friend of his," Shelokov, who took the call, tells us. "He doesn't want to reveal the name."

Shelokov copies the information down and then he, Matthew, and I go over it. One of the victims was treated at Hospital 40, which means I might be able to link that case with the autopsy data from Abramova and Grinberg, should we ever get it. Three other victims died early in the epidemic, two at Hospital 24 and another at Hospital 20. A quick check of the Yekaterinburg map shows that all five home addresses are on streets in Chkalovskiy rayon. For the first time I am hopeful I might have real work to do, that I haven't hauled along a hundred questionnaires for nothing. Yampolskaya and I discuss going together to the district tomorrow afternoon, to start looking for the families of these five victims. I write out their names: Anna Komina, Mikhail Markov, Aleksandra Chizhova, Nikolay Khudyakov, and Dimitriy Vinogradov.

That night, I have a dreadful nightmare about Dr. Abramova. Still wearing her pink sweater, she metamorphoses into a vengeful demon intent on destroying me. I wake in terror. Matthew is sleeping soundly across the room, and our dormitory area is completely silent. I try to reason why I should be afraid of Dr. Abramova. Finally I decide it is not the woman herself, but the grisly slides of sliced jejunums, cecums, lymph nodes, lacerated intestines, enlarged spleens, and lung tissue, all suppurating with disease, that have frightened me. Although I know it is essential, dissecting the victims' bodies is for me the least humane way to understand the outbreak. And I am not confident the autopsy data by itself will lead to certainty or truth. How does one know anything for sure, I keep wondering. Is the faint, determined scratching I hear beneath my bed a cockroach or the product of my imagination?

What I am going to need are cross-checks on any information I get. In the darkness, an old memory surfaces. It is about my first fieldwork apprenticeship in 1968, in Antigua, in the British West Indies, when I studied a beachside village community. An inexperienced fisherman didn't have buoys to mark his lobster traps and had not thought to triangulate, that is, to identify their location by multiple points. Had he put them a mile from shore, two miles? We spent hours one morning circling in the emerald water in search of the lost traps. Practiced navigators in the Western Caroline Islands in Micronesia can sense with their bodies their positions between land, sea, and sky.[7] But not us. And now when I think of Antigua, I also have to include what I have since learned about the tests that the British conducted there in 1948, when on that same emerald water transport ships, their decks stacked with caged animals, were sprayed with aerosols of deadly diseases, including anthrax.[8]

Tonight, I have no sense of position; lost traps and deep waters prey on my mind. Investigating the 1979 anthrax deaths will require triangulation, the cross-checking of multiple trustworthy sources of data. But in our evening discussion of the day's events, primary importance was placed on Grinberg and Abramova's data, even before it was examined. Walker, without any review of the autopsy data, was adamant that the mystery was solved.

"There are two ways to find out what happened," he said. "One is the pathoanatomy. The other is someone tells us. We have both. I'm convinced it's inhalatory."

Nothing will ever be that simple for me. I contemplate another reason for my nightmare about Dr. Abramova: that she is a pathologist. I realize that because she is a woman I am projecting onto her my own ambivalence about the way pathology objectifies the body, literally reducing it to pieces. I cannot imagine having the kind of emotional restraint required to incise a corpse from sternum to pubis and to investigate it with an objectifying clinical gaze. I have witnessed only one autopsy in my life, at a Boston hospital where I was doing field research. It was of a full-term newborn with multiple congenital anomalies, and I nearly passed out. Still, I know pathology is essential to medical science and that its long history is based on a rational drive to remove death from "the metaphysic of evil."[9] Yet I want a balance between the dispassionate autopsy and the compassionate understanding of death, a perspective that takes into account both the disease and the human experience of illness and pain.

As these thoughts chase through my head, I come round to the old Freudian formula, that the people in our dreams are merely ourselves in other guises. Perhaps the demonized Dr. Abramova I dreamed of is only a version of myself that I reject, a woman who has retreated to cold, clinical resolve, as if science were without feelings. I toss restlessly in my narrow bed. I need to find the families, the human experience in this story.

Awake at dawn, I am worried about exactly when and how I can get to the five addresses we now have. It's Saturday and the morning has been set aside for a visit to the cemetery while Walker and Yampolskaya work with the two pathologists at the Pulmonary Unit. Much of the afternoon has been set aside for clarifying appointments with still more public health officials and physicians. If Yampolskaya becomes involved in a full day of reviewing autopsy data, how will the two of us break free to search for the families of the victims? And what about a driver? Who will take us to Chkalovskiy rayon if we are supposed to be at some office? Doing the family interviews, it has dawned on me, is in direct competition with the rest of the investigation.

Before breakfast, I tell Matthew about my nightmare.

"You know," he replies, "I had a dream last night that my glasses were cracked. I had to have them to see, but it was terribly difficult, and my eyes hurt."

It is a comfort to know I am not the only one in confusion. But no easy answer arises for getting the interviews done. A priority has been put on the autopsy data and on speaking to people in authority. I feel the rest of the team could just as well do without contacting the families of the victims. The effort is, after all, labor intensive. It means knocking on doors, putting oneself on the line with people who have not counted much, who have no offices and no titles, with people whose relatives may be a source of shame or guilt, the way victims often are to survivors. Memories of the deceased may have faded or been repressed, and relatives might prefer they stay that way. People move on with their lives, as we say in America, and we mean it in the most positive way, that they have dispelled immobilizing grief.

Yet only by discovering where the victims were in the days and nights preceding the outbreak can we construct the epidemiological map that may reveal a conclusive pattern. If the tainted-meat hypothesis is true, then the whereabouts of the victims might be widely scattered, with links back to where the meat was obtained, for example at the ceramics factory. If an aerosol emission came from Compound 19, the locations of the victims would be strung out downwind along its path, whatever they were doing, on the same shift at work, or just at home, awake or sleeping. Even though the victims are no longer here to tell us, their close relations might remember.

The person who has been most enthusiastic about these family interviews is Dr. Alexander Langmuir, the epidemiologist who in 1949 founded
and then ran the Epidemic Intelligence Division at the U.S. Centers for
Disease Control in Atlanta. There and at Harvard University and Johns
Hopkins, he taught generations of students what is called "shoe-leather
epidemiology," the practice of collecting data in the field, while directly
experiencing the locale of the public health problem under investigation.
He conveys a detective's sense of drama about his work. Years ago, in
fact, he often helped essayist Berton Roueché with his medical detective
stories in *The New Yorker* magazine. In the introduction to one of
Roueché's volumes of collected essays, Langmuir summarized the three
essentials for fixing the pattern of a disease: the single patient located in
time and space with vividly described symptoms, the verification of the
diagnosis, and the answer to the main question, "What is the source of
infection and the mode of spread?" So, he continued:

> The investigator proceeds in an orderly fashion. A single case presents many
> frustrations; there are too many compatible possibilities and no way to dis-
> criminate among them. Then, with the recognition of additional cases and
> the performance of appropriate tests, the possible choices of a common fac-
> tor are progressively reduced until all of the pieces of the puzzle fall into log-
> ical place and the problem is solved.[10]

Now retired from CDC and teaching part-time at Johns Hopkins,
Langmuir became involved in the question of the Sverdlovsk outbreak
in the mid-1980s, before the Soviet physicians came to the United States
in 1988. Unable to join us on this expedition, he nonetheless remains
close to our efforts; we have been sending him e-mails of our daily exploits, such as they have been. I know his face will light up with joy if I
can return with good information from the victims' families. I promised
him I would wear out my shoes trekking door-to-door, the way he still
teaches epidemiologists to solve medical mysteries.

6

The Community of the Dead

VOSTOCHNIY CEMETERY

Saturday morning, June 6, eleven o'clock. A light snow is falling when we arrive at Vostochniy Cemetery. Matthew, Shelokov, Hugh-Jones, and I have been driven there by Professor Borisov. The city of Yekaterinburg curves north to south in an inverted S, with easy borders to open fields and countryside. This modest cemetery is located on the northeast bend (hence its name, the Eastern Cemetery) off a main highway. Its front entrance is gated and walled, but its other borders, like the city's, disappear into stands of trees and meadows, with nothing of the pristine neatness of most American graveyards. Within the cemetery, dirt roads wind randomly among clusters of stone and metal markers. In the distance a woman on her knees, oblivious to the chill, is weeding one of the grave sites. With no list and just five cases to go on, we have come looking for the names of the dead.

At the guardhouse, the burly, cheerful custodian, Nikolay, explains that a fire in 1991 destroyed most cemetery records, including those from 1979. We have heard a lot about vanishing documents in Yekaterinburg— that it is normal to destroy old hospital files, that the SES records were confiscated by Deputy Minister of Health Burgasov and his team. More ominously, according to Dr. Abramova, the KGB confiscated the clinical records at Hospital 40 even as she was completing autopsy reports. She tried to save at least the first drafts, but these too were taken.

Nikolay offers to guide us toward the special sector where the anthrax victims' bodies were buried. Around us, most of the graves, some with low iron fences, bear black-and-white photoengravings of the deceased, women and men, the old and the young, that are typical of Russian and other European cultures. These images create the illusion of communities of the dead on watch amid the weeds and wildflowers. Not a few monuments are decorated with plastic flowers. Some are crowned with a red Soviet star or, less frequently, an orthodox cross.

As we approach the eastern border of the cemetery, Nikolay hesitates. He is, he confesses, unsure exactly where the special sector is. Thirteen years have passed since the epidemic, and he himself is a fairly recent employee. More than that, he explains, most people know where the graves of their relatives and friends are located and do not need directions. His implication is clear. Visitors like us, with no personal grief, are rare. Even as Nikolay speaks, we see small groups arriving to pay their respects. One couple carries a basket, obviously planning to have lunch here, where the atmosphere is heavy with nostaglia and the photographs of the deceased are, as Susan Sontag would say, "incitements to reverie" that preserve both the presence and the absence of loved ones.[1] Russians, unlike Americans, choose intimacy with the departed. Many still maintain the tradition of washing and dressing the body of a deceased relative in preparation for burial, a custom long gone from American culture. Russian cemeteries, I am learning, are social spaces, where the living assemble to incorporate the dead into their lives. For a country where nearly every family can count a member lost to war, famine, or political terrorism, this continued embrace of the departed seems like a positive force, a holding on to life to spite death.

Nikolay and his two assistant grave diggers, one a tall rosy-cheeked teenager, the other somewhat older and stockier, regard our team with good-humored curiosity. People from the United States are a novelty here. We look nothing like the glamorous stars of American soap operas that are enormously popular now in Russia. Matthew and Shelokov are in belted trench coats that have seen some wear. Hugh-Jones wears a tweed cap and a parka that have probably been around the world several times. Having miscalculated June in the Urals, I am dressed in a cotton suit with sandals. As we scurry about with cameras and notebooks on our search among the grave sites, we must seem odd indeed, like the man in Gogol's *Dead Souls* who collected the names of the dead.

Vostochniy Cemetery is divided into numbered sections; depending on the source of information, the anthrax victims are buried in Sector 13, 14, or 16. The layout of the cemetery is almost too unruly to distinguish divisions. The graves are scattered under trees and between random juttings of rock, in rows that break down and reform. In 1979, the victims were reportedly buried at the outskirts of the cemetery, but this area has since been overtaken and surrounded by newer graves. The only way to discover the right sector is by reading the dates inscribed on each monument.

We disperse and, after twenty minutes of checking markers, we have located a grouping of grave sites for April–May 1979, within the six-to-seven-week time period of the epidemic. Granted, we are assuming that the dates in the official Soviet report are accurate. Certainly they appear to be confirmed by this shaggy square of land, outside which the dates of death shift markedly to the late 1980s and early 1990s. This turns out to be Sector 13, one border of which extends at right angles to the main path. The two other boundaries have been eroded by more recent grave sites, as if after a decade or so the stigma of the outbreak was forgotten and sheer convenience ruled the placement of new graves.

Our task is to record the name and the dates of birth and death for each victim. One fact we may never clarify is exactly how many died in the outbreak, whether it was the thousands claimed by some Soviet dissidents or the sixty-four reported by Deputy Minister Burgasov. Still, this topsy-turvy Sector 13, about twenty meters square, is at least a start. The young grave digger with rosy cheeks takes off his nylon jacket with its fur-trimmed hood and offers it to me, with a sympathetic smile. I thank him but refuse. Now that we have work to do, I don't mind the cold.

Dates of birth and death are either chiseled on the stone or engraved in metal. They give us the age of each person and, in the aggregate, the age and sex distribution of the victims. Also important is the evidence they give about the epidemic's temporal profile: when it began, when it crested, when it diminished and ended. Matthew, Hugh-Jones, and I begin taking photographs of each tombstone. With no expectation of getting our film developed quickly in Yekaterinburg, we also help Shelokov copy down the inscribed names and dates. This way, we can quickly construct our own temporal graph of the epidemic and also compare it with the 1988 Soviet graph.

These dates of birth and death are more than epidemiological data. They reveal the generation of each victim, the phases of Soviet history each experienced. Some of the deceased lived through and perhaps fought in the Great Patriotic War, as World War II is known, and would have remembered Stalin. The younger ones would have better remembered Khrushchev and his failed economic policies, the swings between relative affluence and collapse, the 1969 "hunger demonstration" by Sverdlovsk citizens, who like others under Soviet rule could protest circumstances but not the system. All of the victims could have told us something about Boris Yeltsin, the Communist Party's leader in Sverdlovsk the year they died.

As we move from one site to another, the photographs on the monuments take us past biographical facts to the individual personalities of the victims. As artless as passport pictures (and precisely because they lack artifice) the photos project each victim's personal uniqueness. Minor idiosyncratic choices—a certain haircut, a thin tie, a flowered shawl, the jaunty cut of a lapel—heighten individuality. But it is the faces, the expressions captured in the portraits, the eyes sad or laughing, the set of the mouth, the curve of the brow preserved in a slice of time and space, that proclaim identity: "This is me! There is no mistake! I did exist!"

The victims' names are difficult for me, an unfamiliar combination of vowels and consonants. Then in a little while, a few rules emerge. Many men's names have sharp consonants, like Boris and Viktor. A woman's name tends to be softened by vowels, like Anna, Valentina, Sofia. A woman's last name (whether from her husband or her father) is usually feminized, given a soft "a" ending, as if it were an adjective. Each name includes a patronymic, a middle name based on the father's first name, and here, too, a suffix identifies the bearer's gender.

Anna Petrovna Komina is a name I heard for the first time last night, from our anonymous source. Now I find her. A strong-featured woman with dark hair, her photo stands out among the others. Her sharp, deep-set eyes and determined jaw say, "Yes, life is hard, but you have to stick with it." She died on April 9, 1979, at age fifty-four, near what is reported as the beginning of the epidemic. She was a child in the 1930s when Sverdlovsk's industries were rapidly expanding and the boundaries of the city were pushing south. She was a young woman, very likely a factory worker, during World War II when the city was producing armaments. Perhaps she married then or after the war. If she had children, they would now be about my age, and, if I am lucky, I will find them.

I search out the other four names, the ones whose families I have at least a chance of meeting. The grave of Mikhail Fyodorovich Markov, the second on my list, is a burnished aluminum memorial, a kind of modernistic pyramid, without a portrait. He too died April 9, at age forty-seven. His monument suits a less traditional postwar personality. Someone, perhaps his wife, has entwined it with lavish red, blue, and white plastic flowers. An iron star painted red, a patriotic symbol, tops the pyramid.

The grave of Aleksandra Chizhova, the third name I have, is nearby, at the edge of the sector. She died at age fifty on April 12, at what has been described as the height of the outbreak, when Abramova and Grinberg were at their most busy.

Nikolay Khudyakov, the fourth name, has a grave with a simple iron marker, just a tripod. To read his name, I lift up a faded bouquet of flowers tied with a white ribbon. Khudyakov was forty-six when he died, but no day or month has been inscribed, as if the living, in grief and haste, had fled. But someone came back, not too long ago, and left those flowers in remembrance.

The fifth and last name on my list is Dmitriy Vinogradov. Like Mikhail Markov, his grave is marked by a burnished aluminum monument with no photoengraving. He died the same day as Markov, on April 9, at age fifty-two. No flowers decorate his monument. Perhaps he was a bachelor or widower or had no children, or his children moved away. A young white birch grows crookedly from his grave, perhaps planted, but who can say for sure?

Dozens of other names surround me: Ivanov, Loginova, Myasnikova, Shatokin, even a stray Romanov (Boris), one of the early deaths, on April 10, at age forty. Many of these victims are in the same generation as the five names I have; they were perhaps neighbors or coworkers, but not, as far as their last names or patronymics show, relatives. The exception is two men named Makarov, with the same patronymic, Vasilyevich, who could be brothers. Aside from them, the two curious features of the 1979 outbreak—that only one person per household was affected and that no children were involved—appear to be confirmed by the grave markers. We know that anthrax is not a contagious disease of the sort that is passed from one person to another, like influenza or pneumonic plague, which can destroy whole families, but we might still expect that infected meat would sometimes affect several household members.

In most epidemics, nature picks off the most vulnerable, the weakest among children and the elderly. In this special sector of the cemetery, older people seem accounted for. But no children or victims in their teens or early twenties are buried here. The official Soviet explanation for this curious feature, expressed by Dr. Burgasov, was based on workers' living conditions during the spring of 1979. That year, in an epoch of bad agricultural planning by the central government, food in general and meat in particular were in short supply. This much was true. In the late 1970s, rationing of staple food products was imposed on Sverdlovsk and other large Soviet cities. Perhaps meat at home, as Dr. Burgasov argued, did go to the men of the house first, and then to women, while children and young people ate their meat at school and escaped the fatal infection.

In the years of discussing the Sverdlovsk outbreak, the idea has now and then come up that, if an anthrax aerosol caused the epidemic, the children might have been protected by being indoors at school. But an anthrax aerosol could easily enter a building just the way safe air does, and the indoor air would remain contaminated long after the lethal cloud passed by, with a total harmful dose possibly equal to the outside air.

Whatever the explanation, I find no children or student-age victims in Sector 13, only a crowd of adults. Here is the grandfatherly Fyodor Nikolaev, dead at age sixty, also on April 9. His face has the cynical expression of an old soldier who has been through many battles, but his eyes are kind. Here is Lilia Fokina, who died April 11 at age forty-nine. In her high-necked black dress, with her hair swept up, she looks like a duchess in a Turgenev novel. The youngest victim's grave is that of Tatyana Kosheleva, just twenty-four when she died on April 12. Another young victim we find is Alexey Syskov, age twenty-seven, who died April 11. In his photo, he looks uneasy and restless, as if ready to speed off on a motorbike. Aleksandr Vyatkin died on April 12, at age twenty-eight, too young. Another twenty-eight-year-old, Yuriy Kramskoy, smiles confidently from his photograph, his whole life ahead of him. He looks witty, as if he has a joke to tell. Was he popular, this charming young man? He died on April 16. The fifty-two-year-old Vasiliy Tretnikov, also died on April 16. In their final suffering, he and young Kramskoy might have exchanged furtive, desperate looks, like two drowning men. Someone has inserted Tretnikov's schoolboy coat-and-tie portrait in the oval frame on his monument. He appears eternally younger than the boyish trio of Syskov, Vyatkin, and Kramskoy. Georgiy Bliznyakov, who looks like a typical Urals worker, died April 18, age forty-three. Was he one of the victims at the ceramics factory?

The women victims in this sector are on average older than the men. Since the proportion of women in most populations increases with age, more older women might have been vulnerable to the epidemic. Here before me is Sophia Bliumova, a grandmotherly woman in a kerchief who died at age sixty-seven on April 10. Aleksandra Volkova, another older woman, her expression gentle and forgiving, died on April 13 at age sixty-five. By Soviet law, these two would have been long retired, but even pensioners then sought other work, paid or unpaid. In Russian culture, the *babushki* (grandmothers) often serve the younger generation. They shop, cook, clean, and care for the grandchildren, as well as tend the sick. In epidemics of infectious disease, like influenza, smallpox, or plague, these traditional caretakers tend to succumb in greater numbers than others.

But anthrax is generally not contagious human-to-human. The older women buried around me here, beneath the light snow, must have been vulnerable to infection in some other way.

A shiny aluminum monument marks the resting place of a man whose name is Mohammed three times over: Mukhametalin Mukhametshinovich Mukhametshin, age forty-five when he died April 22, late in the epidemic. A Moslem, in his photograph he looks as much an ethnic Russian as everyone else. In another portrait, Pyotr Pilyasov, age forty, wears an open shirt and leather jacket. He is handsome and looks as if he knows it. He died April 24. So too did Nikolay Vostrykov, age forty-one, a brawny fellow in a turtleneck. By that time, the hospital beds in Sverdlovsk were almost empty of anthrax patients, and most of the graves in this sector were dug and filled. The epidemic had begun to taper off. They must have seen or heard about others getting sick before they were stricken. Maybe they thought they'd beaten the odds. A day later Nina Yasinskaya died at age fifty. In her photograph, her expression is serenely content, the way her family chose to remember her.

I circle Sector 13 a second time before I notice the portrait of Pavel Retnev, who died April 9 at age forty-one. A serious man, he is dressed in his military uniform, with many medals shining on his chest. No red star adorns his grave, though he surely was a soldier and patriot. What, if anything, did he know about Compound 19? Nearby is an unidentified grave whose iron trapezoid is topped with a red star. The little plot is untended, the iron rusted; here is a nameless soul.

We work until it is past noon, locating about forty graves, some with illegible markers worn away by time. The sky is beginning to clear, but the temperature hovers around freezing. My hands are wet from pushing back foliage from some graves to get a better photograph. My feet, as pink as some of the plastic flowers, are also wet from the snow. In turn we take breaks, sitting in Professor Borisov's car, which he has kept running with the heater on, and drink tea from a thermos.

Before we leave, we quickly inspect other nearby sectors with graves dated April and May 1979. These other sites and their portraits have an innocent air, simply by their place in the social topology of the cemetery. Their deaths were most likely explained by ordinary diagnoses, like heart disease and cancer and the other modern killers in industrialized society. The graves of the victims of the 1979 epidemic were physically segregated for reasons of public health. Yet their disease and its circumstances also set them apart. Anthrax is a throwback. It evokes past centuries when annihilating plagues scoured medieval landscapes or attacked fifteenth-century cities befouled by infected carcasses. In this century, because of rational science and public sanitation, humans are never supposed to die of this disease. Sector 13 tells us and everyone who visits here that in 1979 the rational safeguards broke down and an old image of Death, with a black robe and scythe, stalked Sverdlovsk.

As the rest of us are still reading tombstones, Shelokov strikes up a conversation with three people hovering at the edge of Sector 13. He is innately gregarious, and being in a new Russian environment seems to make him more so. He talks easily with almost anyone, at restaurants, at the dormitory, in corridors at the university or city offices—and his brief translations of these conversations are like reports from a civic disaster center. Since our arrival, he has kept us up to date on hazardous radiation levels south of the city, about increased rates of theft and assault, about Russian mafia gangs, about a Chinese student with a knife who yesterday went berserk in the elevator of our dormitory building, about our concierge's suspicions of foul play concerning our several exploding light bulbs. After Shelokov finishes conversing with the three visitors and they have left the cemetery, he tells us they are relatives of one of the victims.

"Did you get their names?" I ask. I am fully prepared to dash after them, but they have disappeared from view. "Do you know where they live? How we could contact them?"

"Nyet." Shelokov's highly developed sense of etiquette kept him from asking such questions. But, he adds emphatically, they assured him there was an epidemic in 1979. I am visibly dejected. In the distance, Nikolay's two helpers are digging a grave. Death goes on. To console me, Shelokov tells me they were not close relatives, just distant ones visiting at the grave of another family member.

This near-miss, or rather this illusion of a lost chance, suddenly deflates my spirits. All the Russians assisting us, Professor Borisov and Sasha Tiutiunnik, Rector Suetin and his fellow administrators, the public health officials at SES, Nikolay and the two young grave diggers, and even Shelokov, an American citizen for decades, always act as though they would like to help, but we shouldn't expect much. The classic fatalism of Russian culture weighs down on me, as if all human endeavors (and particularly ours) are exercises in the absurd. Life is a glimmer, human nature a wasted experiment. What does the material world matter? What does life matter? This fatalism is the real reason why the light bulbs burst, why our shower has sprung a leak to the floor below, why there are thefts and crime, and why the elevator at the dormitory is permanently temporarily broken, a fact that perhaps tipped the Chinese student over the edge of lunacy.

Standing in the middle of Vostochniy Cemetery I write in my notebook:

> I see propped against a grave two broken spades, the handles gone; they are rusted. What is it about them that is so Russian? That the shovels are broken in the first place? That the spades are propped up and left to rust. A German would have repaired them. An American would have thrown them away. But here someone has positioned them, artfully, like two old hearts.

My fit of melancholy, I reassure myself, is just the result of accumulated fatigue. In three days, we have traveled nearly halfway around the globe, careening through Moscow to the Urals. Here, culture shock aside, we have to climb up seven flights of stairs to our meager rooms, where we sleep on broken-down beds. These obstacles are merely physical—or maybe they are symbolic of a deeper reality. Shelokov considers the barriers to our research to be political and formidable, though not readily apparent. He believes the *naushiki*, the "earphones" or informers of the Soviet era, remain a decided influence in Yekaterinberg, making people afraid to talk to us. Why else, he argues, are the pathologists Abramova and Grinberg reluctant to share their autopsy data, if not out of fear of the repercussions of divulging what they know? Why else did officials at SES present conflicting stories about the animal outbreaks, thereby throwing sand in our eyes, if not out of some conspiracy of disinformation? Why else did last night's source of names and addresses convey them anonymously, if not out of dread of exposure? I begin to wonder if lingering Stalinist influences explain why Sasha, Professor Borisov's son-in-law and our second driver, has trouble with the city map, although he is in every way cordial and obliging. Maybe the local map we purchased at a store yesterday (more clearly printed and detailed than the one we copied from Harvard's Pusey Library) is intentionally inaccurate, to confuse us and all foreigners who dare come here. Shelokov believes that this, too, is a possibility.

As we get into the car to go back to the university, I feel as if glasnost has never happened and that invisible forces of repression still weigh. Yet this visit to the cemetery has brought me new, undeniable certitudes. The photoengravings have given me a vivid sense of the individual personalities of the victims. Their faces do not lie. The segregated sector where they are buried affirms that their death was a collective one. No missing bureaucratic forms, no verbal games, no malicious maps can obliterate the cemetery's proof that April 1979 in Sverdlovsk was a time of sinister tragedy.

Over a quick lunch at a small restaurant near the university, I confide in Professor Borisov that I need my own interpreter, someone to help me while Yampolskaya assists Walker and while Shelokov interprets for Matthew and Hugh-Jones. As a small quid pro quo for the university's hospitality, several biologists want Matthew and Shelokov's assessment of an outbreak of "stamping-foot" disease among students who harvested a state-farm potato crop. The students are claiming serious damage to their nervous systems. Blame is being laid on pesticides or, alternatively, on the students' overconsumption of vodka. This responsibility to confer, as well as the on-going negotiations about appointments with officials, plus attempts to communicate with the military at Compound 19, mean that Shelokov is working more than full-time. And if Grinberg and Abramova allow full access to the autopsy data, Yampolskaya may become completely immersed in that review. Borisov understands my concern and says he will make inquiries at the university.

While we are talking, a well-dressed Asian man from another table approaches with a smile and hands me an incredibly large orange. He bows and disappears. "It is because you are a woman," Borisov explains, with some embarrassment at the man's behavior. "He is a Tatar and Tatars will make these spontaneous gestures." He is not disapproving, but he makes it clear that he does not act this way. The orange reminds me that Yekaterinburg. although technically in Asia, is Russian, a science city, not to be identified with the irrational or the exotic, which is how for centuries Russia has identified its Asians.[2] Yet I cannot help asking myself how rational the city was in 1979.

After lunch, my next stop is the pathology laboratory. Revived, I am trying to look on the bright side. If relations with Grinberg and Abramova, the two pathologists, have reached an impasse, Yampolskaya and I will find a way to set off in search of the five families whose addresses we have. If the city had a freely available telephone directory, we could have started with telephone calls, presuming the families had telephones. But we have no option—this inquiry will be door-to-door. If all goes well, the people who open those doors will have much to tell us about the victims.

7

Abramova's Treasure

In the meeting room of the Tuberculosis and Pulmonary Diseases Unit, Dr. Faina Abramova is seated at one end of a conference table with Olga Yampolskaya, while at the other David Walker is looking at slides under a microscope. As Walker examines each slide, Abramova reads from her 1979 case notes and Yampolskaya translates. The cases are designated by number. Abramova's notes are handwritten and suit the surroundings, which are spare and simple. The main area is like a locker room. In an adjacent laboratory black marble benches are set with sinks, but the benches are bare and look unused. I have come in the back entrance because of a large, rather ferocious dog tied near the front. He was tied there yesterday, too, when we came for our introductory meeting with Abramova and Dr. Grinberg, who is Chief of the Pathology Department here. Dr. Abramova, today in pale blue, maintains the look of a fairy-tale grandmother. After my nightmare, I feel some relief, but I know her soft look is deceiving. In 1979, she took responsibility for hiding her materials when she knew the KGB wanted the autopsy records. She has told us she placed the jars of gross organs preserved in formaldehyde in the hospital's pathology museum, on shelves among other such jars, like so many purloined letters. She hid the tissue samples in an innocuous corner cabinet near the autopsy room. When I asked her why she did this, she replied proudly, "It was my work!"

The photographs of tissues and organs we saw yesterday are put aside. Now it is a question only of what the slides under the microscope, the real tissues, may reveal about portal of entry, whether by inhalation or by eating tainted meat.

Walker appears almost gleeful about the quality of the material he is seeing. Lev Grinberg, serious as a general at war, comes from his office to greet me. He misses nothing of Walker's satisfaction. The autopsy slides Walker saw in Moscow made him think the outbreak could be either gastrointestinal or inhalation anthrax. It is too soon for him to make a judgment here. He shows me several microscopic examples in which the black rods of *Bacillus anthracis* are clearly evident. One tissue slide, he feels, demonstrates their presence in the thoracic lymph nodes and indicates inhalation anthrax, although some others show infection in the mesentery nodes around the intestine as well. I ask if the lung tissue looks especially compromised, for example, by pollution or smoking or disease. He is only on the eighth case, but so far he thinks the lungs look no worse than those of any modern city dweller in the United States. He is confident that in a day or two he can finish reviewing these cases and leave for Moscow, where he plans to meet with colleagues who study his real love, diseases caused by *rickettsia*, tick-borne microorganisms named after the nineteenth-century American pathologist H. T. Ricketts.

"I'm happy with what I am seeing," he says, "and lunch was delicious."

Dr. Abramova, he tells me, brought in roast chicken and potato salad and served it up on one of the laboratory benches. She and Walker, with Yampolskaya's help, work smoothly together. Trust on both sides is crucial in this review. Despite the difference in age and gender and the divide of culture and language, Abramova and Walker are professional colleagues, and they share a framework for analysis, the case approach. She reads the case number, identifies age and sex of the patient, and tells the date of death. Then she describes the bacteriological results, whether positive or negative for *Bacillus anthracis*. This methodical communication almost makes one forget that we are referring to autopsies, that the diminutive Abramova, assisted by the stalwart Grinberg, cut open the victims' bodies and sawed off the tops of their skulls. Walker has made his living the same way, but his technology for exposing the secrets of the human dead takes him far away from the blood and guts of the autopsy room. At his Texas laboratory he has sophisticated methods of analysis—powerful microscopes, computer technology, and laboratory techniques—that Abramova has probably never dreamed of and about which Grinberg has only read.

Walker is perhaps too delighted with what he is finding. Twenty minutes after I come in, Lev Grinberg positions himself at the end of the conference table. He announces in a deep voice that he must have two guarantees from our team. Walker's data review stops cold. Grinberg has our attention. As he demanded the day before, he wants Matthew to write Dr. Semyonov, the chief of SES, and ask permission for a complete review of the autopsy data, which must be recognized as the property of Abramova and Grinberg. Second, he wants Dr. Walker to guarantee that he will not take advantage of his access to this data. Yampolskaya quickly translates Walker's assurance that he respects Abramova and Grinberg's ownership of the data and that later this afternoon Grinberg should talk to Matthew, who is at the university.

Grinberg's uneasiness about the use of the autopsy data is justified. On the basis of their uniqueness alone, the tissue samples saved by Abramova are a medical treasure. Nothing remotely like them is available from any other outbreak and no other modern outbreak matches the dimensions of the one in Sverdlovsk in 1979. Cases of inhalation or intestinal anthrax in humans occur so infrequently that mysteries still abound and will do so for years to come. Indeed, since the late nineteenth century, medical scientists have been trying to discern how inhalation anthrax takes over the body. One school held that after inhaled spores reach the air sacs (the alveoli) in the depths of the lungs, they are phagocytosed (meaning literally "eaten up") by policing cells of the immune system and transported by these cells out of the lung to the lymph nodes. Only then and there do anthrax bacteria first begin to multiply and enter the blood stream. By this view, inhalation anthrax is not a true pulmonary disease—that is, it is not initiated by a pneumonia—since the infecting bacteria do not begin multiplying inside the lungs. The opposing school argued that the primary lesion (where the anthrax bacteria first multiply and do harm) is inside the respiratory system. Swelling, bleeding, and ulceration start, according to this conjecture, at the tracheobronchial tree, near where the airway splits on its way to the two lungs. In both views, systemic infection, called septicemia or sepsis, occurs only at a later stage, after the anthrax bacteria enter and multiply in the bloodstream.

The phagocytosis school now dominates, in part because of Russian science. To begin, Ilya Metchnikoff, the scientist who worked with Pasteur, discovered that anthrax bacteria and other organisms that gain entry into the body can be engulfed and digested by other special cells. He gave these cells the name we call them today: macrophages.[1] This work gained him a Nobel Prize in 1908. Animal experiments conducted under U.S. and British military auspices in the 1940s and 1950s conclu-

sively established that anthrax spores reaching the alveoli do not ordinarily multiply there. Instead they may be engulfed by phagocytic cells,
which, failing to digest them, transport them out of the lungs to the thoracic lymph nodes, where they first begin to multiply. Then, if the multiplying anthrax bacteria succeed in overcoming the defenses of the lymph
node, they wash with the lymph into the bloodstream and cause massive
sepsis, including the possibility of secondary anthrax pneumonia.[2] Evidence that this process also takes place in humans came when Wilhelm
Albrink and his colleagues autopsied three of the four Manchester, New
Hampshire, mill workers who died from pulmonary anthrax in 1957 and
found that inhalation anthrax did not cause ulcers in the respiratory
tract.[3] Soon after, in Philadelphia, the analysis of two additional inhalation fatalities also weighed against the primary lesion interpretation.[4]

Still, these five human cases constitute precious little medical information, perhaps not enough to say what never happens in the human lungs
or where a primary anthrax lesion must always be. Albrink and his colleagues had the advantage of knowing that the cause of death for all five
patients was inhalation anthrax. Today, Walker's task at the microscope
is more difficult than theirs was. He has to use tissue samples selected
and prepared by someone else with only rudimentary pathoanatomical
notes and assess whether he is looking at intestinal or inhalatory anthrax.
With each case, he must attempt to judge which set of lymph nodes looks
more infected, on the presumption that the lymph nodes in the region
where infection is primary will be the most damaged. If, under the microscope, the case presents the involvement of just one set of nodes, judgment may be simplified. If both sets are involved, the conclusion has to
be tempered. If, for example, the body of a victim was overwhelmed with
sepsis, thoracic and mesentery lymph nodes may both show signs of infection. In fact, Grinberg has already indicated that nine of the forty-
two cases have both thoracic and mesentery node infection. As he sees it,
infection was more severe in the former than the latter. In addition, thirty-
nine of the Abramova-Grinberg cases have intestinal lesions. How will
Walker determine that these are not primary lesions when so little is known
about intestinal anthrax and its mechanisms? Grinberg and Abramova
have made their interpretation. Walker will have to make his own.

Grinberg and Abramova are understandably anxious that Walker's
review of their materials reach the same conclusion as their own. They
want their findings broadcast to the world of science and have been making efforts in that direction. In April 1991, they presented a summation
of their work at a pathology conference held in Yekaterinburg. In Feb-

ruary 1992, they were in Moscow at a pathology conference at the Academy of Sciences. They have also submitted a three-part article presenting their autopsy material from 1979 to the Russian journal *Archives of Pathology*. The problem with that submission, they tell us, is that few Russian science journals have any money to publish; issues are running years behind. They want the results of their work acknowledged. Publication (at least in English) is the one area where we might be able to help them.

Meanwhile, their voices somewhat subdued, Walker, Yampolskaya, and Abramova continue their review of case material, which is organized chronologically by date of death. At one point Abramova mentions that a patient worked at the ceramics factory. While trying to be discreet, I crane my neck to see what else she has in her notes, but it is useless. She is keeping them literally close to her chest, not revealing the patients' names. Looking at the notes Yampolskaya writes as she translates, I wonder if these patients are some I have just encountered, their images fresh in my mind from the cemetery. The dates of death, gender, and the patients' ages give hints. The first case, a forty-year-old man who died April 10, could well be Boris Romanov. This patient's cardinal's cap and laboratory tests confirmed the diagnosis on anthrax. Another case, a woman aged twenty-four, could be Tatyana Kosheleva.

By around four o'clock, after Walker has reviewed the first ten cases, Grinberg again suddenly calls a halt to the process. He insists he must talk with Matthew before he will let Walker see any more material. Abramova looks consternated by the interruption, but does not contradict her protégé. I immediately put through a phone call to Matthew at our dormitory suite, where he and Shelokov are translating the veterinary documents that Dr. Burgasov gave us in Moscow. I urge him to come over right away.

Meanwhile a pale and intimidated Walker hastily scrawls a note: "I, David Walker, will not use or otherwise publish the materials of Dr. Faina Abramova and Dr. Lev Grinberg pertaining to the 1979 anthrax epidemic in Sverdlovsk and will ask their permission to use them for presentations at conferences or in selective publications." He reads it aloud and then pushes it across the table to Grinberg, who accepts it in impassive silence. Walker, perhaps expecting a more appreciative reaction, turns stony-faced. Grinberg is signaling that Matthew is the person with whom he wants to deal. Dr. Abramova pushes aside her notes. The tension is palpable, and worst perhaps for Yampolskaya, who is caught in the middle as interpreter and Russian colleague.

When Matthew arrives, Grinberg again lays out his demands, with specifics. He emphasizes that Matthew's letter to Grinberg's superior, Dr. Semyonov, should include the phrase, "because of financial reasons, we want to familiarize ourselves with this material." Matthew's calm but concerned response is to ask what financial motives Grinberg is contemplating, since he himself has none in mind. Grinberg has no answer. Matthew continues by assuring him that he will write Semyonov if necessary and also do everything he can to get the Grinberg-Abramova paper published in English, with them as authors.

Since in my phone call I mentioned wanting access to Abramova's notes to get family names and addresses, Matthew adds that our team needs Grinberg and Abramova's help in carrying out our epidemiological study. At this Grinberg, who knows enough English to leap ahead of Yampolskaya's interpreting, grows stubborn. He insists that his superior would have to get permission from the Sverdlovsk Oblast Health Department for any cooperation in that venture. Thus Grinberg positions himself both as an employee within a hierarchical state bureaucracy and as a potential scientific colleague. As the former, he warns us that this autopsy information could "make difficulties" for his superiors, so Matthew should offer *bona fides* that this data is unique and valuable. He wants the letter to state that this review of the materials is a "preliminary scientific contact"; the implication is that Grinberg will garner professional connections from this agreement.

Abramova, not about to be left out of the discussion, adds that the two pathologists should be referred to as "highly competent." She wants Semyonov to be told that the American team contacted them because these data are already in manuscript form and have been submitted to a journal. Matthew responds that he did not know about the manuscript until now, but otherwise has no problem writing the letter. Then Abramova asks that the letter also state our agreement with their conclusion, that the anthrax was inhalatory. This Matthew says he cannot do until the team has finished its own inquiry. Abramova and Grinberg concede this point and seem satisfied.

In an about-face, Grinberg then proposes tea. The notebooks and materials are put away, and, as we convene around a marble work bench, the mood lightens. Abramova remarks that she recognized Yampolskaya immediately from the days of the epidemic and that she is delighted to work with her again. "Even though we always wore masks," Yampolskaya says, in reference to the clinicians' autopsy garb, "she still recognized me!" This remembrance across the years, along with the hot tea and sugar cookies, has us all feeling more convivial.

The atmosphere becomes so relaxed that Grinberg takes out Walker's "intellectual property" note and tears it up, proclaiming to us in English, "I trust you." He invites us all to his home for a meal at 3 P.M. the next day, Sunday. I have the feeling he is looking forward to a happy, prolonged collaboration, without understanding that our goal is the analysis of the autopsy samples, not necessarily professional exchange.

It's Saturday night and our team's dinner this evening is with Professor Borisov and his wife Natalya at a Chinese restaurant called Harbin. Harbin is, by coincidence, the Manchurian city where Alexis Shelokov was born and his family persecuted after the war. Although I try not to think about it, Harbin is also where Japanese scientists in the 1930s began experimenting on biological weapons. The notorious Unit 731 was established soon after at Pingfan, just south of the city. There Japanese scientists used as subjects a minimum of three thousand local Han Chinese, along with stateless White Russians, Harbin Jews whose families dated back to the city's late-nineteenth-century Russian colonization, Mongolians, Soviet prisoners-of-war, and Europeans of various nationalities. Unit 731 researchers kept records as if the laboratory were a lumber mill and referred to the thousands of victims they injected, sprayed, or exposed to bomb tests as *marutas,* or logs. The Japanese assaults with typhoid, salmonella, plague, and cholera on Soviet forces and on civilians in Manchuria were equally vicious. By the end of World War II, Unit 731 experts developed an anthrax bomb using tests conducted on Chinese captives staked to the ground in groups of ten.[5]

The restaurant serves good Chinese food and, by American standards, the prices are reasonable. Actually, Harbin is Yekaterinburg's top dining spot, set in the old park of a classic nineteenth-century mansion built for the Urals' Head Forester. By any criteria, the meal is a big improvement over last night's peanut butter on crackers.

That evening in the dormitory lounge, our team meets to mull over our commitment to Abramova and Grinberg. The consensus is that Matthew should draft the letter to Dr. Semyonov at SES and that the two pathologists should be heartily assured we wish to continue the collaboration— and he should do it without delay. Who knows, Shelokov points out, how quickly the political scene might change and make scapegoats of people who, like Abramova and Grinberg, put the old government and especially the military in a bad light? Meanwhile, with complaints about military overspending commonplace and the need for defense conversion widely accepted, rumors abound that the laboratory at Compound 19 will be converted to peacetime production, of vitamins, of pharmaceuticals or, as the commander there, General Kharechko, has told the press, to manufacturing bacteria to combat pollution.[6] Despite these hints of reform, Matthew has heard nothing back about the request for our team to visit the Compound that he sent via Rector Suetin weeks ago.

On a practical note, Hugh-Jones suggests that the first publication from this project should be joint and include Abramova and Grinberg. But it could also be that the first paper will be solely theirs, on the autopsy data. The second would be a team report. I find it difficult at this point to envision a second paper. Three days in Yekaterinburg, and I haven't done any interviews. It also looks as if I will lose Yampolskaya for several days more while Walker reviews the autopsy material. Distracted, I try to listen as Matthew enthusiastically goes over the schedule of confirmed appointments that start Monday. They include meeting with public health officials and the chief of Hospital 20, which in 1979 referred patients to Hospital 40.

The most promising venture ahead is our Wednesday trip to the five villages southeast of the Yekaterinburg, in Sysertskiy rayon, to investigate the animal outbreaks. The villages are off the southern highway described as the main artery for conveying the tainted meat into the city. Our goal is to interview the families who owned the anthrax-infected animals and to speak with local veterinarians. The necessary names and addresses of owners are listed in the documents Burgasov gave us in Moscow, which Shelokov and Matthew have spent this afternoon translating and transcribing. This quest is essential, because it can settle the question of whether the animal outbreaks preceded the human ones or happened later. According to the reports Burgasov gave us in Moscow, a sick sheep was slaughtered on March 28. This was followed by a series of animal deaths confirmed as anthrax by bacteriological tests: two sheep died on April 5, followed by two more on each of the next two days and another on April 8. On April 10 a cow reportedly died of anthrax.[7] Many more animals than this must have died, if the official Soviet statement and Dr. Romanenko's recollections are accurate.

The cemetery grave markers suggest that the first human deaths occurred April 9, the earliest date we found. To calculate back in time to when victims were exposed, we need the dates for the onset of the victims' symptoms. Luckily, we are getting some data from Abramova as the series of autopsy cases is reviewed. In today's ten cases, for example, the earliest onset of symptoms was April 7. We know, too, that in her first ten cases, deaths from anthrax followed in one to four days. Is it conceivable that an epizootic broke out in late March, that affected sheep were butchered locally, and that infected meat was soon sold in the city, after which people began to sicken and die? This was the scenario Dr. Burgasov proposed when he gave us the veterinary documents. But are the documents accurate? We can disprove or prove the epizootic explanation only by investigating in the affected villages. We need to find people there willing to talk to us, just as we need to find families in Yekaterinburg who can tell us about the victims' symptoms and whereabouts.

Monday and Tuesday Yampolskaya will stop her work with Walker at 3 P.M., so that afterward she and I can begin our search for families. There is no telling how many days the autopsy data review will take. Our welcome here runs out in a week, when we take the plane back to Moscow. Walker is already confident he has seen enough. "It's inhalatory, no question," he says. In reference to Burgasov and Nikiforov, he adds, "The goddam liars!"

But Matthew counters that we should try to keep several hypotheses in mind, or else we will fail to ask important questions. Although it is well past 9 P.M., the bright sky outside gives the illusion of an unlimited evening. A student down the hall plays a mournful "Hey, Jude" on a flute. Lounging on old Danish-modern couches upholstered in orange vinyl, we mull over some of those hypotheses. We consider whether the burning of infected carcasses could create a lethal aerosol. It might take a lot of fresh carcasses and a great rise of steam to propel anthrax spores into the air, but burning may still be worth considering as an aerosol source. Suppose then we took the ceramics factory as a source point, just as the train station in the Yaroslavl epidemic was the source for the disease. Some fifteen infected carcasses might have been sold there, as the 1988 Soviet statement maintained. But maybe these infected carcasses were incinerated there, as part of a clean-up effort, and spores from that burning infected workers and nearby residents. Or maybe infected meat was burned along the highway south of the city, after being confiscated by officials. Matthew has already obtained wind data for late March into mid-April, with the thought it could provide critical information, and it is clear that the wind direction was highly variable during those days and nights. The source of an anthrax aerosol plume could have been anywhere in the southern area, and the plume itself could have taken a variety of directions as it blew over the city. There is also a meat-packing plant in the southern area, not far from the ceramics factory. Could it have been involved in the outbreak?

Drinking tea, we review some of the descriptions from the dissidents' accounts and from the press that seem to support an airborne source for the 1979 outbreak: that buildings were washed and roads repaved; that thousands died; that there was a second, late wave of cases during the washing and paving phase as spores may have been rereleased into the air. But this second aerosolization is an improbable cause for the late deaths in the last weeks of the outbreak. Anthrax spores in an aerosol would cling to whatever surface they hit; a significant force would be needed to release them again. Even then, the dose of spores would be minute compared to the one inhaled from the initial aerosol.

If there was a 1979 anthrax aerosol, an important variable is the amount of aerosolized spores released over the city. What we know least about is the quantity of anthrax it would take to kill some number of people among thousands who may have been exposed, either in their homes asleep or going about their daytime routines. Albrink experimented with massive doses of 35,000 to 100,000 spores in his research; various levels were aerosol tested on strapped-down chimpanzees in face masks. The results were far from uniform. One animal survived two doses, one of 40,000–65,000 spores, the other of 100,000. Others died quickly. Was that one surviving chimp a kind of super ape, or had it outsmarted the mask with a clever disconnection? In the 1950s, researchers at Fort Detrick used only around 4,000 spores to achieve an LD_{50} (the dose fatal to half the population) with hundreds of monkeys in Fort Detrick's enormous million-liter and now abandoned "8-Ball" test chamber.[8]

In a populous city like Yekaterinburg, a whole range of resistance to anthrax would be represented, among men and women, the old and young, the healthy and unhealthy. Demographics, too, count; Dr. Romanenko at SES has promised to give us 1979 statistics for the city. Even without them, fewer men than women in the over-55 age category can be predicted, both because of the shorter life span for Russian men and because of the great number of World War II battle deaths. This difference might have resulted in older women appearing overrepresented among the Sverdlovsk victims. Still, the amount of spores and where they blew would have made the crucial difference in determining who died.

My mind circles back to the puzzle of the missing children and youth. If a twenty-four-year-old woman died, why not an eighteen-year-old or a ten-year-old or, for that matter, a toddler? Professor Borisov has explained that Russian children complete secondary school when they are seventeen or so. While in school, they go in two shifts and may even change schools at midday, from an academic program in the morning to sports or vocational workshops in the afternoon. Are there primary and secondary schools in the southern area? Maybe in 1979 the children were all safe in some other district, eating untainted mutton stews in sunny school cafeterias and breathing uncontaminated air.

Then there is the unanswered question of the peculiarly extended duration of this epidemic. Seven weeks seems too long for a single release of anthrax to exert its lethal effect. Were victims of pneumonia inadvertently included late in the epidemic as victims of anthrax? Burgasov, in defending the official Soviet explanation, emphasized that spring was a bad time for influenza and pneumonia and that physicians were at first confused in their diagnoses. But toward the end of the epidemic, that confusion should have disappeared. Will Walker discover something unique about the later cases as he continues the autopsy review?

As my final question for the evening, I wonder if out there somewhere is an official list of victims, like the one Borisov mentioned Friday. Even without it, tomorrow, Sunday, will be a bonus for me. With no work scheduled at the Pulmonary Unit, Yampolskaya and I can start hunting for the five addresses passed on to us last night. While we look for families to interview, Matthew and the others will return to Vostochniy Cemetery to finish checking names and dates. Then at one o'clock, Matthew and Hugh-Jones will make their own trip to the southern area of the city. With his global positioning device (which resembles an oversized metal detector), Hugh-Jones hopes to get precise geographic locations, longitude and latitude. I wonder if he can intrude on the community with such a cumbersome instrument without creating a stir. Matthew will photograph the house and building types, which interest him, and the ceramics factory. We all want to see the two military compounds.

Shelokov cautions us not to be disruptive or we will be detained and ousted. As a first impression, though, I find Yekaterinburg more civil and less agitated than Moscow, but even in Moscow I have enjoyed exploring the city on my own. Inaction feels a somewhat greater threat to me now than being arrested.

8

To Chkalovskiy Rayon

The Russian map of Yekaterinburg turns out to be perfectly accurate, much better than the Harvard version. Sunday, at ten o'clock, Professor Borisov drives Yampolskaya and me to Chkalovskiy rayon. We decide to begin just off the boulevard Selkorovskaya that borders the eastern edge of the district. (Selkorovskaya translates as a country person who writes in to a newspaper, a kind of local commentator on events.) Borisov waits in the car, reading, as we try to orient ourselves in the unfamiliar neighborhood.

Unlike the natives of a neighborhood, whose understanding of their space is complex, visitors like us see only unfamiliar and unconnected locations.[1] Naming becomes the key to understanding new spaces in a city. Chkalovskiy, a name I find difficult to pronounce, is a common place name in Russia, one associated with heroism and a certain manly bravado. The aviator Valeriy Pavlovich Chkalov, the most celebrated of "Stalin's Falcons," headed the team that first flew over the North Pole to the United States in 1937. The journey of nine thousand kilometers from Moscow to Vancouver, Washington (where he is honored by a monument), was intended to show the world that the USSR could compete with other industrial nations, especially Germany.[2] Valeriy Chkalov has been called the Russian Charles Lindbergh, but unlike the meticulous Lindbergh, Chkalov was an aerobatic daredevil with a generous, impulsive personality. His career as an experimental pilot was marked by unauthorized flights (for which he was once discharged from the Air Force) and by risky aerial stunts. For thrills, he would fly under the bridges of Moscow.

His heroic exploits, especially the famous Arctic crossing, were used by Stalin to divert attention from the brutal policies and purges of the late 1930s. Chkalov, a team player who generously shared credit for his successes, added the glory of aviation technology and skills to Stalin's list of Soviet successes. And Chkalov was a patriot. In 1938, after a visit to the Soviet Union, Lindbergh dismissed its aviation capacity as a "cardboard reality," criticized Stalin's purges of the Red Air Force, and praised the superiority of the German Luftwaffe. Chkalov joined with ten other Soviet pilots in a letter denouncing Lindbergh as a fascist. Yet soon after, at the height of his fame, while he was serving as an elected Peoples Deputy in the Supreme Soviet, Chkalov publicly spoke against the purges that had killed many of his aviation comrades. He died later in 1938, testing an aircraft so badly designed that his closest friends long suspected that Stalin (who would serve as one of Chkalov's pallbearers in the lavish state funeral) had orchestrated the hero's demise. The official explanation was that he had taken one risk too many, and this may also be true.

Many of the industries that mark Sverdlovsk as a testimonial to Stalinist modernization are located in Chkalovskiy rayon: metallurgy, meatpacking, materials for road building and construction, machinery for the lumber industry, and ceramics. It stands in contrast to the central city of Yekaterinburg to the north, where the university is located. The north has shops (some specialize in minerals and precious gems), museums, monuments, government buildings, the historic Iron Works and nineteenth-century mansions painted in soft pastels, and the better apartment buildings. There the streets are full of automobiles; crowds bustle along its sidewalks and jam its trolley cars.

Despite its factories, whole parts of Chkalovskiy look like a village. The majority of its dwellings are one-story Ural cottages, often surrounded by high wooden fences. Some houses have small bathhouses behind them, for the saunas and steam baths that are integral to Russian life. Garden tracts can also be seen behind the houses. Plots like these all over Russia, allotted to Soviet citizens during the famines of the 1930s and 1940s, supply a substantial amount of the food that gets them through the cold winters, including potatoes, turnips, onions, beets, and cabbage. There are almost no sidewalks in this central area, and few cars are in evidence. In the distance we see an elderly woman tending goats on a vacant lot. The German philosopher Walter Benjamin commented in the 1920s that Moscow's complex urban terrain played hide-and-seek with him, with modern edifices often disappearing behind peasant enclaves and then emerging again.[3] So, too, in Chkalovskiy. A busy highway is within sight, as are Khrushchev-era apartment buildings, and those enormous factories are part of the landscape. Although we cannot see them from where we stand, the two military compounds, 19 and 32, lie only some two kilometers to the northwest, on a low bluff.

We ask the first passerby, a middle-aged man in overalls, for directions. He seems to know exactly what we are interested in and has no hesitation in speaking. He was a worker at the ceramics factory in 1979, he tells us, and was inoculated three times with a "pistolet," a jet-pistol injector. After the first shot, a huge ulcer appeared on his upper left arm. For bad reactions to the first injection, the workers got time off from their jobs, but for subsequent shots, they didn't. Everyone, he assures us, learned to use vodka to reduce the reaction. This account, the first I hear from a member of the local community, validates the official Soviet description of the vaccine program they initiated after the outbreak began. The description of the reaction to the vaccine also rings true. The traditional Soviet STI vaccine is known to produce ulcers and other side effects in a percentage of those who receive it. But was the vaccination program itself a good faith public health precaution or a sham? This worker thinks he was duped.

"At the time," he volunteers, "the authorities said it was for anthrax. But now I know it was bacterial warfare from Compound 19." But he "knows" only because he has heard rumors that the military was at fault.

He wants to show us the ceramics factory, but we are looking for the home of Anna Komina, on Ulitsa Lyapustina, the street named for a local but now almost forgotten Soviet hero called Lyapustin, who in the 1960s was killed defending citizens set upon by hooligans. The worker points us in the general direction and we move on, searching in vain for street signs and trying to find order in the house numbers. We find that some dwellings for which we have addresses have been torn down, leaving vacant lots. Others are divided in two with only one number posted. The high fences sometimes obscure the house entrance. After circling several blocks, we again encounter the man in overalls and take up his offer to see the ceramics factory, which is close by, due south of us. Although we still have no certain figures, both Soviet and dissident versions of the epidemic agree that workers at the ceramics factory were disproportionately affected by the outbreak. We don't exchange names with our guide, as we might have done in the United States. I take my cue from Yampolskaya who, as I begin to understand, is selective about introductions. She, a Moscow physician and an educated woman, is not about to give her name or to shake hands with an Uralski workman on the street, nor would she have done so in Soviet times.

The ceramics factory itself is a huge gated complex of buildings, with paths leading from one to another. On the map posted in front, the different production divisions are illustrated in primary colors. Our guide leads us past the gate, explaining that this plant, which has a Sunday shift, is where industrial pipes, bathroom fixtures, tiles, dishes, and teapots have been made for decades. Economic change has shut down some divisions, including the huge pipe shop. Yet the factory is almost a city tradition, and it keeps on producing. There is even a ceramics factory story about Boris Yeltsin in 1976, when he first governed the oblast. In an experiment in public communication, he went on the radio to encourage his constituency to write him about their dissatisfactions with life in Sverdlovsk, promising he would address their concerns. One problem that surfaced was that the ceramics factory sold only entire tea sets, no individual tea pots. When your teapot broke, you had to buy a whole new set with sugar bowl, pitcher, and tray. Yeltsin solved the problem by ordering the ceramics factory to produce eight thousand individual teapots to sell to the disgruntled customers—not a big step toward democracy, but certainly a crowd-pleasing gesture.

Our guide pushes open a side door and leads us to the enormous company cafeteria, now empty. He knew a woman who worked here who died in the 1979 outbreak, but her family has since moved away. I imagine this woman, maybe one whose picture is in the cemetery, working behind the stainless-steel counter. I imagine her feeling sick, perhaps leaving work early, maybe worried for herself, maybe suspecting she's caught influenza or something worse.

Outside, to the left of the ceramics factory entrance, is the deserted three-story, block-long pipe shop, with a high smokestack. On the top level a long row of large windows faces northwest. Adjacent to the cafeteria is a loading platform and a large open area where, if the official version of the epidemic is correct, a truck from the south brought the contaminated meat that was sold to victims of the epidemic. This area, too, is deserted. I feel time sweeping over Yekaterinburg, gradually eradicating all the scenes and physical traces of the epidemic, the segregated graveyard sector, the houses where families once lived, the ceramics factory and, though we have yet to see it, the military laboratory, now reportedly converting to peacetime manufacture.

Our guide sees us beyond the factory gates and takes his leave. On my own and in my own country, I would have detained him to find out more about the factory and the neighborhood. Instead, Yampolskaya and I thank him for his time and head northeast into the nearly rural center of Chkalovskiy rayon. Staying in the middle of the street, which is equal parts packed dirt and macadam, we continue our search for numbers and signs. Our shoes are covered with whitish dust. It is chilly with gusts of wind; the bright sun seems incapable of generating warmth. I cannot help but think that if in 1979 the military biologists at Compound 19 were truly working on an improved vaccine, as we have heard, they might have helped inoculate the community when the outbreak hit. Or, to take speculation further, if the lethal anthrax was emitted from their laboratory, wouldn't a sense of honor compel their leadership to admit its role in the disaster? After all, during the 1991 coup against Gorbachev, soldiers at the Moscow White House refused to fire on civilians. Could the army be indifferent to civilian deaths it itself caused? But Dr. Burgasov is adamant that in 1979 the military stayed completely out of the picture.

As we trudge along, dust from the road covers my sandals and feet. And what about anthrax spores in this ground where we are walking? Dr. Romanenko told us that tests done in the city yielded no positive results, that Yekaterinburg is safe, but is he right? Do any spores still linger here in the soil? Those goats that old woman is herding, are they healthy?

At the far end of the block, Sergei Borisov appears in his car and waves jubilantly. He is trying to tell us that we are where we want to be, on Ulitsa Lyapustina. We easily find the home of Anna Komina, a small cottage like the others on this street. Through the unlocked gate, we enter a muddy yard, with a garden straight ahead and the house entrance on the left. Mounting several steps, we knock on the door. We have formulated a brief introductory speech. Yampolskaya will explain that we are from the university, that we know about the loss of a family member in the 1979 anthrax epidemic. Then, so as not to put people off with the possibility of a long interview, she will follow with, "Is it possible for us to ask a few questions?" We also decided that my being an American, which will not be obvious at first, is best unannounced. In all, Yampolskaya and I look alike, blonde, neatly dressed, not especially threatening or intrusive. I know enough Russian to follow the interview, after which, if the question arises, my nationality can become a topic. Despite these preparations, I brace myself for the swing of a door that, once opened, might be quickly slammed.

Instead, Anna's son, Yuriy Komin, dressed in a factory worker's rough clothes, welcomes us inside. Before we enter we energetically scrape our shoes on the doormat and even offer to take off our shoes, as is customary. Komin, a pale, soft-spoken man in his thirties, tells us not to bother. We do our best with the doormat and follow him to the parlor.

Both his parents are now dead. Komin and his wife have continued to live in the family cottage, as they did before. The little parlor has two day beds in it, a table with four chairs, and a breakfront with china displayed behind glass. A small French door to another room reveals two more small beds. The house is well kept but an indefinable gloom hangs over it, and the sad expression on Komin's face seems more than the usual Russian solemnity.

Komin and his wife, Tatyana, are employed at the ceramics factory, like his parents before him. In fact, his wife is now at work, at the same job his mother had when she died, checking the temperature and pH value of the water supply. Checking equipment is a fairly good job for a woman factory worker. The majority of Soviet and now Russian women have been concentrated in areas of unskilled work, where the physical labor can be brutal and the pay is subpar.[4]

We proceed methodically through the questions on the interview form, establishing first that the tombstone information is accurate and that Anna was indeed a victim of the epidemic. We learn, too, that she neither drank nor smoked nor suffered from any serious illness. "Her teeth were stronger than mine," her son says, with the glimmer of a smile. But no more than a glimmer. The sadness never leaves his eyes.

We then ask him to describe the two main scenarios: first, the onset of the disease and, second, his mother's hospitalization, death, and burial. He reckons back six days from when his mother died and gives us the date of April 4 for the onset. He details the beginning of her symptoms—faintness, dizziness, trouble with breathing. But, he remarks, she seemed to get better after that. We understand: this brief period of apparent revival is characteristic of anthrax. And then, on April 8, his mother completely collapsed. The first doctor who came to the house lacked intensive care equipment, so he called the emergency medical center, Stancia Skoraya, for an ambulance. Komin described how two medics worked for five hours to bring his mother's blood pressure up to a level where it was safe to transport her to the local Hospital 20. The next day, she went into failure, as he put it, and within twenty-four hours, on April 10, she was dead.

Anna Komina's death took place quickly and behind closed doors, without any family witnesses. For five days, her body was held at the hospital, which prevented her relatives from performing the usual Russian washing and dressing rituals and from holding a wake. In the interim, public health workers came and gave tetracycline pills to Komin and his wife, but not to their son, who was only an infant. On the fifth day, Anna's coffin was transported by truck directly from the hospital to the cemetery and buried in Sector 13. The family, on a tip from the hospital staff, went to the cemetery but was not allowed inside the gate. There were police, Komin says, but no soldiers, and certainly none with weapons (as some newspaper reports had claimed).

Later in April, he remembers, the vaccination campaign began, and he himself received a series of three shots at the ceramics factory, as did his wife and father. Then, around the first of May, firemen began hosing down buildings and trees right in this area, near the ceramics factory. Some asphalt roads were put in, but, as he points out, much of Chkalovskiy remains unpaved today.

Komin searches in the breakfront and brings out his mother's death certificate, dated April 10. Under "Cause of Death" is written: "Bacterial pneumonia," a diagnosis he knows is inaccurate. On April 10, though, a clinician, not knowing the name of the killing disease, might have put down pneumonia based on symptoms: the difficult breathing, the high temperature, the obvious signs of infection. Nonetheless, the misleading entry irritates me. After April 12, the certificate could have been changed to read "anthrax" and specifically, "gastrointestinal anthrax" if that was the cause of death Nikiforov believed in. Anyone who has ever read a mystery story knows that cause of death matters. It matters all the more in real life, where we have to understand the physical threats to our existence, even if we choose to ignore them.

As sociologist Anthony Giddens has argued, we modern people are so inevitably engaged in calculating the risks to our well-being that the process forms our very identities. Our technologies have improved and prolonged our lives with efficient sanitation, farming, manufacture, and transportation. The result, paradoxically, has been not to eliminate our sense of hazards, but to pitch it to a new level—away from childhood diseases to the diseases that befall people as they grow old; from starvation to pollution; from bows and arrows to advanced weapons of mass destruction. To navigate these hazards, we have to be able to recognize "fateful moments" when they confront us. The death of a loved one is one such crucial confrontation with risk. But whole groups can also face such events: "There are, of course, fateful moments in the history of collectivities as well as the lives of individuals. They are phases at which things are wrenched out of joint, where a given state of affairs is suddenly altered by a few key events."[5]

Collective deaths in a group's history make for "a tottering world in which all known harmonies threaten to dissolve—those of nature, those of society both at the level of formal governance and at that of intimate human relationships, and those of body and mind."[6] But if the cause of death is misrepresented, as on a death record, how can an individual or a society assess true risks and negotiate real hazards? Without knowing why death has occurred, how can one reckon the potential source of danger and do something to avoid it?

But my thoughts are leaping forward. In this community, whatever the death certificates stated, anthrax-infected meat was the official explanation broadcast to the community. Perhaps that sufficed. But Yuriy Komin tells us that his family bought no meat from private or black market sources. At that time, they were raising two pigs in their yard, animals with no trace of disease. The family ate all its meals together and never suffered from food poisoning.

"My mother often walked home," he says, with a gesture toward the street, "to fix the noontime meal for us, instead of having us eat in the cafeteria." Though they all ate the same food, only his mother became ill. He pauses on the unspoken question, "Why her?"

On her tombstone, he tells us, the family put the Soviet star, not a cross, because Anna Komina was a patriot, not at all religious. As Komin speaks of his mother's grave, his face grows more pale and fills with anxiety. Without our asking, he tells us what happened to his father: crushed by his wife's death, he died shortly after her, of a broken heart.

"So it was a double tragedy," he explains. Now his eyes are filled with tears.

Before we leave, I ask him what he now believes caused the epidemic.

"It came through the air," he responds without rancor, "from Compound 19." He believes this now from what he has read in the Russian press. But in 1979, he and his family had only suspicions and no real idea of why this disaster befell their family.

Once back out on the street, Yampolskaya and I hold on to each other, our own eyes filled with tears. Both of us are familiar with tragic deaths, she, as an active clinician, much more than I. During the 1979 epidemic, she also cared for dozens of patients, nearly all of them fatalities. I have spent years researching newborn intensive care units, where illness and death are the norm.[7] But the story we have just heard is especially heart-wrenching. Komin has described the devastation of a family, a fact missing from autopsy data, missing from epidemiological graphs, and missing, too, from the records of intensive clinical care. The grief of this son, years after his mother's death, and his father's, is as freshly bitter as if the tragedies happened yesterday.

After we leave Komin's cottage, Yampolskaya and I crisscross Chkalovskiy rayon looking in vain for the other addresses on our list. We have one for Nikolay Khudyakov. He died late in the course of the epidemic, on May 21, when he was forty-six and lived at a worker's hostel on Ulitsa Voennaya (Military Street). The lobby of the hostel is run-down and charmless. We comb the halls of this dilapidated building where the doors are plated with iron to keep out thieves. The concrete stairs are eroded and the hall plaster is cracked, but the smells of Sunday cooking are good. A dark-haired woman in a housedress, with two young children clutching her skirt, unlocks one door.

"Khudyakov? Never heard of him. We've been living here for six years. Maybe he had the place before us."

We search on. Either the addresses from our secret source are wrong or the houses no longer exist. At one wrong address, a man and woman volunteer the name of a Lydia Tretnikova, who used to live in an apartment on one of the main boulevards. Her husband, they are sure, died in the epidemic. Yes, we saw Tretnikov's grave in the cemetery; his photo showed an earnest schoolboy in jacket and tie, though Tretnikov was fifty-two when he died. But now we cannot find the building, let alone the numbered door.

At last we locate a second address on our list, a cottage on Ulitsa Eskadronaya (Squadron Street), near the ceramics factory. It was the home of Mikhail Markov, like Komina one of the earliest victims of the outbreak.

Markov's brother Nikolay and sister-in-law Prosovia still live there. At the time of the epidemic they shared the cottage with Mikhail, whom they call Misha, and his wife, and they are willing to talk to us. Their parlor has a plain wood floor without rugs, and a wood partition divides the room in half. Still, there is the obligatory breakfront, with the good china stored behind glass. They politely offer us tea or something to eat, but we decline. We sit on kitchen chairs and they on their couch, where they take turns recounting the story of Mikhail's death. As they speak about their Misha, their faces fill with the same anxious grief as Yuriy Komin's. In talking with us, they are reliving Misha's last days and can do nothing to prevent his inevitable doom. Yet they want to tell the story.

Misha's illness, his sister-in-law begins, started on April 6, when he came down with a cough. He went to the local clinic, where the doctor said that he might have the flu and should go to the neighborhood hospital if he felt worse later. Instead, the next day, feeling a little better, Misha went back to work. The false revival characteristic of anthrax made him optimistic. Then on the afternoon of April 8, as his brother and sister-in-law were preparing to take a pig they had raised to the state slaughterhouse, Misha complained of feeling cold. When it came time to help his brother load the animal into the car, he stood aside, shivering.

"I'd just had abdominal surgery," his sister-in-law says. "I asked him, since he was a big man, 'Why don't you help with the pig?'"

Misha tried to help, but he was on the verge of collapse and shivered all through the expedition. When he got home, he went straight to bed, still shivering but feeling feverish, too. His brother went out and bought vodka as a remedy, but when Misha's wife offered it to him, Misha took just a sip. He grew weaker until, finally, they called the Stancia Skoraya to have him transported to Hospital 20. When his wife telephoned there the next morning, someone told her her husband was doing fine. But later, when she went to the hospital, she discovered to her shock that he had died during the night and that his body had been taken away.

Did the Markov family eat meat? Yes, Misha in particular was a big meat eater, but they bought only from state shops or ate meat from animals they had raised themselves, which were certified healthy pigs. He smoked heavily and was an average drinker, which by Russian standards means vodka every day but not drunkenness. He worked in the ceramics factory, in the pipe shop, where he drove a small electric forklift.

"There were so many deaths in that division," his sister-in-law adds, "that they stopped posting the pictures they usually put up on the bulletin board when someone dies."

This couple has some bitter stories to tell—about the ridicule heaped on Misha's wife, a worker at the local meat-packing plant, for feeding her husband bad meat, about how angry his family was not to have his body back for preparing for burial. They brought Misha's good clothes to the hospital for him to be buried in, but these were refused. "They wanted a new sheet from us instead," his sister-in-law complains.

At the cemetery, a policeman guarded the special coffin; the city, not the family members, paid for it. Nor did they pay for the plot in the special sector. Yes, they were given tetracycline by local medics after Misha died. Yes, a vaccination program was begun later in April. Yes, some local streets and buildings were hosed down by firemen. But why? They did not know. Misha's wife, who still lives next door, kept the death certificate, which indicated only that he died of sepsis. And yes, it was his wife who had draped the grave with the garland of red, blue, and white plastic flowers we saw yesterday at Vostochniy Cemetery. She is not at home now, but we know where to reach her next time.

I ask directly if the Markovs know of any other victims' families we could contact. I ask the question with trepidation. I am in a culture where informing was once a weapon, a way to eliminate someone from an apartment you coveted or to destroy a coworker. The sociological method of "snowballing," of using personal contacts to generate more respondents for a sample, would have been ludicrous in a Stalinist context. Would it be the same here and now? Just an hour before, only around the corner, a man and woman spontaneously volunteered the name and address of a possible anthrax victim. They didn't seem malicious. But as it turns out, the Markovs say they have only vague recollections of other afflicted families. The epidemic obviously brought them no friends, and being in the community of survivors seems to have brought them little collective solace.

It is nearly two o'clock when we leave the Markovs. We have completed only two interviews, and our leads are exhausted. Professor Borisov must get back to his family, and our group has to be at Lev Grinberg's home for a three o'clock meal. Yampolskaya thinks that Dr. Abramova will be there and that she may have information about victims' addresses for me. I am already plotting how to leave the Grinbergs after an hour and return to Chkalovskiy to knock on more doors. I am thinking we might locate the Tretnikov family. Or we could revisit our first contacts to interview both Yuriy Komin's wife and Misha Markov's. Just by walking around and asking, we might find other people affected by the outbreak, other families and friends who suffered losses. Why not? Daylight lasts until ten at night. Now that I have found the human experience I wanted and discovered where the ordinary people are, with their extraordinary, unmasked, credible stories, I cannot afford to waste time.

9

Constraints, Fears, Frustrations

Sunday dinner at the Grinbergs (which I swore I would leave after an hour) lasts for six hours, from 3 to 9 P.M. There are good reasons why I succumb to this hospitality. First of all, I am hungry for good food. Our breakfast at the dormitory cafeteria was tea and rye bread, a hard-boiled egg, and some indeterminate gray meat. Since the cost was the equivalent of two dollars for the six of us, we have no real cause for complaint. Still, we Americans are disgruntled.

In truth, more than food and accommodations are involved in our discontent; we are discovering that teamwork is a trial and, perhaps by unspoken agreement, make the most of this diversion. None of us is particularly a team player, and except for Matthew's and my earlier efforts, the members of this group have not worked together before. At odd moments, visions of other teams dance in my head, the ones Matthew tried to put together in past years. In July 1983, for example, after ongoing negotiations with a high official in the USSR State Committee for Science and Technology, Matthew recruited Joshua Lederberg, Paul Doty, and David Baltimore, another Nobel Laureate biologist, to go with him to Sverdlovsk for a week-long investigation. The trip was supported by U.S. officials, but on September 1, 1983, when the Soviets shot down Korean Air Lines Flight 007 for intruding into its air space and 269 passengers and crew members were killed, the already tense relations between the superpowers broke down. Planning for this Sverdlovsk expedition was then canceled by the Soviet side.[1] Soon after his 1986 trip to

Moscow, Matthew wrote Dr. Pyotr Burgasov to report that, as they had discussed, he had organized a small group to visit Sverdlovsk. "A most distinguished and respected individual has agreed to participate and take overall responsibility for arranging and conducting the visit. He is Dr. Lewis Thomas, President Emeritus of the Memorial Sloan-Kettering Institute in New York." Attached was a list of suggested luminaries willing to go, including a towering figure in U.S. veterinary medicine and public health, Dr. James Steele. Matthew excused himself from the group because of his heavy work load at Harvard, but left an opening for joining in, should Burgasov think it essential for him to participate. "In that case," he wrote the deputy minister, "I would make every effort to come."[2] That trip fell through for want of Soviet response.

Yet another team began to take shape in September 1988, after the Soviet physicians had visited the United States and presented their tainted-meat explanation. In 1985, Dr. Bernard Lown, the Boston cardiologist, and his Soviet counterpart, Dr. Yevgeny Chazov, had received the Nobel Peace Prize on behalf of International Physicians for the Prevention of Nuclear War. Matthew contacted Lown and convinced him of the importance of investigating the 1979 outbreak. Lown, in Moscow on a visit to Chazov, then minister of health, asked permission for a U.S. team of experts to visit Sverdlovsk. This time the team members on the list were America's two foremost anthrax authorities, Wilhelm Albrink and Philip Brachman, along with Martin Crumrine, chief of the Bacteriology Division at Fort Detrick, veterinarian Arnold Kaufman from the Centers for Disease Control, Alex Langmuir, Alexis Shelokov, and me. In late October 1988 we learned from Lown that Chazov had approved the visit. But in December, a letter arrived from one of his deputies bemoaning the lack of any data to be gathered in Sverdlovsk: "Due to the negligence of staff responsible for keeping medical records in Sverdlovsk and unfortunate events with people involved in combating the outbreak [probably a reference to the death of Dr. Bezdenezhnikh] we have not now [any] material for real scientific analysis." Matthew, not to be put off, wrote back that the team still saw considerable scientific value in making the trip.[3] But the Soviets held back. None of these dream teams ever materialized. As time went by, potential participants died, grew ill, or were diverted to other projects.

Among the present recruits, everyone (except Yampolskaya) wants to do it their way and is ready to tell the rest of us how the trip arrangements could be better. We have learned, for example, that a contingent of German historians in town for a conference on World War II usurped our reservations at a superior hotel, built in the mid-1980s for Communist Party bosses, which is why we have ended up at the university dormitory. Exactly what could have been done to head off the Germans is unclear, but grumbling erupts. And there are frustrations quite apart from those of trying to work together. Spending days being herded about from one unfamiliar setting to another is wearing. The language barrier and cultural differences add to the strain. Russian officials can be devastatingly stiff and impassive in formal meetings, which Americans resent, probably as much as Russians resent our glad-handing and easy smiles. So who among those who have spoken to us is telling the truth? Are we being given the runaround? Wouldn't everyone here rather we leave?

In all this, Yampolskaya is strong and patient, the way Russian women are supposed to be. She works terribly hard, has unflagging good spirits, and never complains. That she once believed the anthrax was gastrointestinal and that Dr. Nikiforov, her mentor, is on record as supporting the Soviet infected-meat explanation never deters her from enthusiastically investigating the airborne hypothesis. People make mistakes, she shrugs; sometimes they lie or they are confused. Yampolskaya insists on just one thing, that she be allowed to have a good hot cup of tea each evening.

But not everyone is so resilient. Alexis Shelokov is hoarse from interpreting, a role that limits his participation in the inquiry, but one that he is reluctant to relinquish in favor of a hired interpreter. Martin Hugh-Jones is understandably restless; it will be Wednesday before he can talk to veterinarians. Also, the Russian language baffles him, and he has a hard time remembering the names of people we meet. David Walker has come down with a bad cold and is impatient to leave for Moscow. Only Matthew, who seems to thrive on the lack of creature comforts, begins and ends each day full of energy and purpose. He's had twelve years to ponder the problem and knows exactly what he wants to accomplish here. The other men are less than compliant. For example, they argue that he should arrange another meeting with Dr. Babich, the former SES director who blushed so deeply when contradicted about animal outbreaks. They think he really knows what happened in 1979. Matthew is uninterested in going over old ground. Rather, he wants to move ahead toward a meeting with General A. T. Kharechko, the current head of Compound 19. It is not so much an issue of getting inside Compound 19, although that would help, as it is putting questions directly to the military, which, save for occasional oblique comments in the press, has been mordantly silent about the epidemic.

I stay out of this and other arguments. I have become fully preoccupied with striking out on my own, which will mean finding an interpreter
who can go with me each day, all day, to secure interviews with families.
Otherwise, if Walker continues his review of the autopsy data, I will spend
my days waiting for Yampolskaya. The lesson here is plain: two inter-
preters for three informational quests—autopsy samples, official meetings, and interviews—are just not enough. On top of that is the problem
of transportation. Chkalovskiy is a good half-hour drive through traffic
from our dormitory quarters. Matthew, Shelokov, and Hugh-Jones need
a car for appointments with public health officials, and we usually have
just one automobile and driver available—either Professor Borisov or
Sasha. Can I afford to spend two hours a day on the trolley? Borisov
thinks he can find a sociologist at the university to help me. But Soviet
sociology was too repressed to develop much as a discipline, and I fear
my chances of locating someone who is both bilingual and knowledge-
able about research methods are slim.

Another anxiety is wearing me down. For years, I've had a recurrent
dream in which I am caught behind the Iron Curtain. In it, I am a professor in my sixties, wearing a tweed suit and sturdy shoes, walking down
a corridor like one of the halls at the Sorbonne, where I was once a student. But the setting in my dream is an East European university, more
gray and massive. The marble floors of its lobby are cracked, student
voices echo tinnily through the corridors, and the smell of overcooked
cafeteria food percolates up the basement stairwells. Physically it is uncannily like the Ural State University. In my dream, I suffer a life of terrible constriction, with none of the easy freedoms I knew before. Now
here I am, deep inside Russia, walking these old academic halls. Is this
trip the prelude to my Iron Curtain dream? Will I be trapped here?

Meanwhile, the Grinbergs offer a delightful respite. Lev and his wife
Natalya have covered the entire surface of their dining room table with
bowls of fresh chopped vegetables and artistically prepared salads, with
platters of blini, smoked fish, delectable meat-filled pastries, and cold cuts.
All this food came out of a closet-sized kitchen. Lev tells us he prepared
a lot of it himself, that he loves to cook. He has grown the potatoes, tomatoes, and cucumbers at their garden outside town. We eat ravenously. A
festive meal in a Russian home tastes just as good as it looks. The vodka
flows freely, especially in the direction of Shelokov, Walker, and Hugh-
Jones, who sit companionably side-by-side on the couch. No one breathes
a word about autopsy data.

Instead, with chairs gathered around the couch, we talk about life. I am particularly interested in Faina Abramova's. I am relieved to see her outside my dream and outside the Pulmonary Unit. She is a beautiful woman, in great measure because of her spirit and intelligence. I wonder why she chose a medical career and pathology. She is younger by a decade or so than Dr. Burgasov, who stumbled fortuitously into medicine. Though she may have had advantages he did not, I have the feeling that her path was not smooth.

"Please begin at the beginning," I ask.

Abramova smiles and responds with the story of a poor village girl with no shoes who, at the age of eleven, of her own will, left her family and came to live with an aunt and uncle in Sverdlovsk. Her uncle in particular encouraged her to get an education; that was her attraction to the city, the chance to learn. When just a teenager, she worked in a pathology laboratory after school, cleaning test tubes, and gained a little experience with the world of medical science. Yet her real ambition was aviation; she wanted to be a pilot. Her idols were Maria Raskova, Polina Osipenko, and Valentina Grizodubova, the three women who in 1938 flew a record-breaking direct flight of 6,450 kilometers across the Soviet Union. Flying seemed to her an ideal life. Her uncle supported her so she could go to engineering school. But it turned out her mathematical ability was insufficient and physics proved beyond her. The pathologist she had worked for encouraged her to go to medical school instead. She did, and here she is!

How ironic, it seems to me, that both Pyotr Burgasov and Faina Abramova came from the same peasant background, enjoyed similar educational benefits, and became physicians, and yet have ended up on opposite sides of this anthrax controversy. Burgasov's path was into the central bureaucracy of public health. Abramova's choice was a medical specialty that led to a secure but modest position, with an emphasis on professional competence. Burgasov turned into an administrator with international contacts. Abramova stayed within the confines imposed on a Soviet woman in medicine, at the same job with virtually no reference to the world beyond Sverdlovsk, until perestroika. Which of them is right in this controversy? We do not yet know.

I have more questions for Abramova, but Lev Grinberg interrupts. He wants to make toasts to Russian-American cooperation. Why not! We all raise glasses to this possibility. Then Grinberg and Matthew retreat to a corner to discuss how the ensuing review of autopsy material will be handled. As Abramova gets up and begins helping Natalya serve dessert, the conversation drifts to families, American families, Russian families, raising children. I see my opportunity. I say to Yampolskaya that, above all, the families affected by the epidemic are owed the truth. "Pravda!" I exclaim with gusto. Abramova, who cannot help hearing, comes over to us and promises that tomorrow she will give us whatever helpful information she has in her notes. She doubts there are full addresses; the notes are rudimentary. When the KGB took the victims' records away, they took not only the autopsy reports, but the drafts for those reports. Abramova, who had been working on them, tried but failed to push them out of view under some other papers, but one of the agents noticed them. Only her working notes survive, so I mustn't expect much. I am elated nonetheless at her sensitivity to the human side of the outbreak. All residue of my nightmare of her has vanished.

The elation is short-lived. When we get back to our dormitory, Yampolskaya gives me the bad news that she and Walker will fly back to Moscow early Friday morning. That leaves us only four days during which we can do interviews, and even then, only when she has spent 9 A.M. to 4 P.M. at the Pulmonary Unit as has now been agreed. The good news that our biologist Dr. Shepetkin telephones to us is that five more names have been relayed by his mysterious source. Still, I go to bed that night almost despondent about the interviews.

In the morning, I complain to Matthew that I am bewildered by how we are getting information about the victims' families. If someone out there has ten addresses, the same person probably has access to more, if not all of them. But we are hardly free-roaming detectives who can go sleuthing the city for evidence. Arrangements have been made for us as a respected group of experts, and we have to stay with our schedule.

That afternoon, D. N. Ponomaryev, a short, dapper man who was chief epidemiologist of the Oblast SES (Sanitary Epidemiological Station) in 1979, meets with us to present an hour-long account of the outbreak, which he tells us will be the first of two parts. We take over the office of the vice-rector, who herds several visiting German historians to another room. Ponomaryev begins his talk with a sigh.

"I could write a novel about this!" he remarks. But he assures us he will resist fiction. "I am an epidemiologist. As you know there is a lot of loose talk about the outbreak, most of it totally devoid of logic and epidemiological basis."

He goes on to describe how in late March 1979 he and Dr. Babich went south into Syserskiy rayon to investigate the reports of an animal outbreak of anthrax. I wait for him to say that they found the reports unsubstantiated. Instead, Ponomaryev consults his notes and states that privately owned sheep and a few cattle died in three villages to the south. "We instructed the veterinarians to institute controls and to discover the cause of the epizootic."

The members of our group exchange glances. If this is true, how can Dr. Babich possibly deny there had been an animal outbreak before the human cases?

Ponomaryev continues, reporting that he and Babich returned to Sverdlovsk on April 1. On April 2, he received a telephone call from the city coroner, reporting that a man and a woman had died "as if by lightning."

"On April 2," he says, "Babich and I looked at each other and asked, 'Could this be anthrax?' Two days later, a pathoanatomist confirmed our supposition that it was anthrax. This was on the fourth or fifth."

These dates sound off. Dr. Abramova told us her first autopsy was April 10 and the samples sent to the laboratory then; laboratory results confirming the anthrax diagnosis were communicated on April 11. Dr. Ponomaryev has placed the confirmation of anthrax a week earlier, with an epizootic preceding the human cases. Then he adds, "By April 15, twenty-eight had died." Our calculations from the cemetery data are roughly the same. But Ponomaryev also contends that there were no cutaneous cases, whereas Yampolskaya has already told us that she herself treated several that had become systemic. And he attributes to Dr. Burgasov the order to wash down buildings, which Burgasov has emphatically denied.

To our surprise, Ponomaryev then proposes that there was a second epizootic from April 1 to 15, again south of Sverdlovsk in Sysertskiy rayon. It affected ten settlements, he says, including the area's largest town, Syserts, and resulted in sixty-eight animal cases, with sixty of these animals belonging to private owners. But this outbreak was not a natural event, he tells us, without stipulating the cause. His overview is complicated: animals die of anthrax in March and then in a second wave in April anthrax strikes both humans and animals. In its complexity, this double epizootic scenario is like the one invoked by the 1980 U.S. working group on Sverdlovsk to explain the long duration of the outbreak, but Ponomaryev still has said nothing about either bad mixed feed or an aerosol. All I am learning is that we must clarify the dates of any and all animal outbreaks.

To finish his presentation, Ponomaryev presents a map of the oblast on which he has drawn a straight line from Compound 19 southeast through the ceramics factory and out into the countryside, to Syserts city and to other settlements where animals died. With some glee, Matthew takes a piece of paper from his notebook, on which he has plotted the same six villages with reported March–April epizootics, named in the Soviet publications and in veterinary papers from Dr. Burgasov. He also has found they fall on a straight line. He, too, has drawn a line from Compound 19 down through the villages. His map, in fact, is the same as our speaker's.

Rather than being pleased, Dr. Ponomaryev appears disconcerted by this uncalled-for contribution, as if Matthew has ruined his talk. He checks his watch, then packs up his notes and leaves, with a vague promise to continue part two of his lecture at a future date.

After he leaves, we discuss his construction of the outbreak. Is any part of it valid? Could there have been multiple epizootics, with one starting in late March and the other later? About the washing down of buildings in Chkalovskiy rayon, he might be right that Burgasov gave the cleanup order. Washing contaminated outdoor surfaces is recommended as a general prophylactic measure in the 1970 book Burgasov edited. According to Ponomaryev, the rayon Extraordinary Commission for Emergencies, a standing committee usually composed of local physicians, balked at the clean-up order, but then agreed that the ceramics factory could be hosed down.

Ponomaryev has also suggested that the workers at the ceramics factory, because of the occupational hazard of silicosis (a lung disease from silica dust), might have lesions in their lungs that made them especially susceptible to airborne anthrax, as might heavy smokers. This idea may have merit, but that speculation doesn't help us now. Anyway, not all the victims worked at the factory, and Russian women, a fifth of the victims, are rarely heavy smokers. In addition, Ponomaryev contends that workers sent up on roofs to clean them also died from exposure to anthrax, an explanation of how the outbreak was prolonged that we have heard before but find doubtful. Maybe Ponomaryev is writing a novel after all.

After this presentation, before Yampolskaya and I go with Sasha to Chkalovskiy, the group reviews the schedule for the coming week. The next day's lists of appointments includes one with another epidemiologist who was on the April 1979 Extraordinary Commission. If we have time, we will go to some city offices, such as ZAGS ('Zapis' Aktov Grazdanskogo Sostoyania), the government archive for birth, marriage, and death certificates, to track down background health statistics for 1979, in particular, the death certificate information for victims. Dr. Romanenko from SES has promised to provide a demographic profile of both the city and the Chkalovskiy district as it was in 1979, with as much detail as he can find in the records. Without figures on population density and demographics, we cannot know what percent of residents were affected and whether age and sex distribution had some effect. The following day, Wednesday, is set aside for meeting with veterinarians in the southeastern Sysertskiy rayon, to straighten out, if possible, the question of the dates of the epizootic. The veterinarians should also be able to verify the veterinary documents from Burgasov which include the names and addresses of the private owners of diseased livestock. I am looking forward to cross-checking any epizootic, if it happened and when, with interviews in one or more of the villages.

After that, I will return to Yekaterinburg and, at four o'clock, Yampolskaya and I will go to Chkalovskiy to do interviews. The day after, Thursday, June 11, is the last day she and I can search for the families of victims. All day I have been discouraged by her leaving, even though another interpreter to help me may be on the horizon. Professor Borisov has arranged a meeting for me with the head of the new social science division at the university (a Professor Marenkov), who has located a young colleague interested in working with me. I don't know if the candidate is a man or a woman, with or without an advanced degree or social research experience. So far the day has been all sharp edges, with little comfort or progress. I think of the poet Osip Mandelstam's wry metaphor: "Today is all beak and no feathers / and it's staying that way. Why?"[4] I am hoping the interviews will help me recoup the day, though it is already late afternoon when we set off for Chkalovskiy with its jumble of cottages, apartment buildings, and factories—and with its family stories waiting to be heard.

10

Knocking on Doors

As Sasha Tiutiunnik drives us toward Chkalovskiy, we are caught in a traffic jam south of the university. President Boris Yeltsin is in Yekaterinburg to visit his mother, who has been hospitalized with a heart ailment. Crowds line the sidewalk to catch a glimpse of the president in the motorcade. The police have placed barriers along the main boulevard and guard the intersection as the black limousine rolls past.

I wonder as we wait what it is like for Yeltsin to come back here, now that he is at the pinnacle of government. Born in an ancient hamlet called Butka, twenty kilometers northwest of the city, he grew up on the western side of the Urals, in Berezniki, in the Perm region, and came to Sverdlovsk to attend the Ural Polytechnic Institute, where he majored in construction. He also became active in the Communist Party. In 1976, he was elected first secretary of the Sverdlovsk Region Committee of the Communist Party of the Soviet Union, a plum position for rising to national politics. In 1977, he supervised the destruction of Ipatiev house where Czar Nicholas and his family were murdered.[1] The order had come from Moscow, where there was concern that the many pilgrimages by monarchists were making the house a shrine. Yeltsin's solution was to send bulldozers to Ascension Avenue in the dark of night. In the morning, the citizens of Sverdlovsk saw only an asphalted lot where Ipatiev house had been the day before. We drove by the site yesterday. Heaps of dead flowers were piled in the middle of what is still a vacant lot, now surrounded by government buildings. Yeltsin, since becoming president,

has ordered that the remains of the Romanovs be taken from Yekaterinburg and buried with ceremony in St. Petersburg. One can almost hear
him say, "It's enough!"

The Chkalovskiy streets are full of people on this late Monday afternoon. Men and women pass by us with shopping bags and briefcases.
Children are out of school; we pass several schoolhouses in the district,
which suggest the children would have been close to home in 1979.

As soon as we are out of the car, Yampolskaya and I locate the little
house where Aleksandra Chizhova once lived. She was fifty when she
died on April 12, 1979, at the peak of the epidemic, and her name was
one of the first five our mysterious source provided. Her younger sister,
Olga M., invites us in; sitting on her couch, questionnaire in hand, we
learn that Chizhova was a cashier at the ceramics factory cafeteria, perhaps, I think to myself, the same person the workman told about on Sunday—if so, then obviously her family has not moved away.

Olga M., now in her fifties, shows us the death certificate; "infectious
pneumonia" is given as the cause of death. The question again arises, as
with Anna Komina: is this attribution in good faith? If by April 12, bacteriological tests had confirmed the epidemic was from anthrax, as Dr.
Abramova attests, then why list this cause of death? If the source of the
infection was bad meat, why designate infection of the lungs? Or is this
a clinician's true understanding of how Alexandra Chizhova died, not
from anthrax but from pneumonia?

"My sister was a strong woman," Olga says. "She drove a tractor during the war, when she was just a girl."

Chizhova did not smoke or drink alcohol. She suffered from kidney
problems, though, and some years before her death, one of her kidneys
was removed. That her sister still considers her a "strong woman" may
be more a judgment about Chizhova's personal fortitude than her good
health. One afternoon, two days before Chizhova died, her sister recounts, she came home ill from work. Olga was working the night shift,
so she was home to care for her. Two or three times the next day, Chizhova
complained of feeling terribly sick. Finally, she was brought by ambulance to Hospital 24. The next evening, on her night off, Olga went to
visit her, even though it meant bringing along her own two sleepy young
sons. But the doctor in charge told her that Chizhova was no longer at
Hospital 24. Later she found out that her sister died that very night.

At this point, Olga begins to cry. Her grief is palpable, a grief that
comes from missed opportunity and loss, from the vision of a sister dying alone, frightened and in pain, cared for by strangers, and with oth-

ers, some her coworkers, dying around her. This is a horrible scenario of death, especially for families whose members are close. Both Yampolskaya and I again have tears in our eyes. But we are confronting something else here as well: households that accept the dying; families who cherish the bodies of the dead, who return each year to cemeteries on the anniversary of a death with food and vodka, gathering together relatives and friends, people whose memories refuse to let the deceased go; people whose lives are shot through with suffering and nostalgia.

Olga continues her story. The public health workers arrived and disinfected the house. They gave tetracycline pills to all the family. She herself did not attend her sister's burial at Vostochniy Cemetery, but Chizhova's daughter went and watched from a distance. Then, later, a campaign began to vaccinate everyone in the community against anthrax.

"On television," Olga M. adds, "they said that the relatives refused to pay for the burial. But it was the other way around. The government paid."

And what does she now think caused her sister's death?

"I heard it was an artificial germ from the military compound," she says. "The windows were open at the factory, and it got in." But she is not sure.

This interview is offset by a fruitless quest for other addresses. Sasha drives us back again to the worker's hostel on Military Street in search of someone who knew Nikolay Khudyakov. We have a new number for the unit where he lived. No one is at the concierge's desk. We go to the door marked 88 and knock. No answer. We knock on neighboring doors. Still no answer. We hear a radio playing behind one door, perhaps a ruse to keep thieves guessing, though the building is supposed to be for factory workers who probably haven't much to steal. In 1979, Khudyakov might have come from anywhere to work in Sverdlovsk. Maybe he left a wife and child behind in a village. Or, more likely, he was a bachelor, or perhaps divorced, which might account for the simplicity of his iron grave marker. And yet someone left the dried flowers I saw on his grave Saturday. How will we ever know who it was? Like the railroad men in Yaraslavl, Khudyakov seems one of those workers all too easy to lose.

As we walk the streets of Chkalovskiy this afternoon, we have no qualms about asking passersby for directions, and they have little hesitancy asking us what we are doing in the district. On Ulitsa Lyapustina, near Anna Komina's house, two neighbors of the widow of Timofiev T. direct us down the street to her home. Timofiev is not on our list of victims, but this street is too close to the ceramics factory to ignore the chance to talk to a resident. Thinking we may have made a discovery, we interview the widow in front of her house.

Her husband was a worker at the ceramics factory who died in December 1979, long after the epidemic, of what was diagnosed as pancreatic cancer. But, according to her, he fell ill in mid-April of that year, during the height of the outbreak, with chills and fever. She gestures across the street. "He got sick the same day as our neighbors, Komina and Vinogradov."

Dmitri Vinogradov was one of the first five names we received, and his house, for which we had searched in vain, we now find is a stone's throw from where we are standing.

Mrs. T. remembers her husband getting ill. The ambulance could find no place for him at the hospital and so brought him back home. This part of the scenario seems unusual. We hear once more the theme of how strong the deceased was, able to work three shifts, which is another way of underscoring the tragedy of death. With a weak or sickly person, one can expect the loss, but when a strong person is struck down, the shock seems greater.

Both Timofiev and his wife were vaccinated later in April. Their reactions to the vaccines were so bad, she tells us, that they couldn't lift the affected arms, and they didn't want people to see the disfiguring ulcers the vaccine produced. After he was vaccinated, her husband wanted to be admitted to the hospital, but again he was told there was no room.

I am beginning to think it unlikely that Timofiev died of anthrax. The seven-week duration of the epidemic is puzzling enough, but an eight-month wait before a victim is struck down stretches the imagination. But then, I ask myself, who knows? The infection or vaccination might have fatally weakened him in some way we do not yet understand.

His widow has more to say. She insists that a neighbor's small pig also died during the outbreak, that dogs in the neighborhood died from anthrax. She tells us that meat that was bought at the ceramics factory had to be returned and that it was burned there. So was meat sold at the factory? Yes, of course. She used to buy meat at Compound 19 as well, she adds, until the Chernobyl nuclear explosion in 1986. Because the radioactive fallout from that disaster blew in the opposite direction from Sverdlovsk, I wonder if she is referring to the several nuclear power station explosions in the Urals in the 1980s. But since news of these events was repressed by her government, how could she have known?

At this point, not simply in the interview but in our research as a whole, anything seems possible. Yes, contaminated meat was sold at the ceramics factory. In addition, it appears that the military also sold meat to the residents of the district. Who knows if it was inspected? And the kilns at the ceramics factory were used to burn contaminated meat, which might have disseminated lethal anthrax spores. But the widow can offer no first-hand account of having bought contaminated meat or of seeing the burning of such meat anywhere. She is only passing on rumors, which might be true.

We ask Mrs. T. about Dimitriy Vinogradov, her neighbor.

"He fell down in the street and died in the hospital," she says. "The body was returned home for the funeral. But at night the police came and took it away. He worked at the ceramics factory. He was a big, healthy man."

We leave her to knock on the door of the Vinogradov house, but no one is home. We will try again tomorrow.

That evening, Matthew briefs me on the team's meeting that day with Dr. Yakov Klipnitzer. It is the first testimony of a direct clinical nature from a local physician. Klipnitzer, a surgeon, is now retired, but in 1979 he was the head of Chkalovskiy's Hospital 20, which serves Chimash ("chemical machinery works"), the smaller, more southern of the two microrayons into which Chkalovskiy is divided; Hospital 24 serves the larger, northern one, called Vtorchmet (literally, "processed ferrous metals"), where in 1979 about three-quarters of the rayon's population of some two hundred thousand lived.

Dr. Klipnitzer was a patient at his own hospital when the 1979 outbreak began. It was, as he remembered, on the weekend of April 7 and 8. In bed with nephritis, he was warned by one of his physicians that first one and then another patient had arrived and died suddenly. The same was happening at Hospital 24 and at Hospital 1 in nearby Leninskiy rayon. The heads of all these hospitals contacted each other. The next morning at 6 A.M., another patient was admitted to Hospital 20 and died quickly. Dr. Klipnitzer then called the health departments at the city and oblast levels to tell them that an unusually hazardous infection, and not pneumonia, had broken out. The Extraordinary Commission for Emergencies at the rayon level was immediately convened. It consisted of the executive chief of the rayon, chiefs of the local hospitals, the rayon head veterinarian, and the chief of the rayon SES. This Extraordinary Commission met daily to review the situation and quickly decided to conduct a house-to-house survey in Chkalovskiy to ask after the health of the residents. Here is evidence that the public health authorities already realized the outbreak was localized.

In line with Dr. Babich's description, Dr. Klipnitzer recounted how in 1979 the provincial or oblast government, where Boris Yeltsin was in charge, and the city and local governments ceded their authority to Moscow. Once the Soviet Ministry of Health was contacted (around April 9), after Dr. Nikiforov arrived (on April 12), and then when Dr. Burgasov arrived (about April 13), decisions about handling the epidemic passed to the Extraordinary Commissions (which existed at each of the three levels of government). Nikiforov, for example, initiated the mid-April vaccination campaign: everyone in the district was to be vaccinated except for old people, children, and the sick. Moscow experts probably intervened as well in handling the epizootics in the outlying villages.

Just when the interview appeared to be over, Dr. Klipnitzer offered a surprising recollection. "One more thing," he said. "Something I did not mention in my earlier discussion with Dr. Shepetkin is that before the outbreak in Sverdlovsk there were cases of animal deaths near the town of Aramil, south of the city. This could be very important." He added that, at his recommendation, a barrier was established on the Chelyabinsk road, the major artery to the south, twelve kilometers outside the city, to check cars and trucks for meat. He could not be sure just when, but he knew it was before the first human cases. As he remembered, animal anthrax had been confirmed, and the SES did its duty in ordering the confiscation of suspect meat. Whether the meat confiscated was infected is unclear, but he felt the measure was warranted.

Shelokov and Hugh-Jones find Klipnitzer's account of the outbreak believable. As a result, the tainted-meat explanation reasserts itself in our group discussions, although nothing to substantiate it has come from the early interviews with families and neighbors of the victims, except Mrs. T.'s recollection that meat was bought and then returned to the ceramics factory. It is crucial, we all feel, to meet with veterinarians and sort out the dates and the extent of the epizootic.

That evening, Professor Borisov stops by our dormitory to review the coming schedule of appointments, which is now shifting. The chief veterinarian for the oblast called that afternoon to cancel his meeting with us the next morning. This is a disappointment. We had counted on getting our first professional assessment of the epizootic. No word has come back from the veterinary offices in the Sysertskiy district to the south, but the trip is still set for Wednesday. The head of Hospital 24, a Dr. Margarita Ilyenko, has spontaneously agreed to meet with us early Thursday morning. Later, the same morning, at 10:30 A.M., we will visit the office of a Dr. Bolshakov, now and in 1979 the head of the Chkalovskiy

SES. A veterinarian, he is the person most capable of verifying local events leading to and following the outbreak.

Borisov also tells us that officials at Compound 19 have received no orders from Moscow about our study plan, although the university conveyed our request to visit there three weeks ago. After Borisov leaves, Matthew stays up late composing a personal letter to General A. T. Kharechko, commander at Compound 19, which Professor Borisov has promised to deliver the next day.

The letter, dated June 9, reads:

Dear General Kharechko,

I write to you as the leader of a group of five scientists from the United States who are studying the medical, pathoanatomic, and epidemiologic and epizootic aspects of the outbreak of anthrax that happened in this region in 1979.

I have read in the November 20 issue of Komsomolskaya Pravda that scientists at your facility, like ourselves, also wish to understand what actually happened. Therefore, I wish to invite you or a member of your scientific staff to meet with us, to hear our findings at this state of our study and to exchange information and views regarding scientific aspects of this matter.

I realize that our hosts at the Ural State University have already made contact with your office on our behalf but nevertheless consider it good that I write to you personally.

In fact, our expectations of getting military information are low. This general has been quoted in a Moscow paper, denying any Compound 19 involvement in the 1979 outbreak: "The rumors . . . that an explosion took place on the territory of our institution and that anthrax pathogen was discharged into the external environment do not have any real basis, primarily because we have never had any explosion of that sort."[2] The anthrax vaccine work that was admittedly done at the laboratory was supposedly dismantled and shipped to Irkutsk by 1986, but that, too, is rumor. Nonetheless, we hope at least for a glimpse of the building that housed it and of any remnants of equipment from the past. With luck, someone might be able to describe to us the methods for testing vaccines used in 1979 and the safety procedures in effect.

Our presumption is that even with legitimate military development of anthrax vaccines (not weaponized anthrax), animal research would be conducted with virulent strains. The ordinary course would be to inoculate monkeys or other animals with the vaccine, put them in a closed chamber into which aerosolized anthrax is sprayed (referred to as a "challenge" test), and then keep them under observation. Afterward, the lethally contaminated air in the chamber would have to be expelled through a filtration system. But what was normal procedure in 1979? Were there Level-3 or Level-4 safety precautions like those enforced in U.S. laboratories? Did the larger enterprise resemble in any way how the United States conducted its postwar biological weapons program, which actually involved testing of agents in open-air environments, including the use of simulated agents at the Washington airport, in New York subways, and over the San Francisco Bay Area?[3] Did the Soviets have the same sense of drama as the Americans when they began their program? At Fort Detrick, the first offensive biological weapons laboratory was called "Black Maria" and, because of security risks, during the war years scientists kept a .45 caliber pistol in easy reach on the work bench. Was there a sense of risks to personnel? In the postwar years, four men working at Fort Detrick are reported to have died from exposure to pathogens, two from anthrax infection.[4] Even as the letter to General Kharechko (translated into Russian by Shelokov) is sent off the next day, we know almost nothing about Soviet involvement in anthrax research and absolutely nothing about what was going on at Compound 19 in 1979.

At this point, on Tuesday, June 9, the beginning of our sixth day in Yekaterinburg, it looks as though the Abramova-Grinberg autopsy data will be the only substantial yield of the trip. Given the difficulties we have had in locating people, my remaining list of unexplored family addresses is barely enough to merit the ride to Chkalovskiy. Although she now relays case names to us, Dr. Abramova has only two addresses to add to the ten we have received from the mysterious source, who we suspect may have other names. But when he visited last night, Professor Borisov also brought encouraging news about the televised report concerning a list of victims' names that we heard about on our first day, in Dr. Romanenko's office at SES. The broadcast featured Larissa Mishustina, a journalist who is a Peoples Deputy in the Supreme Soviet, discussing an official list of the 1979 anthrax outbreak victims and possible government compensation to their families. She is, unfortunately, visiting in the United States, with an official delegation to Washington. She is due to return soon, but how soon Borisov does not know—perhaps before we are scheduled to leave.

My solace is that the four interviews we have done (I discount the one with Mrs. T.) have produced some information on the onset of the disease. Among the four victims we have traced, Anna Komina is the earliest case, not by the date of her death, but by the date of the onset of her illness, April 4. If her son's account is accurate, her exposure to anthrax cannot be later than that date and is most likely sometime in the preceding week. The list of names we have compiled from the cemetery indicates others who died in that first wave, April 8–10: Vera Kozlova, Pavla Loginova, Fyodor Nikolaev, Boris Zheleznyak, and Dmitriy Vinogradov, the big, strapping neighbor of Mrs. T. who fell down in the street. Dr. Abramova's notes also offer clues about onset. The single common event to which the first group was exposed has to have been in the same time frame, the last days of March to April 4. Though it remains puzzling why the outbreak went on for more than six weeks, the approximately two days of acute illness before death that the four victims experienced fit the standard virulent pattern of anthrax reported in Western case reports and in the best clinical summary we have about Russian cases, K. K. Averyanov's article from 1940.[5]

What else have I learned? That the emergency ambulance service brought patients to Hospital 40, a central facility located north of Chkalovskiy, is substantiated by multiple accounts. In mid-April that service must have been in operation around the clock. People in the rayon have also attested to the community-wide vaccination program in 1979, but this indicates nothing about the source of the outbreak. Dr. Nikiforov, who ordered the vaccination, must have thought the population was vulnerable after the epidemic began. But what was the nature of its continued risk? Did Nikiforov and Burgasov know that Compound 19 was generating a hazard and might again emit lethal spores? Was it feared that contaminated meat would again infiltrate Chkalovskiy's market from the countryside? Or did some other state of mind—for instance, that an inquiry into the true risks for this population would not be allowed—determine a frenetic implementation of all sorts of public health measures? The efforts were undeniably diverse, from antibiotics to roadblocks. But curiously enough, they reveal little about the cause of the outbreak. Was there a conspiracy to obscure the source of the anthrax or just politically ordained ignorance? The question may be unanswerable. More important to me now is finding out about the dates when victims fell ill and about where each was in late March and early April. To do this, I will have to knock on a lot more doors.

Public Health
and Private Pain

The Sea Dyaks tribe of Borneo had a ritual called *tugong bula*, "the liar's mound." Each member of the community would contribute to a heap of twigs, leaves, and tree branches outside the house of a wrongdoer, gradually creating a conspicuous monument to the deceiver. The more massive the pile, the greater the sum of public judgment and the harder it was to ignore or destroy. The pile was sustained for years, as long as the misdeed was in public memory.[1] When the 1979 anthrax outbreak hit, the stoic population of Chkalovskiy made no public accusations. Its officials and health care workers and its local residents seem to have weathered the storm and then retreated to routine. No activists protested. No physicians or epidemiologists used their expertise to raise public concern about risk probabilities. In a free society, the clamor about the anthrax deaths would have been deafening, and the accusers would have invoked the force of law against those who caused the deaths.[2] Contenders on either side would have become aware that new rules were needed, that the officials who were responsible (whether city officials, the SES, or the military) and the local residents had a relationship, that they lived in the same moral universe.[3] Nothing remotely like that happened after the 1979 Sverdlovsk outbreak.

From our days divided between garnering official accounts in the north of the city and excursions to Chkalovskiy in the south, our data have started to accumulate like piles of twigs. But where, at whose doorstep, do we place them? Veterinarians, public health officials, the meat industry, the military? We have asked officials to consider the possibility of different burning sites (the ceramics factory, dumps along the southern highway, the meat-packing plant) causing an anthrax aerosol, but no one so far has firsthand information. It might have been that the military compound was the source of the epidemic, but through the sale of infected meat. Suppose, we conjecture in our team discussions, the scientists there had been conducting anthrax experiments on livestock, and some entrepreneur decided to make a little money selling the tainted carcasses. We have acquired random accounts of meat being sold at Compound 19, yet for the explanation to be plausible, many victims should have eaten from that supply. But to date, some families deny they ate anything but inspected meat and home-grown, healthy pork, and others tell us they had no meat at all that spring. But, again, we have to balance these statements against other reports that some meat from homes tested positive for anthrax.

If an emission from the Compound 19 laboratory is directly to blame for the anthrax outbreak, we are still left with the question of whether it was an escape from a massive level of anthrax production, enough for weapons, or of a minute but virulent quantity that might plausibly be emitted if vaccine testing had been in process. I wonder why the Soviet government, with eleven time zones at its disposal, would jeopardize a major city of 1.2 million people by large-scale production in a biological weapons facility (for anthrax or anything infectious). Engaged at some level in biological weapons activities, the military at Compound 19 obviously counted on the stoicism, if not the complacency, of the local population. Yet whatever the risks that emanated from its laboratory, not all Sverdlovsk citizens shared them equally. Those in the adjacent working class district and soldiers and their families at the compounds were in more jeopardy than, for instance, the city's brain trust and more privileged people who lived in the center city. This same burden of risk was carried by the little communities near U.S. and British BW facilities during World War II and after, in places like Vigo, Indiana; Pine Bluff, Arkansas; Frederick, Maryland; and the Scottish village across from Gruinard Island.[4]

Our team talks about both biological weapons production, entailing huge fermenter vats and drying devices, and about typical vaccine experiments. Tests "challenging" monkeys with deadly aerosols might have been going on at Compound 19 in 1979, just as they continue to go on wherever anthrax vaccines are being developed. During the post-experiment phase, when the contaminated air must be filtered or sterilized, is when an accidental aerosol emission would have been most likely.

As the history of technological disasters warns us, no guarantees exist that even simple procedures will always be carried out correctly, even in contexts where the risks are at the level of life and death. Fatigue, carelessness, distraction, inattention, hastiness, poor communication between work shifts—all are commonly associated with accidents in the most advanced industrial and high-technology settings. In complex work settings, as illustrated in the events preceding the ill-fated 1987 Challenger launch, people deny hazards even when they are clearly warned, and warnings themselves are often not clear enough to mitigate risk.[5] Add to these obstacles the common psychological problems that affect decision making at work, such as feelings of depression, reactions to family crises, and substance abuse. (Alcoholism was a major workplace problem in the Soviet Union.) Compound these again with dubious Soviet production standards. The result is Chernobyl and other industrial disasters.

So, too, it is possible to imagine the Sverdlovsk outbreak as the result of a work-place accident. Suppose there was an aerosol test chamber at Compound 19, and suppose in late March or early April 1979 a worker fails to notice a malfunction of its ventilation system. A lever is pulled and the chamber's lethal content is spewed over the city. Or spores of a virulent strain of anthrax are in drying or milling equipment in a room with similarly defective ventilation. Either is a possible scenario, but if the military does not offer substantiation, it all remains conjecture. If such an event was falsely denied in 1979 or inadequately investigated, what incentives are there for officials to take responsibility now?

Very few, it seems. In the new Russia, the military is undergoing tremendous reorganization and quickly casting off the past. In the aftermath of the 1991 White House coup, nearly four hundred generals who supported the Soviet leaders and opposed Yeltsin's Russian democracy were "retired." From Gorbachev through to Yeltsin, from the Supreme Soviet down to the ordinary citizen, it has been agreed that overspending on the military brought the Soviet economy to its knees and that the military ranks cannot now be spared attrition. As our group conducts its research, planned cutbacks in personnel have a third of its officers and half of its troops scheduled for dismissal. A family that lost a member to the 1979 anthrax epidemic might hold tight to memories. Top military officials on the other side of the compound wall and in Moscow might well want to forget.

On Tuesday morning, June 9, a mid-level public health official, Dr. Viktor Arenskiy, offers us a detailed account of the first days of the outbreak. His version takes us not only through the bureaucratic responses of the public health service, but out into the countryside to animal deaths, with a special Moscow visitor, Dr. Bezdenezhnikh. Now head of epidemiology at the Sverdlovsk Medical Institute, in 1979 Dr. Arenskiy was an SES physician concerned with tuberculosis. He greets us with the familiar apology that he has no written records, and I mentally brace myself for grand theoretical elaborations. But Arenskiy has a sense of irony about himself and others involved in the epidemic. His logbook of the epidemic was confiscated after the "Moscow guests" (he means Burgasov, Nikiforov, and Bezdenezhnikh) arrived in mid-April. At that time, the authority of the Extraordinary Commission at the Sverdlovsk city level was taken over by the oblast-level commission, under the direction of Dr. Burgasov. After that, the SES records about the outbreak were appropriated by this higher commission, and they subsequently disappeared. This story corroborates what the young, shaggy-haired Dr. Romanenko at SES recounted the first day we were in Yekaterinburg and what Dr. Klipnitzer and others have told us since.

In the first days of the epidemic, around April 7 or 8, Dr. Arenskiy was attending a national conference on gastrointestinal diseases being held in Sverdlovsk. He points out the irony of that coincidence, as if he were being cued to the infected-meat explanation of the outbreak. He was in a postgraduate workshop when he and two colleagues were summoned by their superior to a high-level SES meeting about the epidemic. As soon as they were outside the classroom, she exclaimed with distress, "Still another fatal case! And no diagnosis!"

The earliest cases, as he remembers, came from Hospital 20 in the southeast section of Chkalovskiy. The autopsy of the third case, which revealed massive internal hemorrhaging, sounded the alarm.

At the emergency meeting, Dr. Babich (the heavy-smoking former head of SES) was the group's chairman. He called for suggestions for identifying the disease. One person suggested plague. Another thought it could be smallpox. Everyone rejected cholera as the answer; the symptoms and fast progress of the mystery disease were markedly different. Arenskiy remembers pointing out recent cattle cases he'd heard of and putting his bet on anthrax.

The group recognized that, whatever the disease was, it could be highly contagious as well as fatal. So it instituted what Arenskiy called "a military approach," for which Babich outlined three goals. The first was to get sick patients to a quarantined hospital ward. They agreed that all adults and older children taken ill should go to Hospital 40, to the infectious disease division. Young children and infants would go to Hospital 4, to its pediatric infectious diseases unit. The morgue conditions and the burials had to be sanitary and segregated. Second, the medical personnel, especially the nurses and primary physicians, had to be warned to take appropriate precautions when treating infected patients. Third, the neighborhoods most affected by the disease had to be canvassed and warned of the danger of contamination. Then the group gave the unknown disease a code number (Arenskiy doesn't remember which) and arranged for notices to be sent to medical stations to transport patients to the two designated hospitals. He and the other SES epidemiologists agreed to check closely with the local polyclinics, where several more patients had just been hospitalized, and then meet again.

Also attending the meeting were the oblast chief pathologist, the medical school's chief of infectious diseases, city and oblast officials, and several veterinarians. At the mention of veterinarians, Hugh-Jones interrupts to ask why they were included at this early stage. Arenskiy replies casually that everyone knew about the animal outbreaks in the Sysertskiy villages and wanted to include anthrax as a possible explanation. Why Dr. Babich bothered to deny these epizootics remains puzzling. Are we just hearing another rumor? We press Arenskiy for information about whether the veterinarians and doctors at the oblast level investigated these cases and if Arenskiy knows the dates of the animal outbreak.

Dr. Arenskiy isn't sure about who investigated, and he hesitates on the dates. "A week or five days before the human cases were noticed. Certainly not longer than a week, not a month, for example." This estimate places the epizootics around April 1 to 3. With Anna Komina's onset date of April 4 as the earliest we have, contaminated meat cannot be abandoned as a hypothesis.

Arenskiy adds that the veterinarians could not explain the appearance of anthrax in apparently well-fed cattle outside the city. "Compared to Chelyabinsk, the Sverdlovsk oblast is not overrun with anthrax. To begin, this region has far less livestock." Before the Moscow physicians arrived, the Sverdlovsk commission considered the problem might be within the city, at the meat-processing plant or with hides imported from Kazakhstan (which is only a few hours by car to the south) or in stores of contaminated feed, but on further inquiry it discarded each of these ideas.

In contrast, when he arrived in mid-April, Dr. Bezdenezhnikh was most eager to pursue the tainted-meat explanation. At Bezdenezhnikh's request, Arenskiy (who knew him professionally) drove him to the southern village of Rudniy. There they talked with an old woman who had killed and butchered two sick sheep.

"She asked a Sverdlovsk relative to help with the skinning," Arenskiy tells us. "Some meat she kept, some she sold. And since, according to custom, the head and feet of sick animals aren't eaten, the old woman gave them to two local drunks. These two and the Sverdlovsk relative came down with cutaneous anthrax." In the same village, Arenskiy continues, another, more careful family disposed of the remains of their sick calf in a deep pit.

Both these cases are familiar—they are described in the documents Burgasov has given us.

When Matthew asks what was done to control the epizootic, Arenskiy replies that he thinks napalm was used to burn the carcasses and also that there was a waste dump near the slaughterhouse, at the periphery of the meat-processing plant in Chkalovskiy. The veterinarians also checked any dead animals within the area and disposed of them. The rayon's local veterinarian at the time is on our list of appointments for Thursday and, with happy nods all around, we are sure he will fill out the details of these events for us.

As for any military involvement in the outbreak, Arenskiy remarks somberly, "The military sat silently within their compounds." When the Moscow contingent arrived, headed by Burgasov, its members also sat silently at commission meetings; their instruction to the local officials was "no further questions." But Arenskiy believes that even in 1979 suspicions about Compound 19 as the source of the outbreak were discussed "on the back porches" around the city.

An important fact we have learned from Dr. Arenskiy is that a local public health response to the 1979 outbreak was already in place when the Moscow visitors arrived and that it, rather than the central government, predetermined crucial strategies, such as the transport of suspected patients, segregated burial, and house-to-house checking in Chkalovskiy. Some of his account (like his early bet on anthrax) might be recollections corrected by hindsight, but most of it matches what we have heard from Dr. Klipnitzer and other officials. Another fact is that Dr. Bezdenezhnikh had a firsthand view of the epizootic. It obviously impressed him.

We follow this interview with an unexpectedly mad dash around Yekaterinburg to three different levels of the local bureaucracy (ZAGS) where births, marriages, and deaths are registered. Shelokov and I have an appointment at the first level, the Chkalovskiy rayon ZAGS. Our hope is that the KGB cleanup bypassed its records, but luck is not with us. No records for 1979 exist here, not for anyone. From the first office, we are directed to the second office, at the city level, which is in another part of town, and off we go. No records for 1979 exist there either. From the second office, we are directed to the third, at the oblast level, which is again some distance away.

In the second two offices, we arrive without prior appointments, as people off the street investigating the outbreak. We never get any higher in the administration than blandly courteous secretaries. Despite our disappointment, I find myself admiring the orderly way women run these offices and their deftness in deflecting requests. No one smiles at Shelokov's genteel yet urgent description of our need for information. We are explicit that we would be content with anything concerning the deaths of victims in the anthrax outbreak thirteen years ago. No one seems to have thought much about it. At the oblast ZAGS, an administrator ventures forth from her office and, waylaid by one of the secretaries, tells her to tell us that we should go to the Institute of Military Medicine in St. Petersburg. Possibly a file of original records concerning the 1979 outbreak was recently sent there, perhaps a month or six weeks ago. No one seems quite sure what happened. I think we should make a stand here and ask for precision. To whom was it sent? Why? Are there no copies? I want to persist with questions, but Shelokov maintains that this is our third brush-off and we should retreat.

Hugh-Jones and Matthew are waiting outside in a park for us. I feel I have just emerged from three levels of a *matryoshka*, the Russian nested doll. Nearby, two lovers on a bench are kissing, a sign of new freedoms or of the universal urges of spring or perhaps of limited privacy at home. I think how much I would enjoy having lunch alone with Matthew, or even by myself, but teamwork prevails, and we go back to the university to mull over our limited accomplishments.

That afternoon, Yampolskaya is late getting back from the Pulmonary Unit, where Walker is making good progress reviewing the tissue samples. It is 6:30 before she and I are again in Chkalovskiy and encountering the usual obstacles. The long summer days make a twelve-hour work day seem feasible. But our two hours yield only one interview, with the parents and sister of Yuriy Sysikov, who lived on Predelnaya (Limit) Street. The family's cottage has the same somber aura as the Komins' home. Sysikov died at age twenty-seven. He worked with his father, we learn, at a construction company right next to the ceramics factory. His mother, a large, imposing woman, sits with us at their kitchen table and takes charge of answering our questions, while her husband and daughter hover behind her. Her son died May 12, 1979, so late in the anthrax epidemic that his case poses a difficult question about when he was ex-

posed to the deadly spores. At the time, the date of his death also confused his family. It had nothing to do with eating meat. But first his mother
tells us about what happened after Yuriy became sick.

"Our house was disinfected," she tells us. "The bed linens were taken
away." She is a substantial woman, a woman with confidence, yet her
face contorts and her eyes fill with tears. What is it about these mundane
details that provokes so much feeling, not only in her but in the two figures
behind her, and in us? A boy lies dying in a hospital, strangers invade
and begin scrubbing the walls of his room. They strip the bed where he
lay down in his last illness, maybe the bed he slept in all his life, the bed
that would remain empty in an empty room while his family got up every
day and had their tea and went to work and came home, all the while
grieving. Yet they hold on. They are still here, in the same cottage. On
the way through the living room to the kitchen, I saw a sparsely furnished
bedroom like those James Agee described in his paean to the dignity of
Alabama sharecroppers, with "so great and final a whole of bareness and
complete simplicity."[6] Was that their son's room?

Sysikova wipes her eyes and continues. "He worked with his father.
Friday he came home and I asked him, as usual, 'Do you want to go
for a sauna?' But he said no. He was feeling sick. Saturday, at half-past
eleven at night, his father had to call for an ambulance. He had lost
consciousness."

She makes a palms-down, pushing-away gesture of finality, and once
again her eyes well up with tears. Behind her, the faces of her husband
and daughter are watchful and full of sadness. At this point, Yampolskaya and I, also moved, stop the interview. Children aren't supposed to
die before their parents; it defies the natural sequence, the regenerative
cycle of our lives. It cuts off the promise of youth. Yet of course young
adults perish every day, in accidents, from disease, in war. Since arriving
here, I have learned that Sverdlovsk was a way-station in the 1980s for
planes bringing back the bodies of young men killed in the Afghan war.
The planes were called "Black Tulips," because of their cargo. The
Sysikovs might have lost their son in that wasted effort, but he died before it began, in an even less explicable way.

On her own, Sysikova continues her family's story. After the ambulance transported her son directly to Hospital 40, they never saw him
again. She has no memory of anthrax as the cause of his death, because
the outbreak was more than a month earlier. And the death certificate
reads "sepsis" as cause of death, which they didn't quite understand.

"Only later did we realize what happened," she says.

Yampolskaya and I both know that her son's body was autopsied by Abramova and Grinberg on May 14 and soon after assessed as yet another case of "classic anthrax." There was no reason the family should not have known. But in the "military approach" that the public health officials took, consideration of relatives was not a priority, and this family was already leery of hospital care. In *The House of the Dead*, Fyodor Dostoevsky describes Russian peasants' traditional distrust of modern hospitals, even as these institutions were in the last century: "But what they fear most is the German routine of the hospital, the presence of strangers about them all the time they are ill, the strict rules with regard to diet, the tales of the rigorous severity of the attendants and doctors, and of the cutting open and dissection of the dead and so on."[7]

Maybe at the time of the 1979 outbreak, other Sverdlovsk workers were more inured to hospitals. Maybe at the local hospitals and at Hospital 40, victims and their families recognized other locals similarly afflicted or maybe they knew some of the hospital staff. Still, in the fearful context of this fatal epidemic, which caused panic among professionals and must have terrified the patients segregated for intensive treatment, these would be small consolations.

Was Sysikov vaccinated? His father, speaking for the first time, replies that he himself got shots, but not Yuriy. We are not about to answer the question in his eyes: would vaccination have made a difference for his son? We don't know. Had the family been given antibiotics? No. It may have been so late in the epidemic that public health measures faltered. About when and how Sysikov caught the disease, we have nothing yet to offer this family, but I am certain that they, like the other families, deserve better than the miasma of misinformation they have so far received.

We knock again at the Vinogradov house, but still there is no answer. His neighbor, Mrs. T., mentioned yesterday that his daughter was a doctor somewhere in the northern area of the city, and we make a note to find her. Meanwhile, Matthew and Hugh-Jones appear around a corner. No concerned citizen has bothered Hugh-Jones about his unwieldy detector or questioned Matthew's taking photographs. I can imagine neighborhoods all over America—whether gated communities, suburban tracts, ethnic enclaves, or ghettos—where any number of people would have protested this kind of intrusion. Because Chkalovskiy residents have not, I ponder what kind of community exists here. In some ways it seems no different than the "urban village" of Boston's old West End, where every neighbor was not necessarily a friend and even the threat of demolition did not mobilize residents to defend their neighborhoods.[8] More than that, there's a quiet here, like the vanished church bells that no longer ring.

The four of us return to the dormitory at 9 P.M. and, having skipped dinner, resort again to peanut butter on crackers. Far from tiring me, the rushing about to the ZAGS offices, tromping around Chkalovskiy, and climbing our seven flights of stairs gives me a sense of well-being that even missing dinner cannot diminish. I have finally put all jet lag behind me and feel at home. Like Yampolskaya, I am satisfied with my nightly cup of hot tea and resting my feet on an ottoman.

At that evening's discussion, Walker has strong words to say to Matthew about the bad-meat hypothesis, which he feels should be totally and immediately abandoned. "It's absurd and it's wasting time." From his perspective, which centers on analyzing tissue slides with Abramova and Grinberg, our tearing around the city from one interview to another probably does seem ridiculous. But it appears that animals did die just outside the city, and we must understand exactly when that happened, if we are ever to untangle the confusion of factual information that surrounds the outbreak. And just how conclusive the autopsy data is, we cannot yet be sure.

"Have we been wasting *your* time?" Matthew asks quietly.

Instead of answering, Walker, his cold still bothering him, goes to bed.

Tomorrow, Wednesday, looks promising. We will travel at last outside the city, to Sysertskiy rayon, and meet with veterinarians there. If possible, we will also stop at villages off the highway and interview the owners of livestock that were infected with anthrax in 1979. We have no doubts now that such an outbreak occurred. We need only, we think, clarify the dates.

At 7:45 the next morning, pandemonium breaks out in our dormitory suite. The concierge bangs on the door and gets Yampolskaya out of the shower to take an emergency telephone call from Professor Borisov. The trip south to Sysertskiy rayon and its veterinarians is canceled. Rather than discuss the matter over the telephone, Borisov says he will come to our dormitory. When he arrives, he explains that the southern region still remains closed to outsiders and that further negotiations are required to allow us to travel outside the city limits. The rector's letter asking for this permission was sent, he says, to the local Office of Security for the Russian Federation. The decision that came back was negative. Obviously the travel to local villages that Donald Ellis was allowed in 1979 will not be permitted to our team, which has more than tourism as a goal.

Shelokov embellishes on this bad news by warning that if we dare defy this refusal, our passports will be confiscated. No one suggests that we be anything but compliant. I don't want to be arrested or detained, and I see no hope of making for a friendly border; the nearest is Finland's, more than a thousand miles away.

As Walker and Yampolskaya leave for another day at the Pulmonary Unit, the rest of us have an ominous sense of doors closing.

12

The Unnatural
Steals the Natural

Unable to travel outside the city, we have before us an open and potentially wasted day. No appointments are scheduled; reception to us has reportedly cooled because we are not official visitors, just a band of foreigners. Dr. Ponomaryev will not be giving us part two of his presentation. Shelokov, his voice hoarse, cannot help me with interviews in Chkalovskiy. Even if he were able, I doubt the families would receive him with the trust they show Yampolskaya. Still, two promising meetings are scheduled for tomorrow. One is with the head of Hospital 24, Dr. Margarita Ilyenko who, like Dr. Klipnitzer, was at the center of the start of the 1979 outbreak. The other is with the chief of SES for Chkalovskiy, Dr. Dmitriy Bolshakov, who assumed his post a mere three days before the outbreak began and has remained in it since. But that is tomorrow.

We revert to tourist mode. Professor Borisov gives us a lift to the oldest part of Yekaterinburg, literally to the high ground, to the Church of the Ascension, the city's only remaining example of early classic nineteenth-century architecture. Now a museum, it is crumbling. On one peeling wall inside is a haunting painting of an angel with outspread wings. Outside, a T-34 tank, the model that saved the Soviet Union and the world from Nazi Germany, sits in the middle of the plaza. Its unusually rough surface is hand-finished by a million hammer blows, like something made in a garage. A drunken man approaches and gives it a new pounding with his fists. He rants about the wretched economy, about how too many tanks were manufactured. "They let this beautiful church fall apart!" he bellows before staggering away. Several schoolboys with backpacks climb the tank and contemplate us with amused curiosity, as if we were zoo animals. To make contact, we give them ballpoint pens, a gesture which for some reason they find even more amusing.

We cross the boulevard to the site of Ipatiev House and have a closer look at the heaps of flowers piled against the foot of the wooden ortho-dox cross. The anniversary of the Romanovs' assassination is July 12, more than a month away, yet the layers of flowers, dried below and fresh on top, indicate a steady stream of pilgrims. New discoveries in Moscow archives have recently revealed the brutal details of the Romanov mur-ders. For example, the assassins marveled when their bullets bounced off the young duchesses' torsos, as if a miracle had happened. Then, with bayonets they pierced the layers of precious stones, diamonds and emer-alds, sewn for safe-keeping into the young women's corsets. The royal remains, buried near a mine northwest of the city, were discovered in 1979, but their existence was not revealed then. It was no time for rev-elations. In that same year, also the year of the anthrax outbreak, more than a thousand bodies of Stalinist purge victims from the 1930s, buried at the town of Kolpashevo in Western Siberia, in the banks of the Ob River, were uncovered by a flood. Many of the bodies were mummified and still recognizable to their relatives. The Soviet government's reac-tion was the same rapid Moscow-KGB mobilization applied to the very different context of the Sverdlovsk epidemic:

> When the bodies appeared in the riverbank, alarmed, high-ranking Commu-nist party officials flew into town. The KGB cordoned off the site. Special crews of soldiers and laborers worked in relays for some two weeks to destroy all traces of the grave—no easy task when the thousand-odd skeletons were lodged in the banks of a large, fast-flowing river in flood. The authorities at first vaguely claimed that these might be cattle bones. Finally, fooling nobody, they announced that these were the bones of World War II deserters.[1]

Those faithful to the Romanov dynasty want to build a memorial Orthodox church here on Ascension Avenue, across from colonnaded nineteenth-century government buildings. They cannot bring back Ipatiev House, but, if successful, they can show that the monarchists have the right to congregate where they cannot be ignored by officials. The view over the city, to the river and beyond, is magnificent.

In the afternoon, Sasha Tiutiunnik is free to drive Matthew, Hugh-Jones, Shelokov, and me to Chkalovskiy. Here we are again like tourists, only at the scene of another debacle, where the victims were more hum-ble and their families less famous than the czars, where the only Romanov was Boris, who did indeed, by his cardinal's cap and tissue samples, confirm that the 1979 outbreak was anthrax. We begin our excursion by driving to the low bluff where Compound 19 sits. Passing its concrete walls, we turn left past the open parade ground and guardhouse in front of the adjacent Compound 32. Through the gate, one sees the signs of routine life, women with shopping bags, small children alongside them, a man on a bench reading a newspaper.

Back near Ulitsa Lyapustina, at Shelokov's suggestion, we jump from the car for a chat with a stout, gray-haired woman herding goats, the same woman Yampolskaya and I saw on our first day in the ward. Picking our way over the vacant, weed-filled lot, we take Dr. Romanenko's word that no soil has tested positive for anthrax in Yekaterinburg. Up close, the goats look healthy; they have been vaccinated against anthrax. One of them immediately smells the cookie from lunch I have in my jacket pocket and insistently nudges me until she gets it. The goat's owner, whose ruddy face is sad, has never met people from the United States before. She just knows about us from television.

"We are so poor," she comments. "America should just take us over."

Another woman, neatly dressed and carrying a canvas shopping bag, stops to talk and commands the conversation while her husband lingers in the background. Shelokov explains our interest in the 1979 outbreak. She replies that she and her husband worked at the ceramics factory at that time. "It was a terrible episode!" she exclaims. At least three people who worked in the pipe shop died. She and her husband sent their children away to relatives in Tashkent. She stayed behind only because their older son, blinded in an army accident, needed care. She herself was vaccinated at the factory and had a terrible reaction. When asked about the washing of buildings and asphalting of roads, she seems distracted, as if she doesn't want to talk about the epidemic. She points instead to a nearby factory, a new-meat processing plant, and complains that a pine woods was cut down to make room for it.

"It's true," the woman herding goats, suddenly angry, agrees. "What right had they to do that?"

"To rob us of that beautiful piece of nature!" the other woman adds, and her husband emphatically agrees. Those in power, this trio seems to say, destroy nature, robbing ordinary folk like themselves of a pleasure that is theirs by rights, that they have a claim to life and beauty.

They tell us where the old meat plant is located, in this same neighborhood of Vtorchmet. Almost as an aside, the woman with the shopping bags mentions that she used to buy mutton at Compound 19, but at some point, she doesn't know when, those sales stopped. Is she describing the nightmare scenario of public sales of experimental animals killed by anthrax? Not likely. The meat was just some surplus, she says, that the army occasionally sold off. Is this another clue?

Matthew, Hugh-Jones, and Shelokov decide we should drive to the old meat factory and ask about burning of infected carcasses in the spring of 1979. I disagree. I have only one minor connection to the meat factory, Mikhail Markov's wife. If we are going to barge in anywhere, I feel it should be the ceramics factory, where we have much more to learn, both about the workers who died and about any bad meat that might have been sold or burnt there. But Matthew would rather work through official channels to get us inside. When we reach the meat plant, I stay in the car with Sasha. A virtual vegetarian, I haven't the will to witness sides of beef reduced to vats of hash and rendered fat. Furthermore, I doubt that humane methods for butchering animals, like the kind developed by Temple Grandin, are in effect inside this large pre-war processing plant.[2] And even if they were, I would hesitate to enter. In any event, three experts constitute enough manpower to handle this invasion.

As we wait, Sasha and I (creatively employing his nascent English and my limited Russian) discuss the film *Moscow on the Hudson*. This leads us to considering New York's Brighton Beach, a community he knows all about, and he marvels that such a reproduction of Russian life is possible in America. How does one explain the American urban landscape, its Chinatowns, Little Japans, its Armenian, Greek, Irish, and Italian neighborhoods or, for that matter, a ghetto community like New York's Harlem, Boston's Roxbury, Los Angeles's Watts, or Chicago's South Side to someone whose city appears culturally and ethnically homogenous, monolithically so? One doesn't.

I ask if he knows the movie by Georgian director Tengiz Abuladze, *Repentance*, in which the body of a Stalin-like dictator's victim keeps emerging from its grave. The film, with its powerful metaphor of the unquiet past, is certainly on my mind. But young Sasha has been wrapped up in his science. I almost ask him if he knows the *Star Wars* movies, but then I remember that in America a few years back the term "Evil Empire" was used quite seriously by our president to describe Sasha's country. We discuss the movies that have recently shown on television here: Arnold Schwarzenegger in *The Terminator* and then in his later film, *Kindergarten Cop*. If one Hollywood actor was the emblem of Cold War villainy for Americans, it was the hulking Austrian, whose harsh accent symbolized Iron Curtain barbarity. The Terminator's submersion of his humanity in technologic body parts gave him the power to annihilate. This ceding of the natural to the unnatural was exactly what we feared from the Soviet Union. It is the same monster formula that applies to *Star Wars'* Darth Vader, the good knight who turns into the ultimate killing machine. Was it also what the Soviets feared from us?

In her book on innovations in military organization, Kimberly Zisk argues that the Soviet general staff maintained a consistent Cold War pattern of reacting to U.S. advances in military technology with upgrades of its own weapons.[3] Here in Sverdlovsk, as in any American city then relying on defense contracts, industry must have kept on producing weapons—missiles, guns, plane parts, trucks, whatever the government ordered to counter the American threat. In the Cold War arms race, the ultimate destructive capacity of nuclear weapons became normalized, as if their power were containable. In 1979, Soviet Chief of the General Staff Nikolay Ogarkov argued that a strategic nuclear war was "winnable," a highly irrational proposition. By 1981, though, Soviet President Leonid Brezhnev began issuing statements about the "madness" of nuclear war, paving the way for the end of weapons competition with the United States. That in the late-1980s Schwarzenegger softened his image to the kindergarten cop, overwhelmed by frisky tots, suits the new era, which began with Gorbachev in 1986 advocating a complete end to the superpowers' nuclear arms race and President Reagan eventually agreeing.

To a student like Sasha, with his future in physical chemistry ahead of him, Cold War scenarios must seem like old film scripts. It is unlikely he will have a career developing weapons systems. Instead, he and his generation will have to adapt to the free market economy. But what about the biological sciences, in the Soviet past and the Russian future? If the Soviets aggressively emulated the American nuclear weapons program, they may also have emulated our old biological weapons program with the same drive. If so, hundreds of their biologists, like our own after President Nixon's 1969 renunciation of biological weapons, must now be part of demilitarization, a difficult and demoralizing process. And their "ghost" plants, like Fort Detrick's Building 470, the forty-four thousand square feet of space where anthrax was the primary product, must be sitting vacant and unused.[4] Or so we hope.

After an hour, my colleagues come out of the meat-processing factory in high spirits, a slight odor of processed meat on their clothes. Hugh-Jones is glad to have had a chance to focus on animals, and the plant director obliged with details. For example, this plant slaughters twelve hundred swine and six hundred cattle a shift (shifts are eight hours, with two days off per week), but not sheep. About half the meat products it distributes come from other regions, which raises the issue of inspection. The plant used to employ 130 veterinarians; now they employ 70; with the new "modernization" even that number will drop. The plant has what the director called a "strong" chemical and bacteriological laboratory and a sanitary slaughterhouse for sick animals, where meat is either classified as fit for human consumption or autoclaved at 120–40 degrees centigrade in a "pressure kettle."

The director took advantage of the interview to vent his ire at SES officials who, during the 1979 outbreak, kept trying to pin the blame on his factory and, more specifically, on a dump it maintained just beyond Uralmach, the site of the enormous machine conglomerate, ten kilometers north. That dump was closed down and never reopened. SES officials searched accounts, records, and the dump site. But no evidence of anthrax was ever found, the director maintains. Nothing like massive carcass burning was going on in 1979. I am ready to strike that explanation (never a heavy contender) from our list of possible anthrax aerosol sources. The director also mentioned that a man who had been laid off from the meat factory died in the epidemic, but he insisted there was no association between his plant and the man's death, that no infection had taken place among workers at his plant.

In the late afternoon, Yampolskaya and I are back in Chkalovskiy. We find the widow of Fagim Dayanov in her second-floor apartment on Escadronaya. Her husband, a worker at a nearby building materials factory, died at age forty-three. Like young Yuriy Sysikov, Dayanov died late in the epidemic, on May 10, 1979. Rema Dayanova, a short, intense woman in her forties, has been quoted briefly in a 1991 article on the outbreak in *Literaturnaya Gazieta*.[5]

Her story of the epidemic begins on May 3, 1979, when her husband was sent to clean off the factory roof. The next day he had a high temperature but went to work anyway. Later in the day, he asked to leave work because he felt sick. He stayed at home the next day, but on the morning of May 6 he was taken by ambulance to Hospital 40, where he was diagnosed with bilateral pneumonia. His wife and their young son were not allowed to visit him until May 9 and only then from behind glass. He was getting an enormous quantity of water intravenously and called for even more to drink. His thoracic cavity was being drained continuously, his widow tells us, and he was receiving frequent injections of antibiotics. This description matches with the treatment of patients that Dr. Nikiforov described in 1986 and with what Yampolskaya remembers.

Although they could not touch, the couple wrote messages back and forth to each other. On May 10, after she had been at the hospital a long time and was getting ready to leave, her husband sent her a note, which she now takes from a drawer to show us. "Rema—don't go home," he scrawled. "We may never look into each other's eyes again."

Dayanova has been on the verge of tears since she began talking. Holding this note on her outstretched hand, repeating her husband's dying words, she weeps—and so do we. Once again we see the tragedy of this epidemic, which cannot be reckoned simply by the numbers who died or the suffering of the dying, but must account for the feeling of unnecessary, unexplained loss that afflicts the surviving families. Dayanov and his wife and son were robbed of years together. This apartment, like the other homes we have visited, is suffused with mourning.

When Rema Dayanova asked the physician in charge if her husband would live, his reply was "We have done everything we can but—"

That evening, after she returned home, Dayanova called the hospital to ask after her husband. The nurse told her to come quickly. But when she arrived at Hospital 40, her husband's bed was empty and a sign was posted to burn the clothes and linens. She asked a doctor in the hallway, "Where is Dayanov?" This doctor rudely passed her by. Another doctor, a surgeon, told her to go to the morgue. She found her way there and saw, to her horror, her husband naked on a metal gurney, already "opened up." Indeed, according to Abramova's notes, she and Grinberg did the Dayanov autopsy the day he died.

His body was kept at the morgue and never returned home. Dayanov was buried in Section 13 of Vostochniy Cemetery, in lime, with a police guard attending. His mother was especially distraught. Never having seen her son's body, she had difficulty believing he was really dead and not taken away somewhere by the government. The supposition is reasonable. Her son's disappearance must seem as cloaked and devious as any she might remember, and she might well hold the state responsible.

In April, Dayanova adds, she was vaccinated, getting the first shot at the factory where Fagim worked, and the next two at the local clinic. But Fagim had preferred not to be vaccinated. She remembers the district was washed with a chlorine solution just before the May 1 holiday. "The streets were white," she remembers, "and the leaves on the trees turned yellow." After her husband was hospitalized, their apartment was disinfected, and she and her son were given antibiotics. She collected compensation for her husband's death from SOBES (the social security office) and the fifty rubles that the national Red Cross gave to afflicted relatives.[6]

"But what is that worth to me?" she asks tearfully, "having lost him."

She shows us a newspaper article about pensions that may be coming to the families of victims of the 1979 outbreak. I remember Dr. Burgasov mentioning pensions when we spoke with him in Moscow. Now I learn that on March 30 Yeltsin proposed to the Supreme Soviet that "in the case of loss of the breadwinner for families of citizens deceased after contracting Siberian Ulcer in the city of Sverdlovsk (now Yekaterinburg) in 1979," yearly pensions will be paid to survivors. The amounts will be decided according to "the rules of substitution" that govern compensation for "injury or health damage related to the fulfillment of work obligations."[7] But when? Whether the funds even exist for this pension is left unclear, but the news helps explain why Peoples Deputy Mishustina was on television describing a list of 1979 anthrax victims.

We leave Dayanova to crisscross the district, returning to several of our dud addresses in the hope someone can give us an interview. Yampolskaya and I knock again on the door of the Vinogradov house, but no one still answers. We knock on the door of a house on Ulmeltsev (handyman's) Street, but get no answer there either. At an apartment on the boulevard Selkorovskaya Yampolskaya and I rouse not the occupants but a next-door neighbor, an old woman who comes into the hallway. She remembers Valeriy Poletaev, a thirty-eight-year-old worker at the ceramics factory who died April 12.

"It happened in one day," she recounts, leaning on the railing. "He lived alone and died at home. The ambulance came, they wrapped him in a blanket, and took him to the hospital."

Our next effort is more successful. We return to an address given to us Monday, our first day in Chkalovskiy, by a couple whose door we knocked on by mistake. They know of a victim, a young man who lived outside the area but used to visit his mother in Chkalovskiy. Now we are on the second floor of one of the Khrushchev apartments. Not knowing the name of the victim, we offer the usual brief introduction. The man who answers the door is the brother of Pyotr Gayda, a name from the cemetery list. In addition, Gayda's name is on the Abramova autopsy list, with a note that he received a single anthrax inoculation on April 21, 1979, and that his arm was scarred by the resulting anthrax ulcer. Yet both his thoracic and mesentery lymph nodes were hemorrhagic, and under the microscope anthrax bacteria were observable in tissues throughout his body. Wherever he had been exposed, the dose was lethal.

Gayda's sister-in-law is also at home, and together the two narrate Pyotr's last days. On April 29, in the evening, he complained of stomach pain and nausea. He had come for dinner with his mother, but couldn't eat. It is true that he often stayed at this apartment (their mother's at the time) for convenience during the work week. He worked at the ceramics factory, driving a forklift. That night, his mother sent for the ambulance to take him to the hospital. He died the next day, April 30.

We pause here, all four of us. Pyotr Gayda was only thirty-two; his family says he was healthy. He had spent four years on a Soviet submarine, proof of his strength. It takes little imagination to understand what his loss meant and still means to his family.

Then we ask if the family had been buying meat from private sources or from any source where they suspected it was contaminated.

"There was meat in the state shops," the sister-in-law answers. "It was good."

And did any animals die?

"Five kilometers away, in the village of Rudniy, two people died, and animals got sick." Or so she has heard. But no animals died here in the city.

"When Pyotr died, they denied it was from anthrax," she adds. "He was buried in an iron coffin, with policemen carrying it."

Pyotr's brother refused to be vaccinated that April. The sister-in-law was vaccinated and became sick from it. She believes the outbreak was from anthrax.

"It wasn't anthrax," Gayda's brother insists, dismissing the story of animal deaths. "It was a poison explosion at Compound 19."

We push on from here, still searching for good addresses. Meanwhile, Matthew is collecting soil samples from vacant lots, from ditches, and from the run-down, grassless quadrangles that pass for yards at the Khrushchev apartments. Hugh-Jones is again attempting to survey this part of the rayon. The people in this neighborhood, many of them behind high fences or already sequestered for the evening in their flats, seem to pay no attention. Having run out of addresses, Yampolskaya and I strike up a conversation with a middle-aged passerby who tells us he was an ambulance driver during the outbreak and worked around the clock during the "madness."

"Were there ambulances picking up patients at Compound 19?" we ask.

"Certainly!" he answers, but has to run off before revealing any details.

No matter. It is a beautiful sunlit evening, with the pleasantly domestic clank and rattle of kitchen sounds drifting from open apartment windows. People appreciate warm weather here. For most of the year, the city and region freeze; the median temperature in the winter is -7 degrees centigrade. I feel unaccountably optimistic, having come here for what sociologist Kurt Wolff would call an intellectual "catch," and I am finding it in the necessary surrender to the experience of being in this foreign place.[8] The pieces from our research are beginning to fit together: what the autopsy records show, what families tell us, what people in the neighborhood observe. For all the frustration with finding the correct addresses, one of the Soviet Union's improbable benefits for research is that families stayed in the same residences year after year, generation after generation. Now with the prospect that people will become more mobile and the Chkalovskiy apartments and cottages sold, and with the city's industries modernizing (another term for drastic reorganization and downsizing), the families here will inevitably become harder to find. In the West, one might theorize on a loss of community, but here the signs of vibrant community life seem lacking anyway, especially in the apartment complexes. Some longtime neighbors were friends; other neighbors were not. Some coworkers remember the victims; others only vaguely recall them. It is the families, behind their high fences and steel doors, that are the cohesive units, where memory lives.

At dinner, Walker reports that by tomorrow afternoon, Thursday, he will finish reviewing all forty-two cases that Abramova and Grinberg recorded. There is the possibility, too, that tissue samples from these cases can be shared, by slices from the paraffin blocks in which they are preserved. Walker is willing to take the 1979 tissue samples to his Galveston laboratory for further analysis by sophisticated techniques not available here. But will Abramova and Grinberg agree to dividing the precious material? Their paper on the outbreak is already written. The plan is to have Matthew submit an English summary for publication in the *Proceedings of the National Academy of Sciences,* of which he is a member. Walker, who will help write the article in English, will also be an author, along with Yampolskaya. Grinberg's special incentive for cooperation is the chance to travel to Texas and participate in the analysis. But Walker hesitates at the idea of providing financial support for him. Will good will alone motivate the two Russian pathologists to share their precious materials, or should we be content with just a few days of review and the publication of their findings? At this juncture, our team knows only that time is running short and our research is far from complete.

13

Resignation

June 11, Thursday. This morning we travel to Hospital 24, which serves the northern area of Chkalovskiy, to meet its director, Dr. Margarita Ilyenko. Before we get in the car, Dr. Shepetkin discloses that Dr. Ilyenko is the mysterious source of our first ten addresses. Nothing else about her is terribly mysterious (we already know her name from Russian press accounts of the outbreak), except that she runs her own hospital. In Russia, women have jobs but not power. The women who work in factories are systematically kept unskilled, not taking courses that men do, being confined to more routine and sometimes more physically demanding work, and working as hard at home as they do on the assembly line. One of the better studies of women's work was, in fact, done in Sverdlovsk in the 1960s.[1] It showed that in a week women factory employees put in almost as much time cleaning, doing laundry, and caring for children (thirty-six hours) as they did at work (forty hours), while men with full-time jobs put in an average of eight hours of work at home. In medicine, the structure is approximately the same; women are the foot soldiers, the obstetric, pediatric, or primary-care practitioners, while men run the high-status specialties and the health care administration. For a Russian woman to be a physician is not extraordinary; to have Dr. Ilyenko's rank is.

Her office is in Polyclinic 1, in a new building that replaced the old clinic some years after the 1979 outbreak. Across the courtyard is Hospital 24, which remains just as it was in 1979. Beyond a small woods, at a distance of about three hundred meters, is Compound 19. The space

Dr. Ilyenko commands, about twelve feet by twenty feet, is banked with the usual tall windows of the administrator's domain and offers the usual outsized conference table. As we enter, she is seated at her desk and several women assistants hover around her. One is presenting her papers to sign, another is clearing away records, a third is checking with her about when to serve the trays of tea, cream cakes, and sugar cookies already prepared in one of the anterooms. She rises and greets us solemnly. In her fifties, with sharp eyes and big shoulders, she has a completely nononsense manner. Still, she is wearing a brightly flowered dress, as if to strike a cheerful note.

In the hours we spend talking with Dr. Ilyenko, she brings one and then another folder from the cabinets that line the office wall, until the table is covered with old records, handwritten notes, inventory slips, and 1979 posters advertising vaccinations against anthrax. Her unique claim among physicians we have met is that she is a native of Chkalovskiy. During the outbreak, she says, she was at the bedside looking into the eyes of people she knew by name, recognizing the black and blue "death spots" of acute pulmonary edema on their skin. She characterizes the episode as a *koshmar*, a nightmare.

The first word she received of the outbreak was from Dr. Yakov Klipnitzer, the head of Hospital 20, on a morning in early April. Her hospital was smaller, and patients from this microrayon were referred to Klipnitzer's hospital. "Two of your people are dead," he told her. The cause he identified was "fulminating pneumonia." The next morning he called to say three more patients had suddenly died. On the third day, three additional patients died at Ilyenko's own hospital. Klipnitzer, Ilyenko confirms, called for help with the diagnosis, which led to Dr. Abramova's identifying the disease as anthrax. But that was not until April 10, she believes, concurring with Dr. Abramova's account.

Before that, the early victims were not autopsied. Dr. Ilyenko describes bodies piled up in the hospital morgue and, because it was too small to handle them, outside in the hall. She believes four or five of these bodies were buried in nearby Isetsk cemetery, not in Vostochniy; they were wrapped in plastic sheets, and the coffins were doused with lime. The staff, relatives, everyone was afraid to go near the bodies. Some families left their relatives' identity papers outside the door of the hospital rather than come in. Two young technical assistants, just girls, and a cleaning woman handled everything. At times, even other patients helped bring the bodies to the morgue. She says there were no storage instructions for four days, which fits with what Anna Komina's son told us.

Ilyenko made a vigorous personal appeal to city officials. "This is no time to screw around with me," she told them. "Get people here." But no extra help arrived, although the order quickly came through to send patients to the Infectious Diseases Unit at Hospital 40. Infected people still came to the polyclinic and Hospital 24. Those with temperatures over 38 degrees centigrade were immediately referred to Hospital 40.

Instead of local reinforcements, Dr. Nikiforov arrived from Moscow. By then, around April 11–12, when the diagnosis of anthrax was confirmed, he called a meeting of all involved physicians to tell them. He won no applause with the announcement. ("He got his tail caught in the door" is how Ilyenko puts it.) The reassurance he gave them, though, was that the disease was not contagious. She shows us a cream-colored piece of paper on which she scribbled random notes during this lecture: "anthrax. hypersepsis. intestinal. rupture of blood vessels. gamma globulin. tetracycline."

At that assembly, Nikiforov presented them with tainted meat as the explanation of the outbreak. "We didn't care about the explanation," Ilyenko says. "We cared about the treatment." But since the explanation was official, people began handing meat over to inspectors, and meat was confiscated from vehicles entering the city from the south. People who didn't understand what was happening threw away what meat they had.

The neighborhood-level mobilization she describes is amazing. To create special brigades to canvass Chkalovskiy, Ilyenko herself helped recruit the volunteers; around fourteen hundred local women workers, led by women physicians. They distributed tetracycline to the affected households (not to relatives outside the household or to neighbors), disinfected the sick rooms, confiscated potentially contaminated sheets and clothing, as well as meat, and also checked for illness among other members of the family. People with fevers were sent to polyclinics for observation; those who were very ill went directly to Hospital 40. Around April 22, a "terminal disinfection" plan went into effect, and firemen and factory workers hosed down buildings with chlorine solutions. That order came from the Extraordinary Commission, by then under Moscow control, and she has heard that Burgasov and another health official went up in a helicopter to survey the process.

On top of all this response came the vaccination campaign. From a file marked 022 (the international code for anthrax) Ilyenko shows us summary records. There were eleven sites where the vaccinations were given, including the Dom Kulturi (the House of Culture), just across from where we are now, as well as the ceramics factory, the meat-processing plant, and other workplaces. The vaccinations, which she describes as voluntary, were for people aged eighteen to fifty-five, and were not to be given to those who were ill, because of possible reactions. Around fifty-nine thousand people in Chkalovskiy were eligible, and about 80 percent of these were vaccinated at least once. Of those who received the first shot, it is unknown whether all or even a majority of them received the second and third shots. As many as fourteen thousand people were considered ineligible because of age or ill health, and another fourteen hundred refused to be vaccinated. Like everything in Soviet society called "voluntary," the latitude for resistance to authority, which Soviet people were adept at gauging and manipulating, is difficult to assess.

As proof of the vaccine used in 1979, Dr. Ilyenko pushes across the table an ampule labeled "STI vaccine 12 June 1964. Tbilisi Scientific Institute of Vaccines and Sera." The institute in Tbilisi, Georgia, was indeed a main producer of Soviet anthrax vaccine. Ilyenko is ambivalent about the vaccine and thinks that the second shot in particular caused serious complications for some people. She refers specifically to her sister, fifteen years younger than she, who after a serious reaction to the live vaccine remains permanently crippled by arthritis.

There was also a second series of vaccinations, she says, after the mid-April campaign. She describes being stopped by police as she drove to a May 1 celebration and told that there were ten new anthrax cases. She shows us a poster that announces, "Respected comrades: We invite you to attend prophylactic immunization against anthrax 11 May, 08–20 hours, Rishky per #9, Polyclinic #1." The special brigades once again went house to house. She attributes this second wave of deaths to the building cleanup effort, as we have heard from others.

As the trays of tea and cookies appear, I realize that more than anything, I want her to hand over additional names and addresses of the victims, everything she has. The easiest way is to ask and I do. In response, from the bank of cabinets that line one wall of her office, Dr. Ilyenko brings out another file on the outbreak. This one contains various handwritten lists of patients' names, some with addresses. Some lists are arranged by order of admission to the hospital. Some names on the lists are circled, which means they died. Of these, a few have 022 penciled next to the name. One list, with the names of thirty-four patients, gives the hospital where each was admitted (not always Hospital 24, but Hospitals 20 and 40 as well), plus an address and workplace. Still more lists emerge from the file, most handwritten. Some are undated. One list of twenty-three names, addresses, and workplaces is labeled "List of Patients Treated at Hospital 40 during April–May 1979." All together 48 of about 110 names are circled. An undated list of streets indicates those most affected by the outbreak; from Lyapustina to Selkorovskaya, they are all in Chkalovskiy rayon. There are two copybooks marked "Sepsis 022." In one of them is the notation, dated April 20, 1979: "358 ill patients, 45 dead, 214 in Hospital 40." The numbers indicate the pool of patients screened for anthrax by that date: how many people admitted to hospital were sick, how many died, and how many with high fever or other symptoms were referred to Hospital 40. She gives us permission to borrow this material so we can copy it.

I have a last question, about how the families endured their losses.

"Oh, the psychology!" she responds, then characterizes the families' reactions as fatalistic. "The man who is head of the household falls dead, and there is no reaction!" But she qualifies this response as "resignation, not indifference."

Just before I leave Dr. Ilyenko, I phrase a polite thank you for her efforts. I tell her that for the sake of the families, I want to find out the cause of the epidemic.

"You will never know," she replies grimly and stares out the window in the direction of Compound 19, a few hundred meters southwest. She believes that the biological facility at Compound 19 extends underground and beneath its walls to her own hospital. "Still, they tell us nothing," she comments, with her own brand of fatalism.

It's time for our team to meet with Dr. Bolshakov, the veterinarian at the rayon SES. Sergei Borisov has driven his car to work, and Sasha's is not big enough for all of us. I elect to let the others go first so I can go over my notes. I am fascinated by Dr. Ilyenko and her narrative, which is long and complicated, and seems authoritative.

Yet my judgment of her account of the 1979 outbreak is measured. In one newspaper interview she was quoted as saying her patients did not have anthrax but were killed by a special microbe invented by the military.[2] And, like some other officials we have spoken to, she never says, "I don't know." Except for the awkward overlap on our first day, when Dr. Romanenko and Dr. Babich disagreed about the timing of the 1979 animal outbreaks, our interviews with officials are all based on solo performances, with no chance for anyone "being in bad face."[3] Bureaucrats in any nation might be just as cautious with outsiders. The ones here can count in days back to when the Supreme Soviet made or broke their lives. Perhaps the miracle is that anyone speaks to us at all. What,

I ask myself, is the price of openness here? Who can afford to recall the past? For decades the Soviet Union was a society where remembering events was dangerous, and, like words out of turn, could get an individual arrested or worse.[4] This past danger of course still affects judgments about when to speak and what to say, on whether to turn on the *vranyo* or turn it off. The public health response of 1979, though, is practically impossible to conceal. To the contrary, the more energetic its mobilization, the better everyone running it appears, regardless of politics. Our problem is to understand the extent to which it may explain one hypothesis or another. What caused these deaths?

But when Dr. Ilyenko describes the resignation of families to the 1979 outbreak, I believe her. We Americans have an entire literature on "the disaster syndrome" of shaken nerves and psychological devastation that strikes communities hit by floods, hurricanes, tornadoes, and earthquakes.[5] Yet community disasters do not occur in a political and social vacuum. As sociologist Kai Erikson has described in a series of cases, disasters disproportionately affect the poor and politically isolated.[6] Similarly, epidemics usually follow the fault lines of social class; through the centuries, the poor and disadvantaged have been the most vulnerable to widespread outbreaks of disease.[7] The larger political context also predetermines how epidemics evolve—who shall be stigmatized, who shall be saved. Even though Western approaches, including medical reports, tend to deemphasize the political structure of disasters,[8] an afflicted community, rather than being temporarily troubled, is likely to be all too experienced with oppression. Erikson makes this point by broadening the notion of the trauma that results from a disaster. These effects can be "from a sustained exposure to battle as well as from a moment of numbing shock, from a continuing pattern of abuse as well as from a single searing assault, from a period of severe attenuation and erosion as well as from a sudden flash of fear."[9]

How then do we estimate the sociopolitical "baseline" for a population in the Soviet Union, for the people in Sverdlovsk, for example, at the time of the outbreak? In 1979 they were thirty years past the worst repressions of the Stalin era and the ravages of World War II, the Great Patriotic War. Their press and other media were heavily censored, and their industrial productivity was declining, although the 1970s saw great increases in the number of households with refrigerators and televisions and more holiday travel for loyal workers. The state's guarantee of stability in work, housing, and nearly all facets of social life came at the price of submitting to its order, to the exclusion of other allegiances—

the community or church or even extended kinship relations, which might challenge state authority. As sociologist Lewis Coser succinctly puts it, "In a totalitarian society the concentration of power on the top requires atomization rather than unification of internal resistance."[10]

In Sverdlovsk and, especially, it seems, in Chkalovskiy rayon, the sudden random deaths of family members and of workers must have affected the local working-class population not just psychologically, with personal grief; it must also have shaken their faith in the state, which had failed to protect them—and not for the first time. The older generation, like Fagim Dayanov's mother, having lived through the purges, might reasonably suspect this was yet another one. For the younger generation, the outbreak must have contributed to their cynicism about government and its failure to maintain a norm of security.

The 1979 public health response was an obvious attempt, from Moscow on down, to restore citizens' confidence in the state. Even physicians who saw themselves apolitically fulfilling their professional responsibilities were involved in rebuilding faith in government and in restoring the preexisting order. But, ultimately, what a sad, chaotic effort it was! A barrage of clinical activity, of programs to distribute drugs, to vaccinate, to wash down the city and pave some streets, to confiscate meat, to shoot dogs. All this commotion signaled the state was trying to reimpose its order; even if local officials determined the public health response, the Moscow visitors imposed their authority and silence, the rule of "ask no further questions."

Yet how could the government be trusted when a "veil" (*vual* in Russian, which was Ilyenko's metaphor) lay over the entire event? If there was uncertainty about the outbreak's cause, what guaranteed the disaster would not happen again? The question seems not to have been asked, at least not publicly. Local people had no option but private grief and quiet resignation, and perhaps no greater hope than a return to the normal routines of work and home.

I am still seated in Dr. Ilyenko's waiting room, writing in my notebook, when Matthew comes dashing up the stairs. Is the interview with the SES veterinarian already over?

"The most amazing thing has happened!" Matthew exclaims. "We arrived at Bolshakov's office and when we were all seated, he announced that he had orders not to speak to us and that we had to leave."

"But why?"

"I don't know, but I said we would like to leave questions about the animal outbreak with him. He said he remembered animal deaths in April but not in March. And then we had to leave. We are stunned. The appointment was confirmed by telephone this morning."

That evening, Shelokov tells us that there were men waiting outside Dr. Bolshakov's office who were, according to Dr. Shepetkin, ready to get rough if our group did not leave quietly. Bolshakov apparently also said that Dr. Romanenko at SES has refused to see us again. We are a bit baffled about this, since we hadn't requested a second meeting, only demographic information. Nonetheless, the closing of doors, first the veterinarians in Sysertskiy, now the rayon SES, looks like a trend. In just a few days, our welcome is quite possibly worn out.

Over tea, as the sky outside begins to darken, Yampolskaya and I discuss today's only interview in Chkalovskiy, the last she and I will do together. It was with the elderly widow of Filipp Dyedov, whose grave we found in Sector 13 and who is on one of Dr. Ilyenko's lists. We found his widow on a tip from a neighbor and entered yet another Chkalovskiy cottage, this one darker and more spare than the others we've seen. Dyedov, a retired man, died at home on April 12 at age sixty. His body, against the protests of his family, was taken away to the morgue at Hospital 40. But apparently there was no autopsy, and the death certificate indicated "arteriosclerosis" as cause of death. His widow, whose own poor health keeps her homebound, told us that her husband used to help their niece, who lives near Compound 19, with her garden. What she describes as symptoms, fever, chills, faintness, and blood on his mouth, might well signify an anthrax infection. The pity of it, she told us, is that he had fought in the Great Patriotic War, and because he had survived that, they counted themselves lucky. They worked, built themselves a comfortable house, and were just beginning to enjoy retirement when he died. Dyedova's son stopped by while we were there and lingered in the background. Touched by the widow's story, we mention Yeltsin's decree for pensions, which neither has heard of. We put this case down for potential inclusion in our sample, knowing that no sure medical diagnosis of anthrax is now or perhaps will ever be possible.

As we were leaving the neighborhood, it struck me how quiet it was, and I wondered what the noises were like here in 1979: the blare of ambulance sirens, cries of grief, neighbors talking, exclamations, a shout as someone staggers and falls to the ground, the muffled hisses and clatter from the ceramics factory. But no velvet-toned bells like the ones Chekhov heard. No call to the community. What depths of fear did the people here experience?

Even though Yampolskaya is leaving tomorrow, I am confident the

interviews will continue, and at a rapid pace. Today, through Professor
Anatoliy Marenkov at the university's new social science division, I have
been introduced to Ilona Nikonova, whose title is Chair of Foreign Lan-
guages and who teaches research methods. We met in Marenkov's office,
beneath portraits of Socrates and Aristotle that hang where, he tells me,
only a few months ago portraits of Marx and Lenin were hanging from
the same nails. Ilona's English is clear and crisp, with a slight lilt. She
was taught by a woman whose own teachers were Irish missionary nuns
in Manchuria; she meets weekly with a book group to practice English
conversation. We have agreed to start work at 10 A.M. and spend the
day in Chkalovskiy. The rest of this evening, as the sky fades to darkness, we spend decoding the information from Dr. Ilyenko's lists to garner a new supply of names and addresses for tomorrow's search.

14

Vulnerability and Chance

June 12, Friday. At 7 A.M., Olga Yampolskaya and David Walker depart for Moscow, where we will see them again next week before the American team heads back to the States. Walker has in his briefcase six tissue samples that Grinberg and Abramova have consented to give him and his notes on all forty-two of Abramova's cases. It looks as though Grinberg will be invited to work cooperatively for a short period of time at University of Texas Medical Branch at Galveston, and perhaps Yampolskaya will go as well.

At nine, Sasha drives me and Ilona Nikonova to Chkalovskiy to investigate additional names and addresses from Dr. Ilyenko's lists. The triangulation I want is beginning to emerge, even if only from fragments of information. Dr. Abramova's autopsy notes, which Yampolskaya copied and translated in their entirety before she left, also give us glimmerings of who the victims were. Abramova's notes pertain to only 42 patients, Ilyenko's lists indicate 48 who died, from a general tally of 110 who were apparently screened for anthrax. From the grave sites, we have acquired 62 names, the most extensive but also the most rudimentary of our lists. Of the names from the cemetery, 37 match those of patients indicated as deceased on the Ilyenko lists.

This Friday in Chkalovskiy is lively, and in the bright sunshine the neighborhoods look splendid. The new Russian government has declared the day a holiday, in its own honor. People are working in their gardens, roosters crow, wildflowers in vacant lots shake in the breeze. We begin looking for addresses in the center of the rayon, between two parallel streets, Ulitsa Lyapustina and Poldnevaya (Midday Street), that lead to the ceramics factory. Our list of addresses takes us back and forth on the cross streets between them, and up and down their dusty corridors.

Maria Moseykina, sixty-nine years old, a pensioner, lived in a small house on one of the cross streets close to the ceramics factory. Today we find her daughter standing in front of that house, looking worried. Earlier that morning, a fire broke out in the shed, and two men are still hacking about in the mud and cinders of her yard. This is a bad time for questions about her mother's death. We apologize. There is no good time, she tells us, and begins. On April 14, her mother was taken by ambulance to Hospital 20, apparently suffering from a heart attack. After two nights, she died, on April 16. Since we have no autopsy record, we might discount this case. But the diagnosis written on Moseykina's death certificate is "sepsis," and she was buried in Section 13 in Vostochniy Cemetery. It was the usual: a closed-coffin burial, with the police in charge.

The story in the neighborhood was that Moseykina had traveled southeast to the city of Syserts and had somehow become contaminated with anthrax there, but her daughter insists this was not true.

"My mother was a gardener who worked outside a lot," the daughter says with distress. "Maybe that had something to do with her getting sick." Then she turns back to the wreckage in her yard.

On Promyslovaya (Industry Street), which crosses Lyapustina and Poldnevaya a stone's throw from the ceramics factory, we look for the house of Mukhametalin Mukhametshin, who died April 22 at age forty-five. His grave site was marked by an elaborate, burnished aluminum monument and an engraved portrait. But his family has moved, a neighbor tells us. Mukhametshin owned two houses, one of them since sold to gypsies. We find them at the address, but they have nothing to tell us except that an old woman, maybe the victim's mother, lived there alone until she died four years ago. The house next door is abandoned.

We know from Abramova's list that Mukhametshin worked at a factory (MEX 44) on nearby Selskorovskaya. That he "died on the street" appears in Abramova's notes. As I have noticed before, the classic stages of anthrax (initial flu-like symptoms, followed by a temporary recovery and then a second onslaught of symptoms) are not apparent in all cases. The question now in my mind is whether we have incomplete narratives or if victims reacted differently to the infection. When I hear about anyone collapsing suddenly, with no warning, I wonder if they have been stoic or in denial about earlier sensations of weakness, chills, fever, headache, or nausea. Or could it be that for some individuals the onset of the illness is truly violent and quicker than for others? Or is it just the lack of a close relative to remember the course of the disease that makes its onset appear that way?

When we knock on the door of a little cottage on Poldnevaya, Aleksandr, the twenty-nine-year-old son of Ivan Vershinin, appears at the gate, tousled and sleepy-eyed. Because of the holiday, he was sleeping late. For me, the name Aleksandr Vershinin has strong literary associations. In Chekov's *The Three Sisters*, he is the dislocated visionary lieutenant-colonel with late-nineteenth-century apocalyptic yearnings: "In the old days men were absorbed with wars, filling all their existence with marches, raids, victories, but now all that is a thing of the past, leaving behind it a great void where there is so far nothing to fill: humanity is searching for it passionately, and of course will find it. Ah, if only it would be quickly!"[1]

This Aleksandr Vershinin is living in a similar epoch, in the post–Cold War void, where all sorts of new paradigms compete for meaning. He was seventeen in 1979 when his father died. His father, forty-seven at the time, worked in the tile shop at the ceramics factory.

"On April 11," his son says calmly, "he came home from work and said he had difficulty breathing. The next morning we called an ambulance. He forgot his razor, and we wanted to bring it to him the next day, but he died during the night." The detail reveals what shows in Vershinin's cemetery photo, that he had dignity. His family knew that he would want to be clean-shaven. What they presumed was that he would be well enough to care. The death certificate Vershinin's son shows us indicates "sepsis" as the cause of his father's death.

According to Vershinin's son, no livestock died in the area, but he remembers that stray dogs in the district were shot "by the hundreds." Dr. Burgasov's 1979 memo to the Ministry of Agriculture also mentions dumps of dead dogs; and the official 1988 Soviet statement describes three dead dogs being autopsied and testing positive for anthrax. The scientific literature suggests that dogs, like pigs, are more resistant to anthrax than sheep, cattle, goats, or horses. But in the general sweep of public health orders, strays that might scavenge in garbage, die from anthrax-infected meat, and be eaten by other scavengers may well have been sacrificed.

The Vershinin house was disinfected, and the family was given tetracycline. Aleksandr remembers hearing that his father's coffin was closed and that the police supervised the burial.

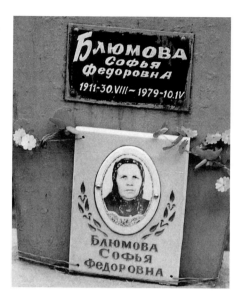

Sophia Fyodorovna Bliumova, age 67.

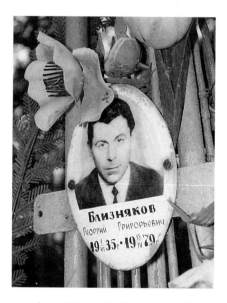

Georgyi Grigoryevich Bliznyakov, age 43.

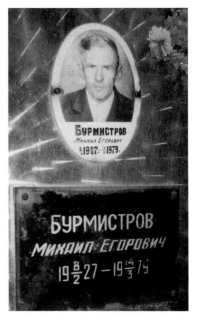

Mikhail Yegorovich Burmistrov, age 52.

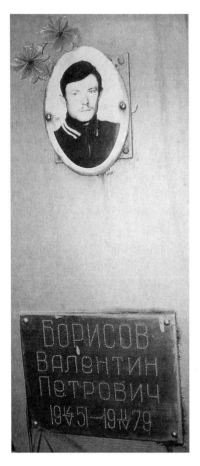

Valentin Petrovich Borisov, age 27.

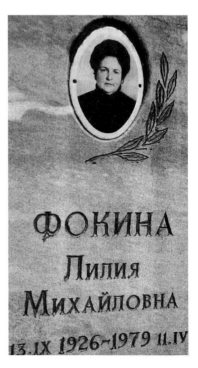

Lilia Mikhaylovna Fokina, age 52.

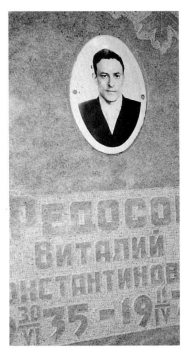 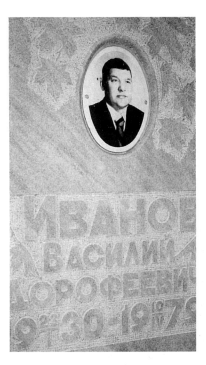

Vitaliy Konstantinovich Fyodosov, age 43.　　　Vasiliy Dorofeyevich Ivanov, age 49.

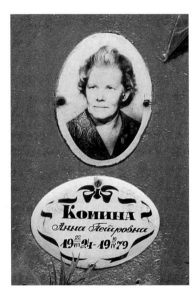

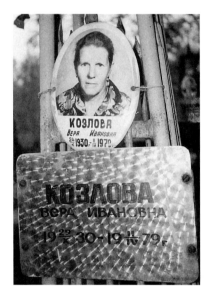

Anna Petrovna Komina, age 54.   Vera Ivanovna Kozlova, age 48.

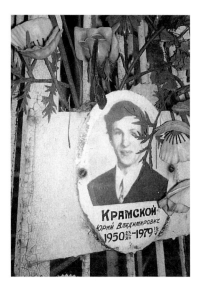

Yuriy Vladimirovich Kramskoy, age 28.

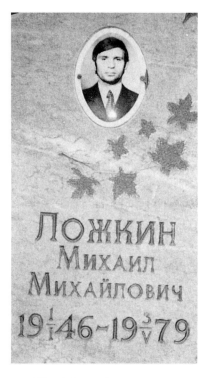

Mikhail Mikhaylovich Lozhkin, age 33.

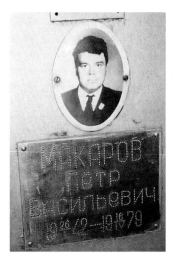

Pyotr Vasilyevich Makarov, age 37.

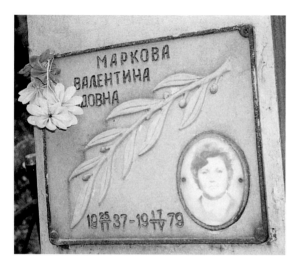

Valentina Davidovna Markova, age 41.

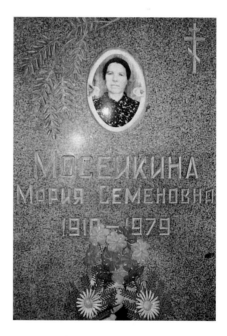

Maria Semyonovna Moseykina, age 69.

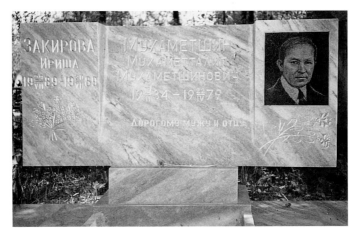

Mukhametalin Mukhametshinovich Mukametshin, age 45.

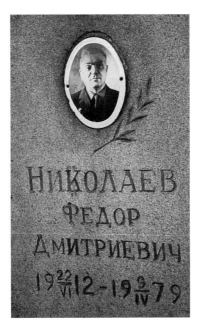

Fyodor Dmitryevich Nikolaev, age 66.

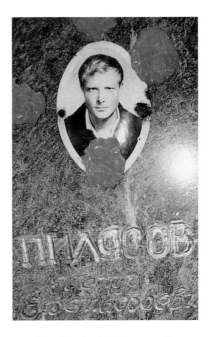

Pyotr Yevstafyevich Pilyasov, age 39.

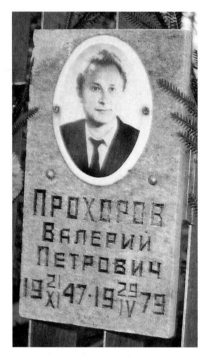 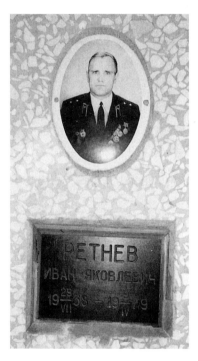

Valeriy Petrovich Prokhorov, age 31.   Pavel Yakovlevich Retnev, age 40.

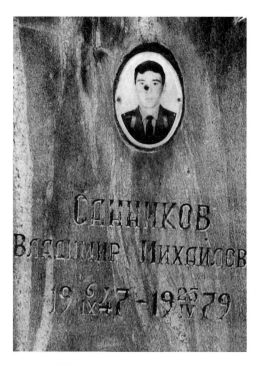

Vladimir Mikhaylovich Sannikov, age 31.

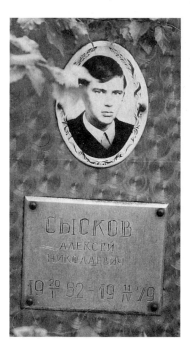

Alexey Nikolayvich Syskov, age 27.

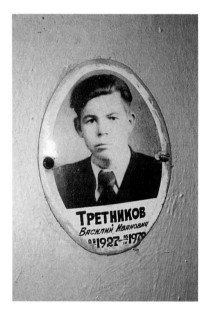 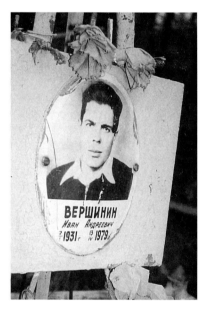

Vasiliy Ivanovich Tretnikov, age 52.   Ivan Andreyevich Vershinin, age 47.

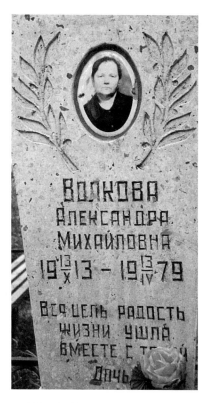

Aleksandra Mikhaylovna Volkova, age 65.

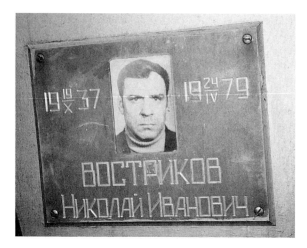

Nikolay Ivanovich Vostrykov, age 41.

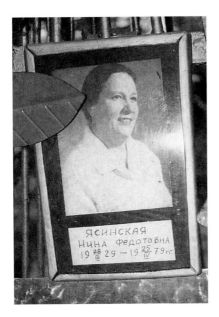

Nina Fyodorovna Yasinskaya, age 50.

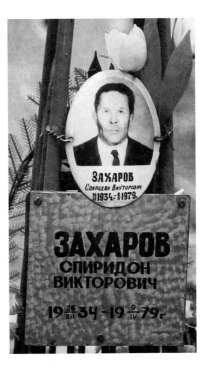

Speridon Viktorovich Zakharov, age 44.

What did Aleksandr think caused his father's death?

"An underground explosion at Compound 19."

We've heard this explanation before. Another rumor in Chkalovskiy, articulated by Dr. Ilyenko, is that whatever deviltry was going on at Compound 19, it was literally buried, taking place in some basement crypt of a laboratory whose terrible contents ultimately could not be contained.

As we make our way through Chkalovskiy, we rely for directions on people on the street or in front of their houses. The community may not be cohesive, but there were obviously friendships among residents. Neighbors know a lot, as we find out when we seek the house of Mikhail Burmistrov, another worker in the tile shop at the ceramics factory, who died April 14, 1979. He was separated from his wife, but they divided their cottage near the ceramics factory in two, with each living in one half. Burmistrov was a heavy smoker and drinker. His neighbors across the street, another ceramics worker and his wife, recount all this after we mistakenly knock on their gate and disturb them at their gardening. When Mikhail got sick, they tell us, his estranged wife was already hospitalized with a problem of her own and couldn't help him. So he died at home, after two days of being sick. Then he was buried in a special cemetery plot, in a closed casket.

Afterward, the two neighbors were vaccinated, with all three shots, at the ceramics factory. The man's reaction to the first shot was a painful ulcer; his wife had little reaction. They know nothing about anthrax-infected meat being sold in the area at that time.

After recounting this information, Burmistrov's neighbors look morose and impatient. The Burmistrov's house was sold in 1984. The family is gone. Here we appear, years later, resurrecting the tragedy of their friend's death, perhaps stigmatizing them with some involvement in the anthrax outbreak. The story, for them, is over, and they have a garden to tend.

No one answers at the former home of Natalya Lyakhova on Poldnevaya Street. According to the autopsy notes, her case is unusual. She became sick on April 15 and was admitted to Hospital 40 on April 17. But, perhaps because of aggressive use of antibiotics and fluids or even the strength of her system, she did not die until April 25. Once again, neighbors fill in the details. To begin, Lyakhova's children recently sold the house and left the area. Natalya Lyakhova, age forty-eight when she died, worked at a brick factory canteen in northern Sverdlovsk. She left each morning before seven and returned around four in the afternoon.

One of the neighbors adds that she is certain Lyakhova was on vacation and stayed at home during the first week of April. Since we want to plot her daytime location on a spot map, this fact is significant for us.

We then move north in the neighborhood to another story of grief and distress. Aleksandra Volkova, age sixty-five, a pensioner, lived in a third floor apartment on the boulevard Selkorovskaya, where electric trolleys run. Her daughter Maria, who lives there now, invites us in and offers us tea and Russian chocolate. She has her mother's death certificate, which lists sepsis as the cause of death and April 13 as the date. Aleksandra's cemetery picture shows a woman whose soft features reflect a forgiving nature. Her daughter resembles her. She turns down the gas under a pot of soup she has been making, and we three sit at a tiny kitchen table.

"It was just after she came back from visiting a friend in Compound 19," Maria tells us. "She called out for an ambulance. 'What's wrong?' I asked her. 'I have pain everywhere.' She felt weak and fell to the floor. But her pulse was normal. She went to Hospital 20. It was the same story. Weak, and no appetite. She could not breathe, but the doctors found nothing wrong. The next day I went to work, but I was called home. A neighbor had telephoned for an ambulance and she was taken to Hospital 40." Volkova died the same day and, according to Abramova's records, her body was autopsied the day after that, April 14, and diagnosed with anthrax.

Again, as for other families, after the patient was transported to Hospital 40, the special brigade arrived. The family was given tetracycline, but Maria disinfected the apartment herself. Some meat was taken for sampling, but she doesn't know the result. As far as she knows, no meat was sold at the ceramics factory, and no burning of meat went on there that she'd ever heard of. No children were affected, again, as far as she knows.

Her mother's visit to Compound 19 still worries Maria. Around that time her mother had also been outside, washing windows. An acquaintance who works in one of the city laboratories told her that her mother died of anthrax, but that the anthrax was artificial, and had been made at Compound 19.

This gnawing anxiety, characteristic in these interviews, is a common effect of epidemics. As if by a roll of dice, the invisible germ strikes down this person and lets another escape unscathed. Thirteen years later Sverdlovsk survivors are still struggling with the unknowns, with questions of vulnerability and fate. In some cases, anthrax is configured like a terrific blow that no one could survive, so in retrospect the victims (even older people with health problems) are represented as extraordinarily healthy but doomed anyway. The point might be that no one expected them, whatever their chronic maladies, to die suddenly. Or sometimes the victims are represented as frail, so that simply being outside in a garden was enough to put them at high risk. As for the specifics about the origin of the disease or about dose and strain, no one knows anything but rumors—maybe there was a special "artificial" microbe, maybe it came from Compound 19.

Still near the boulevard and the trolley lines, we search out the address of Lazar Korsayev, age sixty-four, a pensioner who nonetheless worked at the ceramics factory. The present resident, there for just a month, knows nothing. We hail a woman across the street, a neighbor who, it turns out, was a friend of the Korsayev family. Lazar Nikolayvich, she confirms, worked at the ceramics factory. He was a heavy smoker but drank very little alcohol and, an industrious sort, he always rose early for work. One day he came home from the factory at eleven in the morning because he felt seriously ill, with goose bumps and chills. His daughter called the ambulance. The official cause of death on the death certificate? The neighbor shrugs. "Maybe it said influenza." She isn't sure, but she wouldn't trust what any official document said.

At the time of his death, Lazar Korsayev was separated from his wife, like Mikhail Burmistrov and maybe some of the other single men. His daughter was a doctor and watched out for him, and so did his sister. The neighbor doesn't know where the daughter lives now. But she tells us that Korsayev's sister lives somewhere over on Lyapustina. We thank her, make another note to follow up on this lead, and move on.

At a rubber factory canteen, where all the food looks gray, we take a break for lunch. I cautiously select fresh bread and a hard-boiled egg. Sasha, slim as a pencil, declines to eat. So does Ilona, who is single and says she is dieting for bathing suit weather. A soft-spoken person who gets right to the point, she is a joy to work with. We spent only an hour going over the questionnaire yesterday, but she knows just what to do. Much younger than Yampolskaya and I, she doesn't weep at the stories we hear. She pays respectful attention and makes careful notes.

When we knock at the door of the cottage where Tatyana Kosheleva once lived, a girl answers and tells us that her family has recently bought it. The ever-ready neighbor, a woman passing by, fills us in. Kosheleva, age twenty-four when she died on April 13, 1979, the youngest victim that we know of, was the kindergarten teacher referred to by Burgasov in 1988. The neighbor points to a nearby building, School No. 385, and suggests that on Monday, when it opens again, we can ask about her there. On Monday, I realize regretfully, I will be in Moscow, but Ilona will follow through. Our agreement is that she will continue with the necessary interviews after I leave. We will communicate by e-mail, fax, telephone, and the occasional courier between Cambridge and Yekaterinburg, whatever it takes to stay in touch.

Our list from Dr. Ilyenko locates the former home of Valentina Markova on Lyapustina Street. The woman who opens the door greets our request with astonishment—and in turn astonishes us. "No one named Markova lives here now. But my brother Lazar Korsayev died in the outbreak." Korsayev's sister confirms and adds details to the account her brother's neighbor has just given us. Though retired, her brother worked at the ceramics factory as a packer and maintenance man. He'd been there only two years when he died. He was a heavy smoker and had been treated for tuberculosis from 1965 to 1976. His wife kept the death certificate, on which the cause of death was noted as "sepsis." When he first felt sick, on April 10, he went to Hospital 20. He had aching bones, chills, trouble breathing, and dizziness. Three days later he was in Hospital 40, and the next day he died.

As Korsayev's sister talks, the victim whose family we expected to find, Valentina Markova, drifts away from us. All we know about her is from Abramova's notes. Only forty-one when she died on April 17, 1979, Markova was officially disabled and probably confined here at home, but it seems no one is left to tell us her whereabouts in 1979.

We finish ten interviews before we quit at dinnertime. No one recounts buying infected meat, but would anyone want to? Would they even have recognized it? In the Soviet explanation of the outbreak, the 1978–79 winter was deemed especially harsh, with food shortages, especially of meat, in the spring. The picture we get confirms that harshness, but many Chkalovskiy workers had some source of meat (mostly pigs but also goats and a few cows) and other food from their own gardens. And as some families have flatly put it, they just did without meat at home.

What is most impressive is how routine ordinary life seems to have been in Chkalovskiy in 1979, at least before the epidemic. Nearly everyone worked, even the pensioners, and they all apparently lived by the clock. People did not travel much, except for government-sponsored vacations and expeditions to Communist Party shrines. As for actually relocating from one city to another, people were not allowed to spontaneously pull up roots. The Soviet state kept its promise of stability built around industrial productivity. This stasis, gray and unrelenting as it may have been, will help us plot an accurate map of the victims' daytime locations early in April. That map could lead us northwest up the two streets of Lyapustina and Poldnevaya to Compound 19. Or it might reveal no pattern at all and augment the enigma of the anthrax outbreak. With only seventeen interviews done so far, nothing is conclusive.

Though Ilona and I will go back to Chkalovskiy tomorrow, we take time this evening to discuss how she will proceed after I leave. To build a map, we want to locate the whereabouts of each victim in the days just before April 4, when Anna Komina first fell ill, and we want a round-the-clock perspective. For this, we need both home and work addresses, and reliable testimony as to where each individual was during that time. Was he at work? Did she work the night or day shift? If retired, did he have another job? Was she on vacation or traveling?

We have yet to locate any outliers, the 30 percent of victims Soviet officials claimed lived outside the southern area. If this contingent also worked outside Chkalovskiy, then we will have to figure out how they contracted anthrax, if it was from the same or a different source than victims in Chkalovskiy. Unfortunately, we must rely on Dr. Ilyenko's lists of patients and on Abramova's notes, both of which lack many home and nearly all work addresses. If all information about the victims were complete and freely available, knowing the earliest dates of onset and the whereabouts of the very first cases could unlock the mystery of whether the animal or human cases occurred earlier. But those complete records have not surfaced. We will have to keep piecing the puzzle together the hard and slow way, and we may find we are missing whole parts of the picture.

Our salvation might be if Supreme Soviet deputy Larissa Mishustina, who we believe has access to the alleged official list of victims, returns to Yekaterinburg and shares that information with us.

Meanwhile, this trip to Yekaterinburg is almost over, and we have learned that, unfortunately, no meeting at Compound 19 will be possible. Today General Kharechko responded to Matthew's June 9 letter with a politely-worded rejection: "I deeply regret that the current circumstances do not allow us to organize our meeting at the time that you have proposed." But he held the door open for further contact, suggesting he would review any written questions and "the materials your group has at its disposal" (meaning the autopsy and interview data) with an eye to involving "in the discussion a broader range of specialists in the area of pathoanatomy, epidemiology, and epizootiology of the disease in question, who are currently absent from this institution." His letter ends with a wish for "fruitful contacts in the future." Compound 19 and the military remain sequestered behind the base's high, concrete walls and ornate metal gates.

In the evening we congregate for a farewell dinner at a restaurant called Okean (Ocean), where the platters of fish and other food arrive in endless procession. The party includes Sergei Borisov and his wife Natalya, Professor Shepetkin and his wife, also named Natalya, Lev Grinberg and his wife, the third Natalya at the table, plus Ilona, Hugh-Jones, Shelokov, Matthew, and me. The rock band is loud. Most of our talking consists of elaborate toasts. The first is by Professor Borisov, to Meselson, Shelokov, and Hugh-Jones for all the effort they have put into this investigation. Seated at Borisov's left, I can hardly conceal my annoyance at being excluded, along with Yampolskaya and Ilona, from this tribute. I want credit for relentlessly combing the streets of Chkalovskiy; I have even worn out my doughty Rockport sandals, which are now in the waste bin at the dormitory. We women have worked hard. But wait, Borisov gestures with a smile. After we have lifted our glasses to the men, he offers a toast to the women. Such women as are at this table, he says, and women in general, as everyone knows, are "superior beings, and tonight exceptionally beautiful!" All the women, I notice, laugh at being put on a pedestal, as if nothing can be done about such nonsense and, anyway, they don't want to think of themselves as drudges. The American men hesitate to join in this effusive generalization about the fair sex. But the three Russian men at the table gallantly stand to salute us, and the others join in.

15

The KGB List of Victims

The next morning, Saturday, June 13, Sergei Borisov brings Larissa Mishustina, the Supreme Soviet deputy who has been an advocate for the victims' families, to our dormitory suite. Petite and energetic, she has just returned from a conference at the Woodrow Wilson Institute in Washington, D.C. Having witnessed up close the current wranglings between Democrats and Republicans in Congress, she worries about our government's potential for destabilization. To her, the way the two parties go at each other hammer and tongs bodes ill for our future, and she doesn't know what to make of Ross Perot. It is true that a new phase of incivility has afflicted our elected representatives and a third party movement seems to be emerging; yet, from the vantage of our old democracy, I see Russia's new one as much more precarious.

Nonetheless I envy Mishustina's position and her chance to have a positive influence on this new Russian government. There are as few women in the Supreme Soviet as elsewhere in the high ranks of government or the professions. And even fewer among them can claim to be from the president's hometown. Today we learn that in late 1991 Mishustina sent President Yeltsin a letter to prod his conscience about the 1979 anthrax outbreak. Composed with the help of Alexey Yablokov, Yeltsin's Counselor on Ecology and Health, it read:

Esteemed Boris Nikolayvich,

*My request has to do with an event of which you are well aware. In April
1979 in the Sverdlovsk district there was an epidemic of Siberian Ulcer.
This was the official version. I think that you, no less than I, know that
the death of 70 people was the consequence of bacteriological weapons,
from the so-called 19th military settlement. I would ask you to familiarize yourself with the articles in Literaturnaya Gazeta (August 22, 1990
and October 2, 1991).*

*I beg you to organize an official investigation into the event, since this
part of our past is knocking on the door of our present. The military continue to deny their involvement in the event. All questions remain open.
The families of the deceased received only 50 rubles each. I think that
the most wealthy institution, whose guilt so far no one is trying to prove,
should at least materially rectify itself before the families of the deceased.*

*Boris Nikolayvich! Today I think it is important to return to this sub-
ject. I understand that this will not be an easy step, but I insist on it.*

I beg you not to leave the request of this deputy unanswered.

Peoples Deputy of the Russian Federation L. P. Mishustina

The articles Mishustina urged Yeltsin to read are both by Natalya Zhenova, a native of Yekaterinburg. The first, Zhenova states, was inspired
by the 1977 American novel *Vector*, by Henry Satton, in which a deadly
cloud ravages an American community. (The book had a certain popu-
larity in Russia; Olga Yampolskaya tells me that she was able to borrow
it from one of the Moscow libraries in 1989.) Zhenova interviewed some
Sverdlovsk doctors who claimed, among other things, that victims died
from an extremely lethal, genetically engineered bacterium that "would
strike down people of a certain [military-duty] age." This article was
quickly reprinted in the *Wall Street Journal* (November 28, 1990), in a
translation provided by the CIA's Foreign Broadcast Information Service.[1] Zhenova's second article appeared more than a year later, after she
had obtained a copy of the summary report—written by Matthew and
published in the newsletter of the Federation of American Scientists—of
the 1988 presentations by Burgasov and Nikiforov in the United States.
"Thus," she wrote, "for the first time, I was able to familiarize myself
with our side's complete arguments."[2] Apparently the specifics of the
official version (how many died, how many were infected, purported
symptoms, and the bone-meal production claims) were unknown to Russian journalists and the public at large until almost three years after be-

ing aired in the West. Zhenova renewed her inquiries in Sverdlovsk and the surrounding region for this and also a third article, which strongly questioned the official Soviet explanation of the outbreak.[3]

Without fanfare Larissa Mishustina presents us with an envelope containing a list of the victims of the 1979 anthrax epidemic. Few moments since the beginning of this quest are quite as sweet as the one in which Matthew passes the four pages to me for my perusal. Here it is, sixty-four full names and addresses tapped out on a manual typewriter with distinctively light M's and p's, in an office somewhere, maybe here in Yekaterinburg or in Moscow, by a clerk who worked from notes or from official documents provided by still another cog in the Soviet bureaucracy, who must have gotten them with help from one or another physician, Dr. Nikiforov probably, who was able to say with some authority, having read the records, having understood the progression toward death, that the cause of death was, yes, anthrax and not something else. At the bottom of the list is typed: "from KGB sources." A reckoning was made and then wrapped in secrecy. But who cares now? I have the city map and I have the list and it isn't too late for progress. Mishustina reaffirms that the list came to her from the KGB, but she assures us that now "the list is no secret." Two KGB agents delivered it to her office a few months ago. With it, the Russian government can implement the pensions that Boris Yeltsin, moved by Mishustina's letter, has decreed will go to the families of victims. The money for these pensions has yet to flow into the community, she admits, but the president's gesture at least acknowledges the wrong done.

Is there more to be learned? Mishustina agrees there are more details that could be added to the story. Despite the claim in her letter to "know" that the deaths were "the consequence of bacteriological weapons," she has, after all, also said that all questions were still open about military involvement in the outbreak. Mishustina's spirited optimism is encouraging. In a phrase becoming as familiar to us as "the documents were destroyed," she looks forward to future cooperation.

Within the hour I am pounding the dirt roads in Chkalovskiy with Ilona. Matthew comes with us to scout the territory while Professor Borisov takes Shelokov and Hugh-Jones on a day trip to the Asian-European border, where one can stand with a foot on each continent. If I could be in two places at once, they would be Yekaterinburg and Cambridge. With the addresses on the KGB list, I could easily spend another month interviewing. But tomorrow morning at 8:15 our group leaves for Moscow, and then three days later we make our journey home, where other responsibilities claim me. As Ilona and I begin to scour the rayon for families, at least we have good weather for my last foray.

A wiser head might have chosen pursuit of the outliers, those fifteen or so victims on the KGB list whose addresses are in the north. But those homes are scattered and distant. I have decided that the time it would take to reach them is better spent in Chkalovskiy, where we can find the family homes in clusters on familiar streets. As a compromise, though, we work the outer fringes of the rayon, away from the ceramics factory. For example, Klaudia Spirina, number 59 on the KGB list, lived at the eastern edge of Chkalovskiy, in a third-floor apartment. She was sixty-seven when she died in late April, 1979. Her daughter answers when we ring the bell. She puts aside her ironing to talk with us, but she leaves the television tuned to an Aleksandr Nevskiy–type drama, with bearded Russians fiercely battling invading Swedes or some other enemy.

Although a pensioner, Spirina had a job at the radio works in downtown Sverdlovsk. The course of her illness was unusually slow and, on the Abramova list, a note has been jotted that the diagnosis of anthrax may be questionable; no bacteria were found in her blood or tissue. Spirina's daughter describes the onset of the disease as April 14, when her mother developed flulike symptoms. Admission to Hospital 40 followed on April 22, and her mother's death occurred on April 30. This sequence matches Abramova's record, but neither proves nor disproves any diagnosis. Spirina's primary symptom was lung congestion. After a week in the hospital, she was coughing blood. Sepsis was recorded as the cause of death, her daughter tells us, but she fails to find the death certificate when she rummages through desk drawers. She adds that her daughter, a schoolchild then, fell ill at around the same time and was home two weeks from school. This, too, she believes, might have been from anthrax, though it was never diagnosed.

"A month later, samples of meat were taken from the refrigerator," Spirina's daughter continues. "They said they found germs. They telephoned me. Then the apartment was disinfected." She pauses, reflecting on the peculiarity of the episode.

Who telephoned?

"Sanitary epidemic officials," she answers briskly.

The whole family, Spirina included, was vaccinated, she said, at the nearby rubber factory. "But my mother died anyway." She pauses again. "And my son was born with a heart defect." Maybe future medical science will discover that anthrax (even in its vaccine form) causes severe side effects—like the arthritis Dr. Ilenko told us her sister suffers from or this newborn's heart defects. Right now, though, we are focused on fatalities.

Leaving Spirina's daughter, we take advantage of the proximity of other apartment buildings where victims once lived. A radio playing loud music and a barking dog are protecting the former home of Vasiliy Tretnikov, who died on April 16 at age fifty-two, but whose schoolboy photo is displayed at the cemetery. The nextdoor neighbors, a man and a woman, come into the hallway, with its cracked cement walls and uneven stairs, to talk with us while the dog keeps barking and the music blares. Vasiliy's son still lives next door, but he must have stepped out. Ilona jots a reminder to make another visit here.

According to this couple (and Abramova's notes), Tretnikov's case was one of the quick, virulent ones. On April 13, he developed a sudden temperature, and the next day he was taken to the hospital. "In two days it was over!"

But where had Vasiliy worked? We need to know where he was, both night and day.

He worked for a farm equipment factory right next to the ceramics factory; the neighbors are sure he was there in the beginning of April. They also have vivid memories of the buildings in their neighborhood being washed down at night with a greenish liquid and their being warned not to leave their homes until after 8 A.M. Again we note how the scenes of crews washing down buildings vary from one interview to the next. Sometimes the liquid is white or it is greenish, sometimes the crew is firemen or just factory workers. Sometimes the leaves wither and fall from the trees like an out-of-season autumn; sometimes they do not. The ceramics factory seems to have been the focus of the cleanup, but maybe other factories and apartment buildings were also sprayed. At the same time, roadblocks, posters, and radio broadcasts publicized the hazards of eating uninspected meat, and brigades of volunteers scrubbed floors and walls, confiscated the victim's sheets, took meat from kitchens, and distributed antibiotics. A massive vaccination campaign began. And, again, some men went around with rifles shooting dogs.

Yes, the couple agrees, this would all seem to be true, but they do not know what any of it meant.

We move on to find the family of Fyodor Nikolaev, age sixty-six when he died. In his cemetery portrait he looked like a war-weary soldier, with kind eyes. According to Abramova's notes, he was, like Anna Komina, one of the first to die in the epidemic, on April 9. She indicates April 7 as the date of the onset of his disease. An early case like this might tell us something important about the source of the epidemic. But the apartment has been sold by Nikolaev's son, who has moved away. The best we can do is to interview a nextdoor neighbor who says he was a friend.

"He fell down as he was leaving work," the neighbor tells us, adding Nikolaev to the catalogue of victims who died suddenly.

Where did he work?

"At Compound 19. But he refused to be diagnosed there. He went instead to Hospital 24."

Nikolaev with his kind eyes proves our first link to Compound 19. He might be one of the several men Burgasov referred to as workers there who died.

Our next interview produces a second link to the military. In yet another apartment in this area, we interview young Vladimir, the grandnephew of Taisa Mochalova, who died at age sixty-eight on April 16. Mochalova was his great-aunt, the sister of his grandmother; both women lived with his family. Vladimir was twelve at the time of the epidemic (thin and fair, he doesn't look much older than that now). He clearly remembers Aunt Taisa's last days. She felt fine in the morning, then developed a headache, stomach pain, and high temperature. The next day she was taken by ambulance to the hospital. "In one day, she was dead." We know from Abramova's notes that Mochalova, who suffered from stomach pains and difficulty in breathing, died quickly; her autopsy revealed she died of anthrax. Was she was another stoic—or do we not know the full story of her symptoms?

"She had a special burial," the boy says, and adds a detail that, once he says it, seems to embarrass him. "Someone we knew at the morgue let my mother in to dress her."

I envision yet another sad and unnerving scenario in this strange epidemic: the dutiful niece smuggled at night into the Hospital 40 morgue, carrying Mochalova's best dress. There she struggles to clothe the old woman's naked, incised body, which was probably among a half dozen corpses in the morgue that night. The necessary ritual is completed—but not really, because her aunt will be buried without returning home and without notice to families.

To get to these apartments we have wandered away from the center of Chkalovskiy, far from the homes of other pensioners who died in the outbreak and from the ceramics factory. Did Aunt Taisa work or visit elsewhere in the district?

"She used to work at Compound 32. She kept an apartment there and went back and forth a lot."

We take special note of this other military connection and ask Vladimir for any other details. Her remembers that local yards were disinfected, stray dogs were shot, and meat was taken from other families to be inspected, but not from his; they had none to eat at the time. His mother was vaccinated; he was too young for shots. His mother took care of disinfecting the apartment. She still has the death certificate, if we would like to come another time to speak to her.

What did he think was the cause of his great-aunt's death?

"Bacteriological weapons," Vladimir replies with assurance. "I've heard rumors about a colonel who committed suicide over it."

Indeed he has, in the neighborhood or from the press. In 1991, the Moscow journalist Aleksandr Pashkov (who also interviewed Deputy Minister Burgasov) wrote that the former commander of Compound 19, a General V. Mikhailov, committed suicide soon after, out of shame over the outbreak. In reality, the commander died of cancer. Apprised of this, Pashkov, one of Russia's more responsible journalists, retracted the story.[4] But the rumor was already broadcast. Today, the myth of the commander's suicide fits current animosity against the military much better than a death from cancer. It also explains away the military's silence about the outbreak. After all, how can the dead speak?

We meet up with Matthew and leave Chkalovskiy in the late afternoon, with two more interviews completed, for a total of six today, and many more preliminary contacts made. Back in the dormitory lounge, with the usual cups of dark tea, we three review the questionnaire. Eventually I pare it down to thirty basic inquiries, with emphasis on the onset of symptoms and also on the victim's whereabouts in the first week of April 1979—whether at home or at work or somewhere else. If she or he was on the job during the day, we will need the exact workplace address to plot it on a map of the city. To cross-check what we have learned, we pick out families Yampolskaya and I have interviewed so Ilona can interview them again.

Our time here in Yekaterinburg has disappeared in a flash. This last night, the sun refuses to set and let us rest. We have packed our equipment and notes. Matthew has wrapped in cotton the tiny plastic vials containing the soil samples he has gathered. Maybe I should have been more worried about him, since he was actually digging in the soil. I toss and turn about this. The year before, with the possibility he might be sent to Iraq to aid with weapons inspections, he received the first shot of an anthrax vaccination. (Fittingly enough, it was administered at the Institute Pasteur, where the first anthrax vaccine was developed.) But the follow-up shots never happened because he never went to Iraq. Did that anthrax injection do Matthew any good or any harm? Was he, is he especially susceptible in the first place?

Healthy mill workers were once reported to carry hundreds of anthrax spores in their noses and throats without incurring any infection.[5] Even before vaccines were developed, many more mill workers were exposed to anthrax than ever fell sick or died. Some two hundred thousand people lived in Chkalovskiy in 1979. Consider how few succumbed to anthrax. These calculations of risk bring me no comfort. I come back again to Giddens: it is the consciousness of jeopardy, not any numerical calculation, that stays with us and shapes our reflections.[6] One out of five children is liable to sexual abuse. Half of all college students drink enough alcohol to seriously injure themselves. More Americans have been killed in automobile accidents than in two world wars. We are living in the culture of risk that has brought us weapons of mass destruction and the ruination of the natural environment. From here it is an easy step for me to begin worrying about the safety record of Aeroflot. I remember the threadbare upholstery and the battered interior; I can almost hear the creaking wings of the plane, the jangle of unseen equipment as the plane rumbles down the runway. I have a sedentary nature; I loathe travel—but I love destinations. As it finally grows dark, I appreciate all the merits of remaining in Yekaterinburg. Running up and down seven flights of stairs and eating a diet mainly of instant soup and cucumbers has made me feel fit and muscular. I enjoy doing the family interviews. I know they are important. I don't want to leave.

Matthew, as usual, sleeps soundly, and at 6 A.M. he is ready for the airport while the rest of us are still stuffing clothes in our suitcases and searching for our plane tickets.

16

Moscow Redux

Sunday, June 14. We fly to Moscow, still on the hunt for information. Having accepted Dr. Burgasov's invitation to visit his dacha, Matthew, Hugh-Jones, Shelokov, and I drive there for a long afternoon meal. Burgasov's daughter and son-in-law are there, along with Dr. Vladimir Sergiev, who was Burgasov's secretary in 1979 and is now director of Moscow's Institute of Medical Parasitology and Tropical Medicine. It was Sergiev, who speaks fluent English, who accompanied Burgasov and Nikiforov on their 1988 trip to the United States. He was just a junior administrator at the time of the 1979 outbreak, the person, in fact, who took the telephone call from Sverdlovsk, probably on Monday April 9, as panic set in, and relayed it to Dr. Burgasov, who was in a meeting.

Now in his late forties, Sergiev is part of the transitional generation that was well-placed before the reforms (his father was head of the Institute before him) and now worries about the collapse in government funding for science research. We have already asked him if he feels Burgasov and Nikiforov were consciously lying when they presented the tainted-meat explanation to the American audience. Sergiev says that if they were, they never spoke about it to him. He thinks they probably believed it.

Burgasov's dacha is in the famous Barvikha enclave on the Moscow River. The family of the writer Alexey Tolstoy, among other celebrities, has a home on one of the rustic streets, where high fences separate the houses. Burgasov shows us around his large backyard, with rabbits in hutches and chickens running about. Two thoroughbred dogs, a brindled mastiff and a pug puppy, have free rein of the house and garden. As we stand outside, a train roars by, not more than fifty feet beyond the fence, and stops conversation. Burgasov comments he never even hears it; I take that to mean that he is alone with his thoughts a good deal and can shut out bad noises. On the menu is fish he has caught that morning and platters of fresh vegetables, dumplings, and fruit prepared by his daughter, a physician who, like Yampolskaya, specializes in infectious diseases. The vodka is local, one bottle has a raspberry flavor, another something like licorice, a third pepper.

For the first two hours, the conversation is nothing but pleasantries. Shelokov, apparently nervous about confronting the old deputy minister with details of our trip, diverts the conversation to Hugh-Jones's entertaining accounts of his veterinary adventures around the world, in many barnyards and corrals.

After lunch, on a walk to the nearby river, Burgasov, Matthew, and I have a chance to discuss (with Sergiev interpreting) the Abramova and Grinberg autopsy data. Burgasov shrugs off any conclusions that could be drawn from the autopsies alone. He still insists the full picture is in the missing manuscript he was writing with his colleague Dr. Nikiforov. While we were in Yekaterinburg, Burgasov telephoned the younger Nikiforov to urge him to return the contested manuscript and slides. The answer was no. Burgasov is disappointed in our failure to check out the veterinary documents, which he believes are key. As we stroll along the riverbank, pink, nearly naked Russians of all shapes and sizes are sunbathing on blankets spread over unruly grass. Children splash in the gray-green water and shirtless men fish from rowboats. It could be the 1930s. The pleasures look simple, but only the privileged enjoy this particular idyll.

Our first task on Monday is a visit to the American Embassy, where we meet up with David Walker and are checked through security to be debriefed about our trip. Matthew has us do this as a courtesy but also because it is an efficient way to communicate with government officials: Washington will soon receive a cablegram reporting about our trip. In a windowless cubicle that must be wired (our interlocutor takes no notes), all five of us review our findings. We are not invited to linger. No one brings in a tray of tea and cookies. The American government, it turns out, has other things on its agenda besides an old mystery set in the Urals. The embassy staff has its hands full understanding the day-to-day tumult of the new Russia.

That evening we dine at the Nikiforov home. The elegant apartment, full of stuffed furniture and bric-a-brac, also looks like a comfortable scene from the 1930s. Young Dr. Nikiforov's special pride is an eclectic collection of weapons: a small cannon from before the time of Peter the Great, a German helmet from World War II, shells from Afghanistan, and his grandfather's sword. "It's Russian steel," he says, pressing it across his lifted thigh, "and does not bend." And as the dinner ends, while we eat sponge cake, he shows us a rare and gruesomely graphic video-tape of a man dying of rabies. At our lunch two weeks ago, Hugh-Jones expressed an interest in seeing it. None of us expected to watch an on-screen death, but then our mission is nothing if not morbid.

After the film is over, Matthew and the young Nikiforov have a pri-vate conversation concerning access to documents from the 1979 out-break. Our host agrees we can have the thick clinical files of five sur-vivors on loan for our overnight reading. His father picked well; these are detailed records of people who went through the advanced phases of anthrax infection—and lived. Historically, they are gold. As the files are bundled up, I notice the grand old desk in his office, where the elder Nikiforov must have reviewed the Sverdlovsk material, where he must have spent some time preparing his 1986 Moscow presentations to Matthew and later to the National Academy group, and for Washing-ton and the American audience in 1988. In such a private retreat, with so many facts at his disposal, had he not a single thought about the pos-sibility of inhalation anthrax? Was it, as his son guessed, that Nikiforov could not speak his innermost thoughts in public, or were those thoughts absent from his consciousness?

The economist Timur Kuran identifies "preference falsification" as the act of misrepresentation under perceived social pressures.[1] It is strategic behavior we all engage in, out of fear of what others think. But in to-talitarian systems, where revealing what one believes can incur severe penalties, the individual may perceive no choice but to suppress private reactions. Moreover, as Kuran argues, living within a repressive system eventually corrupts critical faculties, bending them to lies and slogans and making some thoughts unthinkable. Standing in Nikiforov's living room imagining his life, I consider the risks had he dared accuse the mil-itary at Compound 19: the loss of his livelihood, the loss of this beauti-ful apartment, the risk of destitution for his family, the destruction of his son's career, danger for his subordinates like Yampolskaya and the other junior clinicians, and, finally, arrest, a trial, and a long imprisonment for treason, which with his physical frailty would have been a death sen-tence? Who in his place would have played the hero?

At the hotel, until very late that evening and then again early the next morning, Matthew and Shelokov transcribe information from those five thick files, the only complete patient records we have seen. Matthew packs this transcription in his suitcase and has the originals delivered back to Nikiforov's son. The files confirm dates of onset and admission (which we have in fragments from Dr. Ilyenko), details of clinical treatment, and the constant monitoring of victims in the special care unit at Hospital 40. The records also make clear that Dr. Nikiforov made repeated bedside visits to these patients. But nothing in them offers any definitive clue to whether the anthrax is inhalation or gastrointestinal. All that is sure is that each of these patients suffered severe systemic infection and somehow beat the odds of certain death. I make a note to e-mail the five names and addresses to Ilona so she can begin looking for these extraordinary survivors right away.

Tuesday, June 16, is our last full day in Moscow. Matthew, Shelokov, Hugh-Jones, and I have a mid-morning appointment at the Kremlin. At ten sharp, one of the side doors on Red Square opens, and we are invited inside by a nameless man in a somber suit. We follow him up two flights of broad marble stairs. The ceilings of the Kremlin halls are almost too high to see; they speak empire. But the stair-runner and hall rugs are threadbare, and the floors have been carelessly mopped. One of the halls leads to the office suite of the Councilor of the Environment and Health, Alexey Yablokov. Another, which we do not take, leads to the office of President Boris Nikolayvich Yeltsin, who is at this moment in Washington, about to address a joint session of Congress with a speech denouncing biological and chemical weapons.

We four visitors sit on the side of a conference table facing the view to Red Square. Such strong light comes from the high windows that I can see almost nothing but the glare off the top of the councilor's desk and off the table. The backlit minister and his assistant, Svetlana Revina, sit opposite us. Although Yablokov's English is good, Revina needs a translation, which Shelokov supplies.

Having listened to presentations from others for a week, I now begin my own by explaining that I have interviewed the families and neighbors of twenty-five victims and I feel that their tragedy—what they went through because of the outbreak—is an unresolved problem. I argue that the actual cause of the outbreak remains without scientific documentation and that the families in particular should know what killed their loved ones.

Unimpressed, Yablokov explains that Yeltsin ordered an investigation of the Sverdlovsk epidemic earlier this year, which Revina carried out. Really, he insists, the matter is settled. A recent decree from Yeltsin entitles the families of victims to extra pensions. Yablokov is personally convinced that the outbreak was caused by an accident at Military Compound 19, where research on anthrax was being conducted. When Matthew asks him why he believes this, he tells us that the only thing Revina's research unearthed was an empty KGB folder concerning Sverdlovsk, labeled, "Order to Confiscate All Documents Connected with Military Activity." That the folder was empty is proof enough for him that the military, despite denials, is responsible for the anthrax outbreak.

Proof enough? An empty folder? Apparently so. In December 1990, Yablokov tells us, the contents were destroyed by a top secret order of the Council of Ministers. He questions Matthew about why he is pursuing information on something that happened so long ago.

"It is important," Matthew replies, "for others to know that if they violate their obligations, they will eventually be found out."

Yablokov appears unpersuaded. His final words to us are, "It is time to close the book on this event."

My frustration with this dismissal lasts down the marble stairs and out into Red Square where tourists are lined up in the June sunshine to see Lenin's tomb. Since 1920, John Reed, who is my distant cousin, has been buried near here in the Heroes' Grave beneath the Kremlin wall. Although he contributed to Lenin's legend, he was suspicious of pomp and privilege. Had he lived, he might well have deplored Stalin's mummification of his hero and would probably approve of the reformers who now want to bury Lenin like an ordinary mortal. Stalin banned Reed's book on the Bolshevik revolution because it barely mentioned his role and made a hero of Leon Trotsky.[2] Now the book is available, but no one cares about the origins of the Soviet state. So much for history.

I am suspicious of presidential decrees. Yeltsin's in April awarding pensions to Sverdlovsk families proves nothing about why their relatives died of anthrax in 1979. What use is it that Yablokov's assistant has found an empty file or that he speculates the military caused the 1979 outbreak?

By decreeing that pensions will go to the Sverdlovsk victims' families, President Yeltsin may just be covering his tracks. As Communist Party boss for the entire Sverdlovsk oblast, he must have known something about activities at Compound 19. The local KGB, we understand, reported directly to him as well as to Moscow. If violations of the Biological Weapons Convention were ongoing at the military base, he should have known that. If KGB agents were confiscating records after the outbreak, he should have been advised and known why. Throughout the epidemic, he was there in his Sverdlovsk office.

Now, with government archives bursting open everywhere, the Russians are discovering and, fairly often, repudiating Soviet history. The process is not uniform, in large part because of the problem of present accountability for past actions. The murderers of the Romanovs, like their victims, are long dead. Reprehensible military activity for which those responsible are still alive and hold government offices is much harder to reveal. When he was the underdog and vying for government leadership, Boris Yeltsin bluntly expressed the dilemma: "One of the chief reasons [for restraining reform] is that a number of party leaders lack the courage to appraise in a timely and objective way the situation and their personal roles in it, to speak the bitter truth."[3]

Or—and this is equally possible—Yeltsin knows nothing except that the KGB file is empty, and he has taken a big broom (the decree awarding the pensions) to sweep away the past.

Either way, no one is taking responsibility for the victims' deaths. The book is closed, at least inside the Kremlin. No prince from Gogol's imagination is urging his officials who "still have a Russian heart" to seek honor. The past will bury the past, and the dead their dead. For now we have finished with Russia, and Russia, at least at the official level, is finished with us. For a nonofficial group, we have done well, and I feel our research has only begun.

Wednesday afternoon, June 17, we depart for the United States via Finland. Helsinki, with its immaculate parks, its healthy citizens boating in the summer sunshine, its unending supply of hot water from noiseless pipes, is by any standard utopian, but especially so compared to Moscow and Yekaterinburg. Yet, at our last dinner together, the team members are out of sorts. The piece of Matthew's luggage containing the crucial notes on survivors and other materials was mistakenly put on a plane to Germany and has only now, a day later, been delivered to the hotel. He is relieved, but the loss rattled him. Was the suitcase purposefully delayed and searched? Shelokov is sure of it, though the contents are undisturbed and nothing is missing. Hugh-Jones seems dejected that he never got to meet with any veterinarians. For someone used to jetting around the world to epizootic hot zones, for him the trip was long and unproductive. Walker is also irritated, believing that we have been repeatedly lied to, except by Abramova and Grinberg. My thoughts are on Ilona, who I hope is having success with the family interviews. And I wonder what explanation of the outbreak they will ultimately give us. As much as I would have liked to stay in Yekaterinburg to press on with research, I now feel relieved to be out of Russia. It was only two weeks, but more than I realized at the time, I felt the constant political tension of the great changes in process.

At the Helsinki Airport, as we wait to board the plane for New York, I pick up a stray copy of the *International Herald Tribune*. A front page article reports that Boris Yeltsin has publicly stated the military were responsible for the 1979 anthrax epidemic in Sverdlovsk. Timely reporting this, I think, perhaps in reaction to our investigation, about which he surely knew. Then, more modestly, I realize that we are in a phase of international agitation about possible Soviet violations of the Biological Weapons Convention. Yeltsin had to say something about Sverdlovsk if he was going to be in Washington. In fact, he made sure he went public on the matter before his meeting with President George Bush.

Unknown to us, on May 27, just before our expedition to Yekaterinburg began, the Russian newspaper *Komsomolskaya Pravda* published an interview with Yeltsin, in which he clearly acknowledged that there had been biological weapons development in Sverdlovsk and laid blame on the military for the 1979 anthrax outbreak:

(Interviewer): You knew about the development of bacteriological weapons in Sverdlovsk. But it was only recently that you first talked about it publicly. Why did you keep quiet all this time?

(Yeltsin): First, nobody asked me about it. And, second, when I learned these developments were under way, I visited [then KGB chairman Yuriy] Andropov. . . . When there was an anthrax outbreak, the official conclusion stated it was carried by some dog, though later the KGB admitted that our military development was the cause. Andropov phoned [Minister of Defense Dimitriy] Ustinov and ordered these production facilities to be completely scrapped. I believed that this had been done. It turned out that the laboratories were simply moved to another oblast and development of the weapons continued. And I told Bush, [British prime minister John] Major, and [French president François] Mitterand this, that the program was under way. . . . I signed a decree setting up a special committee and banning the program. It was only after this that experts flew out specially and stopped the work."[4]

Yeltsin's befuddled rendition of the cause of the outbreak, that "it was carried by some dog," suggests that he has not immersed himself in the details of the official Soviet explanation of the 1979 epidemic, which mentions dogs but nowhere has them as the cause of the epidemic. His so-

lution to the Sverdlovsk problem, to establish a committee and write a
decree, indicates good bureaucratic reflexes. President Yeltsin's interviewer, equally unclear about the official version, failed to have him clarify his understanding.

The Sverdlovsk incident raises the whole issue of the role of the military in Soviet (and now in Russian) politics and, by extension, its mandate to protect civilians. During the 1991 coup attempt the Soviet military's refusal to fire on the gathering crowds was pivotal in stopping
the takeover of Gorbachev's government and propelling Boris Yeltsin
to power. Who will forget the first democratically elected president of
the Russian Republic climbing on a tank in defiance of the Soviet government that had attempted to incarcerate its own president, Mikhail
Gorbachev?

But Yeltsin was cultivating the military even before the coup, when
he was jockeying for power with Gorbachev. In September 1990, Yeltsin
created an office for coordinating Russian defense and security affairs
with other Soviet Union ministries. "This gave him," political scientist
Robert Barylski writes, "a formal excuse to begin building political relationships with the senior military and KGB personnel."[5] And Yeltsin
made a point of contrasting his empathy for the military with Gorbachev's firm commitment to defense cuts. The date of the destruction
of the KGB file on Sverdlovsk is December 4, 1990, just when authori-
tarian forces in Moscow, in reaction to military unrest in the Baltic and
other Soviets, threatened to overwhelm Gorbachev. It is at this juncture
that Soviet Foreign Minister Eduard Shevardnadze resigned, with the announcement that democracy was failing and "dictatorship was coming."
As chronicled by reporter David Remnick, Shevardnadze's efforts to bro-
ker new relations with the west were undercut by the Supreme Soviet
and the KGB, which were reluctant to give up the Baltic States or otherwise accept reform, and the Soviet army was their agent in the field.[6]
The month after Shevardnadze quit, on January 13, 1991, Soviet tanks
rolled into Lithuania and soldiers attacked and fired at demonstrators in
Vilnius, killing 14 and injuring hundreds. Russians had already deserted
the Communist Party by the millions; those still members who were expecting a humane socialism were disillusioned. President Gorbachev never
recovered the political ground lost by the use of force against Lithuania.
Yeltsin, who accused him of precipitating a military dictatorship, called
for a public pro-democracy demonstration on March 28 that reactionaries tried to prevent with threats of armed intervention. But Yeltsin
carried the day peacefully. It was in this atmosphere of contention be-

tween reactionaries and reformers, with Yeltsin still as an outsider, but nonetheless a real contender for power, that the incriminating Sverdlovsk documents were purged.

Yeltsin's appreciation of the military would stand him in good stead in the August 1991 coup. With tanks positioned around Moscow, Yeltsin took to the radio and exhorted the troops: "At this difficult hour of decision remember that you have taken an oath to your people, and your weapons cannot be turned against the people."[7] The army ultimately backed him against the leaders of the coup, which included the minister of defense, and during Yeltsin's three sleepless days under siege in the Moscow White House, his supporters behind the barricade were in active communication by phone with military and with KGB allies.

In the aftermath of the coup, although Yeltsin instituted two committees to review military culpability, his real goal was to shield its leaders from prosecution and gain their gratitude, after making it clear that he had the power to terminate their careers. Thirty generals from the high command and 334 other officers were moved into retirement without scandal. Only the minister of defense, Dimitriy Yazov, and two other plotters suffered public disgrace.[8]

But the post-Soviet relation of the Russian military to President Yeltsin keeps evolving. Yeltsin cannot afford to antagonize his army, which is an important base of his power. He has promised its officers better salaries, better housing, and more professional status. At the same time, Yeltsin and his advocates for democratic reform are determined to reduce army personnel by half in three years and to use every other means to slash its budget, while at the same time keeping it at the ready against insurrections and coups. Politically he cannot afford to call army leaders into account about the Sverdlovsk outbreak.

No one individual or set of individuals has, in fact, been held responsible for the outbreak of anthrax. No officer has bowed his head in shame that such a tragedy, even if accidentally caused, took place on his watch. No one has come forward and taken blame for a violation of the Biological Weapons Convention at the Compound 19 facility. Is it because the military is innocent or because no one inside the base knew when or how the accident occurred? Did the Compound 19 commander, General Mikhailov, who died of cancer, take his secrets to the grave with him? Or is the silence from the military based purely on self-interest?

On June 10, the day after Yeltsin was in Yekaterinburg to visit his ailing mother (the same day we were denied travel outside the city), another article in *Komsomolskaya Pravda* reiterated the Sverdlovsk story.

An unnamed representative from Minister Yablokov's office tells the press what we were to hear a week later, that secret documents from Sverdlovsk were held in the KGB archives until December 1990, when a decree issued by the Soviet Council of Ministers ordered their destruction.

Still, as we finish our trip, it appears the Russians are willing to be more open about their military science capability. On June 12, *Izvestiya* reported on the first-time visit of a group of journalists to the Russian Ministry of Defense Microbiology Research Institute in Kirov. But the article also notes that one-third of the institute's employees have left because of its lack of funding. Not just the problem of no salaries beleaguers the enterprise; no money exists for the most fundamental necessities: heat, electricity, and research equipment. The situation is more difficult than a shift to peacetime production. The system is bankrupt and scientists skilled in BW research and development, and perhaps even production, could go to countries seeking a biological weapons buildup. The price of American assistance for demilitarization is sure to be that Russians become ever more open. But such revelations may not extend to the past or to the Sverdlovsk incident, which is a shame. Burying those civilian deaths under a presidential decree is too much of a Soviet-style strategy to bode well for future relations with Russia.

As we fly home, Boris Yeltsin's address to the United States Congress, guaranteeing that the Russian Federation will be completely forthcoming in its declarations of past biological weapons programs, is on the television news. "No more lies!" he swears with stolid dignity. But, as Supreme Soviet member Mishustina phrased it, the Sverdlovsk past is still knocking on the door of the present.

17

Names Go to Places

MAP BUILDING BEGINS

Soon after we arrive back in Cambridge, Matthew and I meet again with retired CDC epidemiologist Alex Langmuir, who has come to the mainland from his vacation home on Martha's Vineyard. Alex's concern about biological weapons goes back to the Korean War, when the U.S. army sought his advice on detection tactics and he publicly advocated civil defense measures against biological weapons. A large man with a great domed forehead, Alex acquired a reputation throughout his career at CDC, as well as at Harvard and Johns Hopkins, as a fierce and ready critic who brooks no fools, and as a distinguished researcher. He was also a member of the Chemical Corps Advisory Council, which oversaw the development of U.S. biological weapons (BW) programs. In the years following the end of World War II, as information about U.S. and British BW programs became public, the news media and members of the government were caught up in a frenzy that led, for example, to members of a congressional committee telling the press that a "germ proposition" sprayed from airplanes could "wipe out all life in a large city."[1] The 1948 Finletter Report to President Harry Truman advised that biological weapons were progressing so rapidly that it was "impossible to predict the future."[2] After the first Soviet nuclear bomb test in 1949, U.S. civil defense efforts focused on the threat of nuclear weapons, but Alex Langmuir hasn't lost his concern about the development of biological weapons or defenses against them.

He attributes his attraction to science to the influence of his uncle,

Irving Langmuir, who won the Nobel Prize in chemistry in 1932. Like his contemporary Dr. Burgasov, Alex found his vocation in medicine—though he never waited in any lines to get into Cornell's medical school. He wanted adventure, which is what public health and the CDC brought him. Along with scotch and late dinners, his stories—about misreported malaria cases, about a dangerously defective polio vaccine he helped track down, and about mysterious anthrax cases—become part of our days as he, Matthew, and I compile our data. Recently widowed, Alex seems to welcome this activity.

In 1986, when he read in the *Harvard University Gazette* that Matthew was still on the track of the 1979 anthrax epidemic, he immediately called to discuss where the project was going. In preparation for the 1988 visit by the Soviet physicians, he helped put together the panels of experts and served as the moderator for each of the presentations.[3] Alex is passionate about all matters investigatory. The three of us spend hours reviewing the photographic slides from Nikiforov and Abramova and Grinberg, which Matthew had copied. The autopsy data, though, is not enough by itself to tell us the source of the 1979 outbreak. To describe the full and complete anatomy of the outbreak, we need to construct the epidemiological map that addresses the essential questions of "when" and "where." Where were the victims, including the five documented survivors, at the end of March and beginning of April 1979? What was the exact timing of the event that exposed them to the disease?

To begin, we turn to the criteria for a case definition: who shall be included as an anthrax victim? We start with the KGB list that we received from Larissa Mishustina, and immediately find independent verification of it in the lists of patients that Dr. Ilyenko gave us. From the list of more than 110 names of people who were admitted to the various Chkalovskiy hospitals in April–May 1979, 47 are circled as having died. All but three of these names are on the KGB list. Other cases, like that of Aleksandra Chizhova, are verified neither by autopsy, the KGB list, or other detailed sources. For her case the interview narrative cannot count by itself. By careful cross-checks, we eventually establish which are our most reliable anthrax cases to map, the individuals who died from that infection and not some other cause.

Alex, Matthew, and I begin building two spot maps. In the first map we plot the victims' home addresses, presumably where they were at night. Home addresses within Chkalovskiy rayon are easy to locate, and the sticky red paper dots go down quickly. I know the streets—Lyapustina, Poldnevaya, Eskadronaya, Selkorovskaya, Patrice Lumumba—because

I have walked them. With our detailed street maps, we can even pinpoint exact house locations. But as many as a dozen streets, like Sovremennikov and Batalionnaya, are not on the map. And some of the addresses on the KGB list are unintelligible acronyms, like MSD34 and NII44. A flow of e-mail begins from Cambridge to Yekaterinburg, with requests to Ilona for clarification of these addresses and for relevant cross streets that will let us designate where on an unfamiliar block a house or apartment building or hostel is located.

Meanwhile, we plot twenty-two homes of victims squarely within Chkalovskiy, in the area near the ceramics factory and stretching northwest to Compound 19. We also locate twenty-one residential addresses scattered outside the district or at its far edges. A nighttime release of anthrax aerosol would seem to be excluded; those "outlier" victims presumably would have been at home. On our first take, it appears that— as Soviet officials maintained—about a third of the victims' residences are outside Chkalovskiy rayon, but we need more information from Ilona to be sure.

The second map we start is to show the daytime location of each anthrax victim in early April 1979. This task is far more frustrating. Using the first set of interviews and fragments of data from Abramova's notes and Ilyenko's lists, we piece together where each person was likely to be during the day, based on what we know about whether that person worked or was a pensioner, was disabled, on vacation, or otherwise likely to be at home. At first cut, six victims can be placed at the ceramics factory, two at construction companies close by; two older pensioners and one unemployed man were likely to have been at their homes in Chkalovskiy rayon. One worker, kind-eyed Fyodor Nikolaev, was at Compound 19. Another pensioner, Taisa Mochalova, was probably at her flat in Compound 32. At this point, still lacking information on many victims, I feel we are fumbling in the dark.

In late July, Ilona sends us a packet of material, brought to the United States by a relative of Professor Gubanov, the physicist who facilitated our invitation from the Ural State University. Her letter jubilantly announces that, using the KGB list, she has contacted or tried to contact relatives of all but nine of the sixty-four victims. The yield is gratifying. She has sent full interviews for twenty victims, including a replication of the one Yampolskaya and I did with Rema Dayanova about her husband, Fagim.

Ilona also returned to the former home of Anna Komina and interviewed her daughter-in-law, which gives us more information on this early victim. According to the daughter-in-law, Anna first fell sick on April 4 (as her son described to us). On April 6 a physician from the local poly-clinic was called in, but could discern nothing worse than a cold or the flu. Later, on April 9, Anna's cough grew worse and she began to spit up blood, and she was transported to Hospital 20, where she died at 6:35 A.M. April 10. We cannot ask for more precision than this.

In addition, Ilona has completed partial interviews at another eleven addresses, including some where Yampolskaya and I had reached an impasse. Through the neighborhood rumor mill, she also located the relatives of a Maria Chapaeva, who is not on the official list, but who is buried in Sector 13 at Vostochniy Cemetery. Despite these accomplishments, gathering the still missing information is vital. We e-mail Ilona our gratitude and send her more details to nail down.

The 1988 Soviet report claimed that thirty-two people (including seventeen cutaneous cases) who caught anthrax survived the 1979 outbreak. We have sent Ilona the names and addresses of the five survivors from the Hospital 40 records that young Dr. Nikiforov let us copy just before we left Moscow. From those records we know that these five patients were diagnosed with systemic anthrax (without cutaneous infection) and that their treatment with antibiotics and fluid management was intensive and prolonged. If Ilona can find any of these survivors and they are willing to talk, we will have unique testimony on the outbreak, from the perspective of the patient inside Hospital 40.

The cross-checks (the triangulation I have wanted) hold up beautifully. Of the twenty-two full interviews Ilona has sent, seventeen concern patients on the Abramova and Grinberg list; twelve of these seventeen are also on Dr. Ilyenko's list as having been patients at Hospital 24. No significant discrepancies appear between what relatives and friends recount and the information in the clinical records. And the dates of death given in both these sources generally agree with the cemetery data. The full and partial interviews indicate that some cases at the start of the epidemic (Komina and Nikolaev for example) did miss being autopsied, as Lev Grinberg suggested and as Dr. Ilyenko described. But nearly all victims, early and late, were buried in Sector 13.

The stories of individuals I thought we had lost emerge more clearly, and more voices of family members are heard. The son of ceramics worker Ivan Klyestov told how his father held off from being hospitalized and then lost consciousness in the ambulance. The son and daughter-in-law of Andrey Komelskikh, a pensioner who lived on Poldnevaya, described how busy the old man was before he became ill, puttying the windows on his garden hothouse. His first flulike symptoms abated, and then a high temperature and dizziness set in. He died on April 14, after being sick for three days.

As we had discovered during our time in Yekaterinburg, everyone worked, which sometimes interfered with care-giving. Ilona spoke with the wife of the young Alexey Syskov, who in his cemetery photo looked restless, as if ready to dash away on a motorbike. A welder, he lived in Chkalovskiy. His first symptoms emerged April 9; he came home after 4 P.M. from his day shift with a high temperature, labored breathing, and dizziness. His wife, who worked a night shift until midnight, called for an ambulance when she returned home. He arrived at Hospital 20 in the early hours of April 10 and died on April 11.

His contemporary, young Aleksandr Vyatkin, was a pipe fitter. He collapsed in the street April 14. His mother told how passersby thought he was drunk and called an ambulance to take him to a "sobering station" (*Vytrezvitel*) to dry out. But he was dead on arrival, and the doctor at the station sent his body to the Hospital 20 morgue.

The important role of friends who were also coworkers is frequently evident. The youngest victim, twenty-four-year-old Tatyana Kosheleva, taught at the ceramics factory kindergarten for four-to-five-year-olds, Ilona writes us. Her coworker, a nurse, was also a neighbor and friend. She called the ambulance for Kosheleva when, near collapse at work, the young woman complained of a high fever and difficulty breathing.

The most touching story about friends is that of Ignat Maslennikov, age forty-nine, who worked in the pipe shop at the ceramics factory. On April 8, he visited his friend Speridon Zakharov (the first name on the KGB list), who also worked in the pipe shop and was home sick, apparently with something like the flu; on Friday, April 6, a doctor at Hospital 24 had found nothing specifically wrong with him. Zakharov died April 9, at the age of forty-four, at Hospital 20 (where Dr. Klipnitzer was chief). Maslennikov helped Zakharov's relatives dig a grave at Isetskiy Cemetery, but authorities wouldn't allow the burial there. His illness was too suspicious. Maslennikov's wife, who gave this account, was a nurse at Hospital 24. When her husband then fell ill on April 11, she gave him aspirin and antibiotics. The next day, while he was at work, he felt worse and went to the ceramics factory clinic. From there he was taken by ambulance to Hospital 40 and died the next day. The two friends and coworkers, Zakharov and Maslennikov, were buried near each other in Sector 13 at Vostochniy Cemetery.

The eleven partial interviews leave us with only traces of those victims. For eight of the eleven, Abramova's cursory notes, cemetery data, and the information on the official list offer just glimpses of the lives lost. And for some of them, the information is strictly minimal. Pyotr Geptin, who lived on Selkorovskaya within a cluster of other victims, died at age thirty-nine. He was, according to the autopsy notes, a "classic" anthrax case and an "unemployed vagrant." We know that Yuriy Kramskoy, whose cemetery picture suggested a witty, charming young man, was a con- struction worker. He was admitted to Hospital 40 after having drunk "much vodka"(perhaps in an attempt at self-treatment) and died after twelve hours of intensive therapy, including a blood transfusion. Like Kramskoy and Nikolay Khudyakov, forty-two-year-old Mikhail Lavrov was a factory worker who lived in a local hostel. He died in the ambu- lance before reaching Hospital 40, perhaps another stoic. Anastasia Myasnikova, aged sixty-three or sixty-four in April 1979, lived alone and died alone, with no medical records left behind; she is barely re- membered by the neighbors in her apartment building. The same is true for Vitaliy Fyodosov, age forty-eight. He lived in an apartment about fifteen kilometers to the north of Chkalovskiy rayon, on the boulevard named for Yuriy Gagarin, the space-age inheritor of Valeriy Chkalov's heroic mantle. So far as we know, Fyodosov has no one left to remem- ber him.

At the very end of this contingent of the forgotten is the "unknown male" autopsied by Abramova and Grinberg and buried anonymously in Vostochniy Cemetery. Found dead on the riverbank in Chkalovskiy on April 18, all that is noted is that he was "not an old man."

Ilona soon informs us by e-mail that MSD stands for the Motor- strelkoraya Diviziya (Motorized Rifle Division) located within Com- pound 32. The address NNI44 refers to Compound 19's Scientific Re- search Institute (Nauchna Isledovatyelskiy Institut); and Sovremennikov street is likewise not on our map because it is inside Compound 19. Now we can place Valentin Borisov (no relation to Professor Borisov), who is on the KGB list of victims and worked or was a soldier at the base, and six other victims (three at Compound 19 and three at Compound 32).

Not all the missing streets can be found. The city's topology has changed in thirteen years, as some areas disintegrate and others emerge. The city's older housing is disappearing as Yekaterinburg begins eco- nomic as well as political reconstruction. One victim, Boris Zheleznyak, who died April 8 at age thirty-eight, lived north of Chkalovskiy. Ilona writes us, "It is impossible to find his relatives, because the street [Bata- lionnaya] itself doesn't exist any more." The houses on the street were torn down, and the two remaining corner buildings were given new addresses on the adjoining avenue. In another example, victim Nina Yasinskaya's apartment was apparently turned into part of the local library. In Abramova's notes, she is described as a "classic" anthrax case, but here too there is nothing that will help us plot her daytime location.

As the summer days go by, we have to exclude some cases whose daytime locations cannot ascertained. For example, Vasiliy Ivanov, who is on the KGB list, is described in Dr. Ilyenko's notes as working at an unspecified meat factory and living near Compound 19. He may be the anthrax victim the director of the meat factory said was laid off at the time of the outbreak, or maybe that wasn't Ivanov at all. Unable to verify his daytime whereabouts, we leave him off the map.

We also hear from Ilona that four names have been added to the official list, bringing the total (including the anonymous man) to sixty-nine. The first addition is Filipp Dyedov, the seventy-two-year-old man whose widow Yampolskaya and I interviewed in her cottage in Chkalovskiy. The widow and her son had not then heard of the Yeltsin pension decree, and our theory is that they applied to Larissa Mishustina's office to be included on the official list. Two other additions are a man and woman from Compound 19, Aleksandr Zhelnin and Valentina Tischenko. Zhelnin was twenty-six when he died. We have no record of where he was buried or what hospital treated him, when he became ill or when he died. Tischenko was thirty-two. Again, her name has not surfaced on any other list or record. Their inclusion brings the total number of anthrax deaths at the military compounds to nine.

The fourth addition is Galina Sergeyeva, who lived in an apartment north of Chkalovskiy rayon. She was fifty-five when she died and might already have retired and therefore been at home in early April. But we have no cemetery marker, no autopsy notes, no date of death for her. All we know is that she is on Dr. Ilyenko's list of patients who died, which is not enough information to plot a daytime location.

As the summer proceeds, the red dots of residence locations for the dead and the survivors form no uniform pattern, although enough cases (thirty-six) cluster in Chkalovskiy to suggest a focal point there (see Map 1). Twenty-four home addresses are outside the area, and we are still unsure where ten victims of the 1979 outbreak (including two survivors) lived.

By e-mail and in packets delivered by travelers from Yekaterinburg, information continues to come from Ilona, who is making steady progress finding information about daytime locations. We ask her to check in each

interview about night-versus-day factory shifts, in case we have to re-
verse a victim's location. So far, Ilona has located just one night worker,
Anna Komina, who according to her daughter-in-law, worked on the difficult midnight-to-8 A.M. shift and also on weekends, with Mondays off.

Again, nearly everyone worked and worked hard. Ceramics factory
employee Vera Kozlova was one of the few women employed in the pipe
shop, where Dr. Arenskiy described the work as "back-breaking." At
sixty-seven, Andrey Komelskikh, the retired man who was repairing his
greenhouse, also worked as a janitor at the ceramics factory. And sixty-
seven-year-old Sophia Bliumova, we learn from Ilona, lived in a apartment on the boulevard Selkorovskaya, well within Chkalovskiy rayon,
and worked as a cleaning woman at the adjacent supermarket.

Two men we thought might be related are not; they just happen to
have the same last name and patronymic. Pyotr Vasilyevich Makarov
lived and worked at Compound 19. He was thirty-seven when he died
on April 16, when the outbreak had reached its peak. Ivan Vasilyevich
Makarov, who died on April 24 at age forty-seven, worked as a pipe layer
for a construction company near the center of Chkalovskiy. Both men
were autopsied by Abramova and Grinberg and judged "classic anthrax"
cases by laboratory tests and pathoanatomical observations. Pyotr may
have died at Compound 19, with his body transported to Hospital 40
for autopsy.

We concentrate on determining what difference there was between the
victims' daytime and nighttime locations. We have to reckon with some
twenty people who appear to have both lived and worked outside
Chkalovskiy. Then there are those who lived outside and who commuted
into the area to work. As the weeks go by and we process the interview
data, the number of anthrax victims known to have worked days at the
ceramics factory reaches eighteen. Of these, thirteen traveled to work from
their homes outside or at the edges of the district. We still need to get
more precise information on the location of other industries where workers spent their days. More e-mails from Ilona clarify some street locations in Yekaterinburg, and we continue plotting the victims' homes and
workplaces dot by dot. Some cases remain ambiguous, like that of Nikolay Vostrykov. In 1979 he lived and worked outside Chkalovskiy, but he
was employed as a driver, making deliveries all over the city. With no better information that this, we plot his location at his outlier workplace.

The survivors Ilona contacts corroborate what we heard from relatives and friends of the victims who died and from public health officials.
From the families' perspective, the system for treating patients was, if

not "German" in its rigor, at times highly impersonal. Galina P., who worked as head of a kindergarten on Selkorovskaya, felt the symptoms of anthrax in mid-April and was admitted directly to Hospital 40. Her husband recounted going there to see her and being told she had died. Indeed, he saw her name on a posted "list of the dead." Fortunately, by asking more questions, he soon discovered his wife was alive. Her records may have been confused with those of man with a similar last name, a seventy-four-year-old pensioner not on the KGB list and not autopsied, but buried at Vostochniy Cemetery, where his grave marker is almost illegible. In Ilyenko's handwritten records, this man's address is the same as Galina's. We add him to the roster of unknowns.

Another survivor, Nikolay Y., also worked in the tile shop at the ceramics factory; his memories of the outbreak are vague. He recalled that out of a hundred on his crew, three died, but he doesn't remember the names. Just twenty-eight when he fell ill, he was treated first at Hospital 24, then admitted to Hospital 40, with a diagnosis of double pleurisy.

While doing her interviews, Ilona discovered two survivors not on our lists. Maria F. and her son Valeriy were ceramics factory workers. Maria worked in the cafeteria (as did Aleksandra Chizhova) and on April 13, at work, she fell ill with chills, fever, and joint pains. She called the doctor on duty at the factory's clinic and was taken home, but then immediately the decision was made to take her to Hospital 40. She was still there three weeks later when, on May 9, her son, who worked in the tile shop, was admitted to the same intensive care division with the same symptoms. His was a curious clinical case. He had received two of three inoculations against anthrax, one around mid-April when the program started, the second ten days later. He took the tetracycline distributed by the public health brigade at the time his mother first became ill. She was in the hospital three months. He remained for twenty-one days, perhaps helped by the antibiotics, vaccinations, and his youth. He was twenty-nine at the time, and his mother was fifty-six.

Another survivor from the ceramics factory, Nikolay K., at first refused to be hospitalized, even when his wife insisted. The second call for the emergency ambulance came when he had a high fever and was vomiting blood. After twenty days of aggressive therapy, he was discharged.[4]

Two more survivors offered stories that placed them well outside Chkalovskiy in early April, adding to our list of outliers. One, Anatoliy S., lives in the rayon very near the ceramics factory. In 1979 he was a metal press worker at TechRubber, a factory outside Chkalovskiy. He fell ill May 12 and was taken by ambulance to Hospital 40 on May 14.

Ilona conducted the interview with his daughter, who said her father remains reluctant to talk about the outbreak. Apparently in March and early April 1979, he and his family had traveled on a vacation to Leningrad. When he returned, he began building a bathhouse in his backyard. But when did he return? The date remains unclear.

Another survivor, Nina T., lived near the ceramics factory, on Poldnevaya. In 1979 she worked as a baker at the Forest Industry Machinery Plant north in the rayon. She left at five each morning and was gone all day. Her early morning departure took her away from the district well before some dozen ceramics workers, who also contracted anthrax, arrived for their 8 A.M. shift.

From Dr. Nikiforov's clinical case histories that we read in Moscow, we know that both Anatoliy S. and Nina T. had near-fatal anthrax. But where did they get it? This and other puzzles about victims' locations continue to trouble our map-building.

With the strong possibility that the outbreak was caused by an emission from Compound 19 always in my mind, I have often wondered during the months of our research about the motivation of the scientists and technicians inside the compound. Anonymous letters, reportedly written by its scientists, to editors of the newspaper *Izvestiya* proclaimed that the work was patriotic and that, regarding Sverdlovsk, "accidents happen."[5] Anthropologist Hugh Gusterson's study of physicists at the Lawrence Livermore Laboratory in California showed that they were able to do research on the ultimate weapon by similarly sidestepping the moral issue of whether such weapons should even exist. They also recast the pain of those killed or injured (for example, in the 1945 bombings of Japan, in animal and human tests, and in workplace accidents) into scientific tabulations of symptoms, as if the pain were not real. In this way, they severed the connection between weapons use and the suffering of those attacked.[6] Scientists involved in developing biological weapons for the United States, that is, before 1969, had the same commitment and worked in the same military science environment. But the BW experimental agenda was of a different order. Nuclear weapons testing sometimes included exposing animal and human subjects to radiation. BW testing was focused entirely on bodies and biomedical reactions. It went far beyond laboratory and open field tests to include simulated attacks on cities and towns, as mentioned earlier. The entire experimental legacy is dismaying, from the hundreds of dead monkeys at Fort Detrick to the spectacle of Seventh Day Adventist soldiers, the vaccinated volunteers in Project Whitecoat, strapped to chairs amid cages of animals in the Utah sunlight as Q fever aerosols are blown over them. Most chilling are the mock scenarios played out in urban areas: light bulbs filled with simulated BW agents being dropped in New York subways, men in Washington National Airport spraying pseudo-BW from briefcases, and similar tests in California and Texas and over the Florida keys.[7] Meanwhile, real pathogens were being produced, "weaponized," and stockpiled, ready for deployment on the real target, the people in Soviet cities.

The offensive intent of the U.S. BW program against civilians was made explicit when its retired commander, General J. H. Rothschild, published his book *Tomorrow's Weapons* in 1964. In it he proposed that in the event of a Soviet conventional arms attack (that is, an attack that did not use nuclear or chemical or biological weapons) on Western Europe, aerosolized brucellosis bacteria disseminated over the Soviet Union could halt the aggression. His plan was to target the Western Urals and assume a casualty rate of 30 percent: "Everything would stop. It would require the maximum effort of the population to take care of the ill, transport sufficient food for its own needs, keep utilities in operation, and maintain sanitary measures, so that the support required by the field forces would be impossible."[8]

Earlier, during the period from January to September 1953, the U.S. St. Jo Program tested versions of this attack scenario in and near three cities—Minneapolis, Minnesota; St. Louis, Missouri; and Winnipeg, Canada. These three areas were selected for "tracer tests relating to the physical aspects of aerosol cloud diffusion" because they were "considered to include the range of conditions as regards climatology, urban and industrial development and topographic features likely to be encountered on the more important potential target areas of the U.S.S.R." The report on the tests goes on to describe the various types of test areas (open fields, riversides, residential clusters, and the densely populated downtown), with distribution of the bacillus from single-point sources, multiple-point sources, and line sources at elevations from about three feet to forty-five feet above ground level.[9] The intended agent was anthrax in bombs.

The morally repugnant aspect of the St. Jo tests is that civilians' lives are the explicit physical targets. Not buildings, not soldiers in gas masks, not battleships or battalions, but ordinary, unprotected people are to be (and would have been, had the order been received) assaulted by invisible pathogens. More than knowledge about biology, aerodynamics, and bombs, BW attack planning by any state program requires a complete suppression of imagination about the medical consequences for civilians, which itself shows the significant loss of a moral compass.

Should the targeting of civilians as if they were "logs," in the terminology of the Japanese during World War II, surprise us? Military technology in the twentieth century seems at times like nothing more than the relentless development of ways to attack defenseless populations. By mid-century, the capacity of powerful nations for massive aerial bombing and the development of nuclear missiles obliterated the on-the-ground distinctions between soldier and noncombatant that were recognized in the wars of earlier centuries. With such indiscriminate lethal weapons, the foot soldier and the civilian are equally at risk and equally devalued.[10]

The American offensive BW program is long gone. The superpowers are reducing their nuclear and chemical stockpiles, and Russia is moving (or lurching) toward demilitarization of the Soviet BW investment. Still, the physical debris of the superpower arms race is massive: the junk piles of old nuclear weapons, dangerous stores of plutonium, abandoned silos, and leaking canisters of nerve gas. Years before that arms race was declared over, a new weapons competition had already begun among other, less powerful nations, vying with each other for either nuclear weapons superiority or chemical and biological weapons capacity. New border wars, religious wars, ethnic wars, and campaigns of terrorism— all have involved civilians as pawns and targets. "Informalization" in the world arms trade, that is, the circulation of weapons through new private markets, is characteristic of end-of-the-century militarism; it is a new, global "second economy" that eludes international control.[11] In the post–Cold War world, biological weapons, relatively easy and cheap to produce, retain the essence of the dreadful phrase "weapons of mass destruction." Its presumption is that humans in the aggregate—with no regard for individual worth or sensibility—are expendable. And the complex processes of life are the target.

Biological Weapons and Political Outbreaks

On July 2—too soon after we are back, I feel—Matthew and I travel to the Brookings Institution, a think tank in Washington, D.C., for a presentation on our work. Elisa Harris, a policy analyst there, has scheduled the event, with the cooperation of John Steinbruner, director of the Brookings Foreign Policy Studies Program. Harris is one of the best critical thinkers in the chemical and biological weapons (CBW) field and has followed the Sverdlovsk case from before the 1988 visit of the Soviet physicians.[1] This meeting, on a broiling day in the nation's capital, brings together the members of the American team that visited Yekaterinburg, plus a dozen experts on biological weapons from a variety of organizations, including the CIA, the U.S. Arms Control and Disarmament Agency, the United Kingdom's Porton Down biological defense facility, the National Academy of Sciences Committee on Security and Arms Control (CISAC), and the National Institute of Allergy and Infectious Diseases.

Alex Langmuir is there, along with Joshua Lederberg from Rockefeller University who has been part of the Sverdlovsk discussion since 1980, and veterinarian David Huxsoll, former commander at Fort Detrick and now dean of Louisiana State's School of Veterinary Medicine (where Martin Hugh-Jones is a professor). Also in the group that day at Brookings is Dr. Donald Henderson, now medical science advisor to President George Bush. At the Centers for Disease Control, he worked for twelve years for Alex Langmuir, who was grooming him to take over his position. Instead, to Langmuir's chagrin, Henderson left to lead the World

Health Organization campaign for the global eradication of smallpox. In 1988, Dr. Henderson, then dean of the School of Public Health at Johns Hopkins, was a generous host to the visiting Moscow physicians and opened their presentation to the university community at large.[2]

At the meeting, chaired by Steinbruner, Matthew begins with an explanation of his own involvement in the Sverdlovsk investigation, from 1980 to the present, and of how he arranged the team's study trip. He then summarizes the series of interviews we had with public health officials and physicians, which indicate rapid mobilization of the public health service but offer no clear evidence for the source of the outbreak.

After Matthew, the team's pathologist David Walker discusses Abramova and Grinberg's materials and shows slides of what he believes are the most important lesions in some of the forty-two autopsy cases from 1979. He argues that the autopsy materials are conclusive evidence of inhalation anthrax, based on two assertions. First, each of the autopsies showed hemorrhagic destruction of the thoracic lymph nodes and hemorrhagic inflammation of the mediastinum, the area between the lungs. He points out that the route the macrophages take in transporting anthrax spores out of the lungs is directly to the thoracic lymph nodes. There is, he argues, no documented spread of B. anthracis to these nodes from the intestines. Second, he asserts, hemorrhagic lesions in the intestines of thirty-nine victims were caused by the spread of bacteria through the blood stream directly from the gastrointestinal tract, not from tainted meat infecting the gut. To illustrate this point, he shows slides of anthrax bacteria in the small blood vessels at hemorrhagic sites in the wall of one victim's intestines. He also compares several slides of infected lymph nodes and thoracic tissue from human and chimpanzee inhalation anthrax cases with several from the 1979 cases, noting their similarity. He explains the lesions in the mesentery lymph nodes seen in nine of the forty-two Sverdlovsk autopsy cases as secondary to—that is, coming after—inhalatory infection. And he refers to the pathology text by Davidovsky (which Abramova and Grinberg also rely on), which states that most such gastrointestinal lesions can be due to inhalation and cutaneous infections.[3]

Following Walker's presentation, I describe the interview part of the investigation. My first assertion is that the interviews are proving remarkably trustworthy, giving me the cross-checks I wanted. The dates and other details we have from families and neighbors accurately match the information from the cemetery and from autopsy and other records. All nine interviews I have for victims who were autopsied closely match what Abramova noted about when and how they fell ill. In nearly all instances, death came within a few days after high fever and dizziness set in. The survivors of systemic infection are, of course, the amazing exceptions. Whether there were, in addition, subclinical cases, we cannot say. Once anthrax bacteria are released in the body, the chances of serious illness and death seem very high.

The interviews also confirm the organized public health response that officials described: the volunteer brigades going house-to-house to disinfect homes, distributing antibiotics to the victim's family, and procuring meat samples, and the use of Hospital 40 as the main treatment center. The vaccination program, the efforts made to wash buildings and to pave roads, and the official appropriation of the victims' bodies were also confirmed by interviews. It was the police, not the army (as mistakenly reported in the Western press) that transported coffins and cordoned off Vostochniy Cemetery. Sometimes the system worked imperfectly. At least two bodies were mistakenly sent home and then retrieved. Some number of victims died at home, in the street, or in ambulances, either misdiagnosed or with a sudden onset of severe symptoms. With this, as with any epidemic, the question of whether surveillance could have been better always arises after the first cases are definitively diagnosed. The fear, panic, and resignation of local residents is implied in this description of the 1979 outbreak.

In the discussion that follows, reactions to the autopsy data, our most important find, are mixed. Impressed but apparently not convinced, a CIA expert comments that with such advanced systemic infections as found in the Sverdlovsk cases, Walker's logic may be questioned.[4] Lederberg raises the question of how solid this new evidence about the Sverdlovsk outbreak is. Could the pathoanatomical material have been fabricated? Could the interpretation of the evidence—that it shows inhalation anthrax—be mistaken? Getting corroborating information from my interviews, he says, will be critical. Thomas Monath, former chief of virology at Fort Detrick and now a vaccine company executive, agrees about the importance of the interviews for corroborating the autopsy and other data.

Of course, Alex Langmuir also agrees that the interviews are crucial, but he has no doubt that inhalation anthrax is demonstrated by the autopsy data. He has confidence in Abramova and Grinberg's materials, in large part because Walker ultimately had good professional relations with the two pathologists: they trusted each other. Langmuir points out that, given what we know now, it appears likely that the victims were exposed either by an anthrax aerosol at the ceramics factory or by an emission from Compound 19. It is important, he believes, to discover if our "outliers" (people who were far from either site) have links to one or the other.

The dates of the animal outbreaks, whether they preceded or came after the initial human anthrax cases, remain unresolved. All we have are conflicting or vague accounts from local officials, accounts from Soviet journals, and Dr. Burgasov's documents.

Afterwards, I ask Donald Henderson two questions. One is whether he thinks Dr. Burgasov would lie about the tainted-meat explanation. He replies it wouldn't surprise him, though in 1988, when he hosted Burgasov at Johns Hopkins, he believed that explanation was plausible. He tells a story about Burgasov. Once smallpox was eliminated in the Soviet Union, the deputy minister had a terrible time getting the health service to stop giving inoculations against it. Lenin himself had decreed them and there was no going against Lenin, even three decades after his death. But Burgasov, by carefully working the system, had eventually prevailed, and the Soviet smallpox vaccination program was discontinued. The point of the story, which Burgasov told Henderson with pleasure, is that one had to work the system.

My other question is whether Henderson thinks we can ever pinpoint the time of exposure to the anthrax spores. He optimistically explains that precise interview data is the key. The answer lies in ascertaining where each victim was in the days just prior to the start of the outbreak—then the pieces of the puzzle should fall into place. Ah, I think, easier said than done.

While we are in Washington, we also get an update from Elisa Harris and other arms control experts on Russian efforts to come to terms with "transparency," that is, with revelations of past and present weapons programs. The new Russia has quickly evolved from a coercive state for which secrecy was essential to every aspect of power to a state struggling with administrative discretion, with what government should or should not disclose. "Every government has an interest in concealment; every public in greater access to information," philosopher Sissela Bok writes.[5] In matters of national security, every state maintains its "Top Secret" classifications. But now, with the end of the Cold War, among former enemies weapons of mass destruction are no longer protected by the shields of secrecy. Transparency with regard to nuclear weapons, though, has been more successful than with chemical and biological weapons, and of these two, BW development in laboratories that have double use (that could be producing pharmaceuticals, for example) present the most difficult obstacles to disclosure. The former Soviet Union may have had a long history of exploring BW, going back to the 1930s,[6] but eliciting historical facts even from the new Russia is a difficult process. And even if the Sverdlovsk epidemic is finally laid at the door of the military, we may never know except by inference whether Compound 19 activities were permissible vaccine research or violated the Biological Weapons Convention (BWC) with aggressive agent testing and munitions development.

In his address to the U.S. Congress in June 1992, President Boris Yeltsin expressed a deep commitment to getting rid of both programs. Soon after he issued a decree, "On Priority Measures for Implementing Russia's Obligations in Destroying Chemical Weapons Stockpiles." The decree created a Committee on CBW Convention Problems and gave it two months to submit proposals for the creation of a phased system to destroy chemical weapons. The first stage is the conversion of several chemical weapons factories to the production of agent-detoxification products. Later, he affirmed, these products will be used for peaceful purposes (e.g., antiseptic, anticorrosion, and fireproofing)—swords into plowshares. The U.S. plan to incinerate its chemical weapons is already underway.

In fact, the loss of chemical and biological weapons to an arsenal may be no great loss at all. Strategically, they present problems that conventional weapons do not. A major one is time delays. For instance, no BW produces the immediate destructive effect of an explosive shell or a bullet. It takes time for a disease to incubate before it harms a victim; the same is true of many chemical agents. Moreover, CBW agents cannot be turned off. They remain active and beyond anyone's control. A lethal aerosol cloud, for example, will continue to travel downwind, whichever way the wind blows. With conventional weapons, if the shell or the bullet fails to hit a target, more might be used. But as Julian Robinson describes in one of his volumes on the subject: "With CB weapons, where there is no such immediacy, there may be corresponding uncertainty about whether things are going ahead as planned. And if there is doubt, the decision about whether to use more weapons is made more difficult by the possible dangers of overdosing a target with CBW agent"[7]—among them finding one's own troops are suddenly downwind. On the other hand, as Robinson also points out, the indiscriminate nature of chemical and biological weapons, what makes them weapons of mass destruction, also makes them especially appropriate if the aim of the attackers is insidious or clandestine.

In the West, Cold War suspicions about Russian biological weapons persist. On July 4, two days after our Brookings' debriefing, the Unification Church's *Washington Times* reports that in secret debriefings in 1990 a Soviet defector to Britain, a high-level scientist in a BW program, "caused Western intelligence to more than double its estimate of Soviet (and by extension Russian) biological weapons production capabilities and the number of BW storage facilities run by the military."[8] The defector is later revealed to be Aleksandr Pasechnik, former director of a Leningrad Biopreparat facility, the Institute of Ultra Pure Biological Preparations. Biopreparat is the massive Soviet archipelago of pharmaceutical laboratories within which, it is becoming apparent, secret work was done on biological weapons.

In late 1990 Mikhail Gorbachev responded to the Western anxiety Pasechnik generated by inviting American and British experts to spend two weeks inspecting four Biopreparat research facilities. By the experts' estimate, the facilities had production capabilities clearly in excess of any legitimate work. The experts also concluded that these facilities had extensive military connections. Biopreparat was held to be a commercial cover for research in violation of the Biological Weapons Convention. In 1992, representatives of Merck & Company, the international biomedical corporation, drew similar conclusions—that is, that the facilities were set up for suspiciously extensive production, though such activity appeared to have ceased by that time.

In sum, in 1992 the United States and Great Britain remain dissatisfied with Russian BWC compliance. Would Yeltsin ever admit to the full scope and size of the former effort? More important, is he sufficiently in control of military officials who might want to keep parts of the Soviet program intact?

On August 31, after we are back in Boston, the *Washington Post* reports at length on more American dissatisfaction with Russia, with quotes from State Department officials. It also quotes a United Nations official's statement that the Russian BWC declaration of information is long overdue. Past offensive BW programs and present biodefense activities should have been reported in February.[9] The United States, Great Britain, and Canada had submitted theirs by mid-April (late but not too late), and some twenty-eight other countries have also filed their reports. The Americans, British, Canadians, and French have all cited previous offensive work and outlined their defensive programs (for vaccines and protective equipment).

But it is soon clear that the UN spokesman quoted by the *Post* made a mistake. The Russian declaration actually was submitted to the United Nations almost two months before, on July 3. Moreover, the Russians claim that this new declaration gives a wealth of details about the Soviet BW program. As submitted by the Russians, "Form F" admits "research and development" of biological weapons after the 1972 convention banned development. It describes a BW program beginning in the late 1940s "as a response measure," and specifically mentions Sverdlovsk, along with Kirov and Zagorsk (now known as Sergiyev Posad), as places where work was done on anthrax and other diseases, such as tularemia, brucellosis, typhus, plague, and Q fever. This work included outdoor aerosol tests on Vozrozhdeniye (Resurrection) Island in the Aral Sea as well as laboratory research. "In the mid-1960s, experimental enterprises were built to investigate the feasibility of mass producing biological agents at facilities in Sverdlovsk and Zagorsk. These enterprises had appropriate divisions: a section to produce culture media, a cultivating, concentrating and purifying section, a sewage treatment plant, and other supporting technical services."

But, the Russian statement goes on, "Military biological agents were never produced or stored at these facilities. If required, and by special government order, these plants could have been used for their production." The report specifically mentions that in the 1970s, the scientific research and testing structures at these facilities, including Sverdlovsk, were improved to "a high degree of biological safety" and states that "All work with biological agents was conducted in strict compliance with required medical and public safety measures. Personnel were protected by immunization, by group and individual protection equipment, and by air purification and sewage treatment systems. The safety of processed air and environmental cleanliness was continuously monitored."[10]

What looks like six pages of detail to Russians is, however, much too vague by Western standards. Confidence-building relies on precise listings of agents, quantitative data about production, facility descriptions with floor plans, and other such detail, rather than general statements. On the plus side are Yeltsin's 1992 announcement that Russia has withdrawn its proviso to the Geneva Protocol retaining the right to use retaliatory BW; the cessation of BW testing at the Aral Sea facility; and a presidential decree of April 1992 "banning any work in the territory of Russia that contradicts the Biological Weapons Convention." The statement repeats several times that conversion to peacetime industry is the goal and mentions that the plan for the former Sverdlovsk facility (Compound 19) is to produce modern antibiotics. Still, there is concern in Washington that the new Russian government—or part of it—may be holding back.

On their part, the Russians complain that the Americans are not responding to their proposals for a mutual verification program, that they have twice proposed to the United States a joint commission of experts that would check the information available on both sides on bacteriological weapons research. But, the Russians say, Washington is not cooperating.

Whatever the cause of the logjam, it appears to be broken on September 11, when a trilateral agreement is struck between the United States, Great Britain, and Russia to reaffirm commitment to the BWC. At this point, President Yeltsin invites outsiders to again visit the St. Petersburg Biopreparat facility named by the defector Pasechnik. The rest of the agreement throws open the doors of former Soviet facilities, at least in theory, in exchange for inspections of Western laboratories.

At a news briefing about the agreement, Major-General Valentin Yevstigneyev, Deputy Chief of the Defense Ministry Radiation, Biological, and Chemical Directorate, expresses the hope that the BWC will become more precise about what is prohibited or permitted at biological facilities. "But were all suspicions about us groundless?" he asks. "I have continued trying to ascertain. Alas, not all. In the mid-seventies, on the orders of the top leadership, well-protected premises were constructed at certain pharmaceutical enterprises. There was no doubt about their purpose. Due to space reconnaissance, their existence at once became an open secret. These are real facts. Nonetheless, what is called 'forbidden activity' was to a considerable extent connected precisely with the military-technical appraisal of work performed abroad, in connection with the potential for producing bacteriological weapons there."[11]

What the general means by "work performed abroad" is the Soviet belief that the United States never gave up its extensive biological weapons program. In 1969 President Nixon renounced biological weapons, and by the time the Biological Weapons Convention entered into force in 1975, U.S. BW laboratories were shut down or converted to defensive research (for example, on vaccines), and stockpiles were destroyed by autoclaving and burning. But the Soviets feared that the program had merely gone underground. In fact, a 1976 Senate hearing made public the fact that the CIA had independently kept some BW capability into the early 1970s, a defiance of orders said to have infuriated Nixon. Project Whitecoat, which used vaccinated army volunteers for tests on a long list of diseases, ended only in 1973. In addition, with every new advance in American biotechnology, with yet another article about the cellular biology of anthrax or other potential BW agents, the Soviets may have seen signs of a weapons breakthrough that would leave them in the dust.

In 1992, another Russian defector, this one formerly a high official at Biopreparat, confirms General Yevstigneyev's statement about Soviet competition with what they believed was an ongoing U.S. biological weapons program. In his debriefings by American Intelligence, Dr. Ken Alibek (a Kazakhstan native known in the Soviet Union as Kanatjan Alibekov) describes his own firm belief and that of his superiors that the United States kept its program alive after 1969 and that patriotic duty required keeping the Soviet program competitive. Alibek held this belief until, in 1991, he headed a delegation that toured Fort Detrick, as well as the former BW production facility at Pine Bluff, Arkansas, and other converted sites, and realized he had been competing with an illusion.[12]

Meanwhile, as scientific exchanges continue, it is increasingly evident that covert Soviet laboratory work on BW was extensive. In November 1992, British and American experts again visit the St. Petersburg facility. The official Russian position is that until May 1992 research was carried out there on a strain of plague but that this research effort was not offensive in nature, just exploratory. The visiting experts refrain from judgment; no offensive research seems in process now. But the Soviet Union had multiple biological facilities, often in remote areas. Whether the former "Evil Empire" has created biological Darth Vaders and Death Stars remains a question. And where unemployed Russian biologists will take their skills in a global market for arms proliferation is a most troubling question. The "Terminator" may still live or, in being dismantled, may prove even more dangerous.

The videotaped interview that Dr. Burgasov was complaining about last June airs in September in Russia. A retired counterintelligence officer, General Andrey Mironyuk, also interviewed, states flatly that a researcher at Compound 19 switched on a ventilation system without switching on the filtration system and caused the 1979 anthrax outbreak. To which Burgasov replies, "Let's believe this counterintelligence agent: the ventilation was not working. But how long was it not working? An hour, two, or three? A day, two days, or three? But not one-and-a-half months! And why would this ventilation [accident] affect only the people outside the facility, and only the doomed Chkalovskiy rayon, where it came down and infected all the people? This is outrageous! Completely outrageous!"[13]

Manifestation

Back in Cambridge, Matthew and I continue building our spot map of the daytime locations of anthrax victims just before the outbreak. We are getting more precise in placing our red dots as Ilona continues to send us better addresses and place names. Correlation of the interview data with conclusions from the autopsy data also affects the placement of dots. Two outliers on the KGB list, Vladimir Lyzlov and Vitaliy Buchelnikov, apparently did not die of anthrax. According to Abramova's notes, Lyzlov, a truck driver, succumbed to a heart attack and Buchelnikov to pneumonia. Maria Chapaeva, Ilona's discovery, was diagnosed as having died of acute gastroenteritis, not anthrax. Her death certificate, issued April 15 from Hospital 40 data, indicates gastrointestinal hemorrhage, supporting this diagnosis.

We also continue to corroborate the public health response as described to us by officials. We have garnered information from thirty-five death certificates and find that those for early cases (April 9–11) were signed either at Hospital 20 or at Hospital 24. Starting April 12, as Dr. Klipnitzer, Dr. Arenskiy, and others told us, the cases shift to Hospital 40, as attested by the later victims' death certificates. I had suspected that giving the cause of death as pneumonia or virus or the like was a cover-up, but these diagnoses appear only in the early cases. Once deaths were being recorded at Hospital 40, the cause is routinely described as "sepsis," a reference to the overwhelming infection from which the patients died. It was well known locally that anthrax was the disease. Dr. Nikiforov, who was in charge of clinical decisions, probably had little difficulty choosing the most general category of infection, rather than a specific kind of anthrax (gastrointestinal or inhalation), thereby ignoring any possible problem about the outbreak's source.

Meanwhile, as our map-building continues, an important fact about incubation in inhalation anthrax comes to light. The presumption that anthrax kills quickly, within days after exposure, has pervaded analysis of the 1979 outbreak, whether the disease was believed to be gastrointestinal or inhalatory. The expectation was that victims either ate infected meat or inhaled anthrax spores and died within at most a week's time. Yet for inhalation anthrax, we now discover, the incubation period can be much greater than has been recorded for gastrointestinal anthrax; for some individuals, it could be more than a month.

The explanation of the extended duration of the epidemic, which had from the beginning confounded intelligence experts, may lie in the capacity of anthrax spores to remain dormant in the lungs for extended periods. A 1956 British article showed that in monkeys anthrax spores can remain dormant as long as one hundred days after aerosol exposure, as revealed in autopsy.[1] Someone involved in the pre-1969 BW program would probably have known about this research, which was published in a prestigious journal, and also about research done in the United States that showed this same phenomenon.[2] Perhaps demilitarization at Fort Detrick and elsewhere affected institutional memory about anthrax aerosols; even the records of the many nonhuman primate studies done in the 1950s and 1960s have been lost. Or the shift to a molecular biology paradigm, starting with the work of Harry Smith in the mid-1950s, may have distracted attention from the primate studies and incubation. In any event, belief in quick incubation lent plausibility to the Soviet infected-meat explanation. While we are working on our map in Cambridge, new monkey experiments by Colonel Arthur Friedlander and his colleagues at Fort Detrick, Maryland, show that inhaled spores deep in the alveoli of the lungs can take as long as fifty-eight days to develop into the lethal bacterial form.[3]

Therefore, no prolonged consumption of meat, no second aerosol emission or exposure is necessary to explain why the Sverdlovsk outbreak lasted for weeks and not days. Instead, the crucial factor would have been the interplay of the dose inhaled, the general state of an individual's resistance, and chance. We understand now that inhalation and intestinal anthrax differ in the potential span of the incubation period. Nonetheless, once severe symptoms begin, both forms are likely to prove fatal within a matter of days.

The process of mapping the Sverdlovsk victims' daytime locations is like developing a photographic print, but very slowly, as if one were stuck in the darkroom for weeks before an image emerges. By late autumn, we know that twenty of our outliers worked in Chkalovskiy, not merely in the district, but near the military facility or the ceramics factory to the southeast. Another twenty-six people were at home or worked in local industries within the same area. While the map of addresses shows a scattering of individual victims, the map of the likely daytime locations of the same begins to manifest a distinctly nonrandom pattern.

In early November, Alex Langmuir is with us when we first see the outline of a discernible band of cases stretching southeast across Chkalovskiy. When I recognize the pattern, the hair goes up on the back of my neck. I have never worked in a laboratory or done any research where visual information emerges to confirm a hypothesis. It has always been words that make the case. But here the words, what we were told in interviews, are being transposed into what may become a graphic image of a specific event in time, and not just an ordinary event, but of violent, collective death.

Alex is the only person I know who can sound both hearty and grim at the same time, as if he relishes tough facts and would rather have them, thorns and all, than easy theory. When he sees the emerging outline, he exclaims, "Well, here it is! You're getting results!"

Matthew, who has been meticulous about placing the red dots, fixes us drinks, and we sit in the living room, slightly stunned, somewhat satisfied, but not what anyone could call joyous.

At this time we are also seeking to correlate the result of our map-building with information on wind directions in Sverdlovsk just prior to the outbreak. Some years before, as part of his early investigations, Matthew acquired this data for March 26 to April 30, 1979. Major airports around the world report atmospheric conditions every three hours to the United Nations World Meteorological Organization in Geneva. One of the reporting airports, even in 1979, was Koltsovo, the principal airport for Sverdlovsk. Matthew was able to obtain the information from the National Center for Atmospheric Research in Boulder, Colorado, which archives the UN data; he arranged to have it sent electronically to his office computer. For most of the days in late March and early April 1979 wind direction in Sverdlovsk was variable; the exception is April 2, when

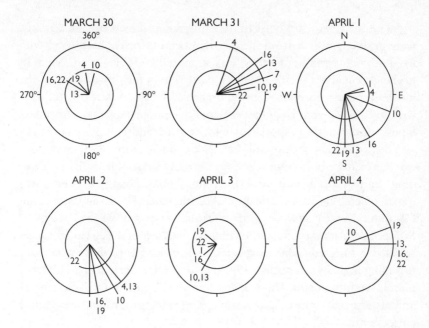

FIGURE 2. Wind directions and speeds reported from the Sverdlovsk Koltsovo airport for the period March 30 to April 4. Numbers at the downwind end of each line are the local standard times on a 24-hour clock. The inner and outer concentric circles designate wind speeds of 2.5 and 5.0 meters per second, respectively. Archived data are from the National Center for Atmospheric Research, Boulder, Colorado.

the wind blew steadily from the northwest. (See Figure 2.) If we are, in fact, dealing with an aerosol, the distribution of the victims' daytime locations would reflect the wind pattern at the time of exposure.[4]

"Liars" is what Alex calls the Soviet physicians who visited in 1988. Knowing the wind data and now seeing this map, he is willing to dismiss any tainted-meat explanations as bunk.

Yet we have the responsibility to be absolutely sure of our conclusion and not ignore any important information that does not fit. For example, as many as twelve victims were outside Chkalovskiy on April 2, 1979. We must explain how they could have contracted anthrax, whether it was the intestinal or inhalation form, or discover if they died of some other cause. Eleven men lived and worked far outside the district. The elderly Klaudia Spirina (whose daughter we interrupted at her ironing) is also an outlier. All, as far as we know, succumbed to anthrax. But how? Again, as far as we know, none of these cases are linked by dates or location or any common characteristic we can yet decipher.

In addition, two survivors of the outbreak, residents of Chkalovskiy, were probably absent from the district in early April. Anatoliy S., who lived near the ceramics factory, was supposedly in Leningrad. Nina T., his neighbor, spent the day making pastries in a factory canteen to the north. Yet their hospital records, preserved by Dr. Nikiforov, indicate without a doubt that both had suffered from noncutaneous anthrax. Is it possible that anthrax spores somehow spread randomly across the city?

The problem of the animal outbreaks, to which more than one official in Yekaterinburg bore witness, continues to trouble us. Did the animal deaths precede and cause the human ones, possibly by the burning of infected carcasses? Did animal deaths caused by an emission from Compound 19 cause later gastrointestinal cases among the citizens of Sverdlovsk? An epizootic in the villages southeast of the city might have resulted in infected meat being eaten by some subset of those who died, including perhaps our outliers. Spirina, after all, reportedly had infected meat in her refrigerator. This scenario appeared logical to Dr. Ponomaryev and also to the 1980 U.S. government working group, and we cannot ignore it now.

On December 2, 1992, Major-General Valentin Yevstigneyev is back in the news, being interviewed about BW programs formerly run by the once little-known Fifteenth Directorate of the General Staff, which he used to head. Once sixty-five hundred people worked for it, he says; now that number is halved. The enormity of the operation, old or new, raises eyebrows in Washington. About biological weapons the general says,

> At times we have reproduced some of them in order to conduct a military-technical evaluation. Before the [BW] Convention was signed, we studied how we could use our delivery equipment and load it with special loads. We called them mockups for biological agents. No special stocks were created. . . . The offensive program did not require a large amount of money—after all, it was not an accumulation of arms but a series of research projects."[5]

Behind the scenes, Russian defector Ken Alibek is telling U.S. intelligence that, even after the 1972 Biological Weapons Convention, the Soviet military was engaged in massive offensive development and production. He himself directed the phantasmagoric facility (six stories high and two football fields long) at Stepnogorsk, in Kazakhstan, where anthrax was produced in fermentation vats of twenty thousand liters each.

Although it is highly unlikely the Sverdlovsk facility ever approached that magnitude of production, trying to calculate a potential dose, the amount of spores that may have been released from Compound 19 in 1979, occupies Matthew and Alex for hours. They consider how best to calculate the amount: whether it should be measured in kilograms, as U.S. intelligence still insists, or whether it was considerably less. At issue here is volume production. Was the laboratory at Compound 19 producing vats of anthrax in volumes suitable for filling bombs? Even kilogram amounts could have no peaceful purpose. Or were their scientists engaged in vaccine experiments with considerably lesser amounts? Was there a violation of the BWC or just routine vaccination research that got badly out of hand?

Alibek also testifies that Soviet military laboratories were experimenting with manufacturing exotic diseases, so-called "chimeras"—for example, combinations of plague and smallpox. By agreement with the World Health Organization, Russia still maintains a reservoir of smallpox at its Vector facility in Novosibirsk, a fact that unnerves all who hear word of Alibek's allegations. After the eradication of treacherous smallpox from the world, will it now reappear as a biological weapon? Alibek's testimony raises other questions that have troubled Western observers. How aware were top Soviet scientists of the requirements of the 1972 Biological Weapons Convention? How aware were past political leaders of prohibited biological weapons research in remote corners of the huge Biopreparat conglomeration? How widespread are BWC violations now?

The other well-known Soviet defector, Aleksandr Pasechnik, offers little assurance that all was or is or will be well in his former homeland. His own laboratory staff worked on improving biological weapons munitions, but he insists that he knew nothing about this being a possible violation of the convention. Apparently, entire Soviet institutes were doing one or another aspect of biological weapons work, but in the absence of the actual hardware for weapons, their scientists may have thought their activities did not violate the BWC. Pasechnik recounts discussions "about the possibility of using biological preparations in various military actions, including subversive activity . . . because it can be produced fairly easily and applied in such a way that it could be very difficult to discover. . . . Terrorists might introduce it into a city and then deny it." At the same time, he characterized the BW enterprise as slow to overcome scientific hurdles and as functioning with "the inefficiency typical of bloated secret bureaucracies in the Soviet system."[6]

There is some suspicion in the West that in the late 1980s Mikhail Gorbachev, even while he was reducing size of the military, tolerated foot-dragging from sectors involved with chemical and biological weapons. Boris Yeltsin is regarded by Western intelligence sources as even less in

control of far-flung military facilities than his predecessor,[7] not an encouraging thought if Russia has inherited a BW behemoth.

While the United States and Russia wrangle over issues of transparency, the United Nations Special Committee (UNSCOM) for investigating Iraq's arsenals is translating piles of documents on Saddam Hussein's biological and chemical weapons arsenal. Anthrax, botulin toxin,
and nerve gas were all being produced for weapons use. The bombs are
described, the missiles intended to deliver them are identified, and the
tests for aerosol delivery (using everything from using vacuum cleaners
strapped to small planes to a more feasible Italian crop duster) are documented. Iraq's 1988 use of nerve gas on Kurdish villages is on the record,
and there is evidence that it was prepared to deploy anthrax in missiles
on Israel during the Gulf War. The U.S. government suspects that other
hostile states, such as Iran, Libya, and North Korea, are also invested in
CBW. The era of biological and chemical weapons as the "poor man's
nuclear weapons" could be in the future, with all its connotations of
destabilization. Even Israel, not a party to the BWC, is suspected of having a BW program at a secret facility at Ness-Ziona, outside Tel Aviv.

The bipolar hostilities of the Cold War were politically simple compared to the numerous sources of conflict emerging in their wake. Although the information is not revealed until later, other destabilizing
forces are at work, each a bizarre offshoot of international conflict. In
the spring of 1992, just before our investigation began, the doomsday
cult Aum Shinrikyo ("Shining Truth") established a base in Moscow,
bought a radio station there, and successfully recruited tens of thousands
of Russians into the sect. The promise of the apocalypse, a great and final
destruction of the world, appeals to post–Cold War Russians who lived
with nuclear threats just as it does to the Japanese converts, whose nation in 1945 was defeated by nuclear conflagrations. Funded by its converts worldwide, Aum Shinrikyo developed ties and training grounds in
Australia, Germany, Taiwan, and the former Yugoslavia. Its agenda included making weapons of mass destruction; it moved heavily into the
production of anthrax spores and botulin toxins and conducted experiments with aerosol devices and radio-controlled drone aircraft for spraying targets.[8] It even sent a contingent of forty members to Zaire to acquire Ebola virus.[9]

The phenomenon that the Central Intelligence Agency calls "blow-
back" is equally unnerving. During the 1980s the CIA, the British intelligence service, and the Saudis covertly supported the *mujahideen* ("holy
warriors") in its opposition to Soviet forces sent to Afghanistan in an at-

tempt to protect Soviet borders after the fundamentalist revolution in Iran.[10] When the Soviets finally withdrew in 1989, the still-armed warriors, infused with the spirit of *jihad*, or holy war, developed a global mandate and vowed to aggressively carry "their message back to the very groups that previously supported their revolutionary goals."[11] Their recruits are legions of impoverished young Moslem men, deracinated by war, with no future but firing AK-47s or setting off bombs. What if, like the Aum Shinrikyo, their leaders should explore the possibilities of biological warfare?

The same destructive, militaristic agendas are evident among members of the United States' own antigovernment cult groups, the Posse Comitatus, Aryan Nations, and scores of small militia and white supremacist groups whose literature glorifies mass destruction. Will their hostility find expression in biological weapons? One group, the Minnesota Patriots Council, is known to have planned the use of the deadly poison ricin to kill government officials.[12] More such attempts at terrorism may be in the offing.

In this atmosphere of potential hostility, loose ends about the 1979 outbreak continue to frustrate us, especially concerning Compound 19. In January 1993 Matthew travels to Moscow for an arms control meeting and is able to arrange an appointment with Major-General Valentin Yevstigneyev and several of his military colleagues, including Colonel Nikifor Vasiliev, who was stationed at Compound 19 in 1979.[13] Matthew shows them a satellite map of Sverdlovsk and asks for a precise indication of where the anthrax laboratory in Compound 19 is located. Without hesitation, Vasiliev takes a pencil and marks a building about one kilometer southwest of the main gate. He tells Matthew that he was working on anthrax. Mainly the research was on vaccines, but some experiments in very small quantities were done with virulent strains. "There were many strains in the Sverdlovsk collection," he says. "All but the vaccine strains were destroyed at the time of the Extraordinary Commission"—around April 12, 1979.

But General Yevstigneyev, who arrived as scientific director of Compound 19 in 1984, has his doubts that the military was the source, although aerosol chambers were used there to test vervet monkeys and baboons injected with STI anthrax vaccine. The maximum used in such a test, he insists, was no more than forty milligrams (0.04 grams, around 40 billion spores), and he believes that no such challenge tests were done, at least according to records, in late March or early April 1979. Besides, as in the United States, the laboratory was maintained at a P3 safety level.

Its rooms were hermetically sealed, with negative pressure recorded by manometers; a special filter and ventilation system controlled the release of any aerosols from the chamber. The filtered air, Matthew is told, was released at roof level, three to four meters above ground.

The general also mentions that six anthrax victims were treated and cured at Compound 19 by using high doses of horse serum. Another, Pyotr Makarov, died (we know that he was autopsied at Hospital 40) and was buried in Sector 13. The military, he says, was never asked to be involved; the public health officials ran their own show.

The general says that he accepts the possibility that there were inhalatory cases and the necessity of considering that Compound 19 could be the source of the 1979 outbreak. But he says that military calculations about the event, based on atmospheric diffusion models, suggest otherwise. These calculations indicate that if the compound were the source, the largest number of cases would be clustered near it, rather than three kilometers away at the ceramics factory. That is, there should have been a much more rapid fall-off of fatal human cases with distance from the compound than was reported. He also believes there is evidence for some gastrointestinal cases. And he is concerned that the burning of anthrax-infected carcasses may have generated infectious aerosols. In all, he regards no explanation of the epidemic as proven.

In the spring of 1993 we put together a working draft of a paper on the interview findings and their match with other records. The line of cases describing what we now think of as a danger zone between Compound 19 and the ceramics factory, extending toward the city limit to the southeast, is enough to suggest an aerosol plume from the compound, probably on April 2. But still the dozen outliers confound this explanation.

In May 1993, Dr. Lev Grinberg brings the entire array of samples from the 1979 autopsy cases to David Walker's pathology department in Galveston to subject them to electron microscope, immunochemical, and other modern modes of analysis. Soon he sends us news that one of our outliers, Klaudia Spirina, may not have died of anthrax and should not be plotted on our map. In 1979, Abramova recorded that no bacteria were found in either Spirina's blood or tissue samples. But *Bacillus anthracis* was difficult to culture in the Yaroslavl cases in 1927 and often eludes detection; therefore, the lack of bacteria in this case was not taken as conclusive. On the basis of autopsy findings, Spirina's case was diagnosed as anthrax and included in the English summary, just published in the March *Proceedings of the National Academy of Science*, although Abramova and Grinberg had some doubts. Alex Langmuir, too, was skeptical about Spirina's case. When he reviewed the 1992 notes Walker made at the Pulmonary Unit, he immediately recognized that a particular lesion atypical of anthrax was found in Spirina and penciled in, "Was this anthrax or some other bacteremia and toxemia?"[14]

Grinberg will be in Texas for six months and may discover other revisions; eight cases, for which culture tests and histology were negative or lacking, were attributed to anthrax solely on the basis of autopsy observations. This news about Spirina underscores the elusive nature of certainty in medical science or any science that attempts to capture complex reality. It also reinforces the importance of our mapping venture.

Matthew and Alex continue to debate the dosage question. And how do we figure the virulence of anthrax strains in this wind-borne scenario? Strains used for vaccines should be attenuated and relatively innocuous, but the testing of vaccines requires truly virulent strains. Were the scientists at Compound 19 working with an experimental, more deadly strain of anthrax? When Joshua Lederberg met Dr. Nikiforov in Moscow in 1986, he asked him what strain affected the victims, and Nikiforov replied it was just the usual "garden variety," which was why, he said, he saved none of it.[15]

Loose ends still abound. In addition to our outliers, who seem to have been nowhere near Chkalovskiy on April 2, we have no accurate reckoning from SES (the Sanitary Epidemiological Station) of the total number of people who might have been in the Chkalovskiy danger zone on that date to compare to the number who died. The veterinary documents Burgasov gave us remain unverified, languishing in a file. We never drove to the villages where animals were supposed to have died. We have never been inside Compounds 19 or 32. As far as we know, only nine people resident at the military bases were affected during the outbreak, plus perhaps the six more mentioned by General Yevstigneyev. But why, when the two bases together had as many as fifteen thousand residents, would so few get sick? Do military officials have anything to tell us now that almost fourteen years have passed? We never made an official visit to the ceramics factory, where as many as eighteen anthrax victims were employed.

Science is forever incomplete, as Claude Lévi-Strauss advises, especially when it attempts to capture complex human behavior.[16] Yet the Sverdlovsk incident is as much about morality and political accountability as science. We want better answers to our questions.

In August, 1993, Matthew and I pack our notebooks and the preliminary draft of our article and head back to Yekaterinburg.

Mirage

THE ANIMAL OUTBREAK

The second trip to Yekaterinburg goes more smoothly than the first, although it begins with an exercise in calamity. In Moscow, our driver picks us up promptly at Sheremetyevo Airport, but as we drive away, an impenetrable fog bank descends, blocking all vision. All other fogs I have seen in my life have a vaporous, wispy quality. This one is thick potato soup; nature (and pollution) are against us. Our driver rams the car in front of us and is immediately rear-ended by the car behind us. Having been in a taxi accident in New York some years before, I feel all the horror of being hurtled forward, but we are only roughly jostled by the double impact. In a few minutes the fog lifts, and we see ahead a line of ten other stalled cars, most of which quickly pull away into traffic. But our driver insists we abide by the law and wait for the police to arrive. An hour goes by. We share Snickers bars (I have brought a five-pound supply for Professor Gubanov's son in Yekaterinburg). Automobiles, buses, and trucks zoom by. The terrain around us has the dreary flatness of outer Moscow. From this moonscape protrudes a giant X, the sculpture of an iron tank trap that is a monument to how close Nazi forces came to invading the city in 1941. Two airport policemen in a car stop to tell us we are over the city line and need Moscow police. After another two hours, with no police in sight, we muster our resolve and drive off. Ten minutes down the road we find a police station, where our driver and one of the policemen light up cigarettes, talk about life, and then get around to filling out the necessary report, which omits our having left the scene of an accident.

Yekaterinburg is more manageable. We know the city, and there are no fogs, except the metaphorical ones around our research. The data we want are specific and, we think, available. Matthew and I check into a suite of rooms in Gastinitsa Oktyabrskaya, the centrally located and relatively opulent "Hotel October" we were bumped from last year. The greatest advantage we have in our quest, as it has been from the beginning, is having academic colleagues who believe in research as much as we do. Our arrival here last year would have been impossible had not a groundwork of cooperation already been laid, for example, by exchange programs like the one that brought Donald Ellis from Northwestern to Sverdlovsk in 1979 and the visit to Fort Detrick where Matthew and Dr. Alexey Yablokov met in 1990. Any group considering a similar verification exercise will have to lean heavily on international colleagues or face tremendous obstacles.[1] Of course, perestroika made all the difference in allowing our team to make its initial inquiry, but as private citizens with a mission, where would we have been without the support of Counselor Yablokov, Rector Suetin, Professor Sergei Borisov and his son-in-law Sasha, Professor Shepetkin, Larissa Mishustina, and Ilona Nikonova? In a parallel fashion, the professional trust between Dr. Walker and his Russian counterparts, Drs. Abramova and Grinberg, made it possible for the 1979 Sverdlovsk autopsy data to gain the wider international audience it deserves.

From Professor Borisov, we have the impression that Yekaterinburg is becoming increasingly open, as Western and Japanese companies aggressively seek deals to capture the region's resources, which include not only its minerals and ores but its technical elite, who have to find new ways to cope with the decline in military research. Meanwhile, the economy is in a period of great uncertainties; institutional salaries at all levels have not been paid for months.

Yet life goes on. In the past year, Ilona has married a young physician, and their baby daughter, Tatyana, was born just a few weeks before our arrival. A new colleague from the university, Irina Belaeva, will help us with interpretation, while Ilona, still on the track of outliers, uses her home telephone to reach the victims' families. Irina's English, like Ilona's, is superb and her specialty is biology, an invaluable asset for our inquiry. Just forty, with a teenage son, she is a comfortable person to be with, quietly perceptive and yet spontaneous, too. As with Olga Yampolskaya and Ilona, I feel quickly confident that we can manage the interviews that still have to be done. The first of these will be in the countryside, at Abramovo, the farthest southeast of the villages where we know animals died of anthrax in 1979.

Before Matthew and I drive south into Sysertskiy rayon with Professor Borisov and Irina, we meet with the present chief veterinarian of the city SES, Vladimir Krasnoperov, at his sparely furnished office on Rosa Luxemburg Street. This is not the rayon chief veterinarian who last year turned Matthew, Hugh-Jones, and Shelokov out the door, but an official at the next highest bureaucratic level. We have a simple request, that he look at the five pages of veterinary documents Dr. Burgasov gave us and tell us if, to the best of his knowledge, they are authentic. From his first words, he distances himself from the 1979 events by explaining that at that time he was stationed in the eastern part of the Sverdlovsk oblast, two hundred kilometers away. "All I know about the outbreak," he says, "is from our radio and television." He seems to chide us for the fourteen-year gap between the event and our present inquiry, to want it impress upon us the uselessness of our questions. The person who could have helped us, he says, was another SES veterinarian, a man who died last November. He reminds us that this past May, former SES Director Babich also passed away, taking with him to the grave the full account of his experiences in 1979. "Today," he comments gravely, "it is difficult to judge; we are not accurate or objective."

Krasnoperov silently studies the Burgasov documents. He has absolutely nothing on his desk, not a scrap of paper or a pen, and his eyes seem equally empty. We sit motionless, like obedient schoolchildren. It is one of those situations in which there is nothing to do but watch the dust motes collide in the morning sun. He might very well judge the documents pure rubbish, and we will be back at square one with the animal outbreaks.

After a full five minutes, Krasnoperov finally speaks. He tells us that he recognizes the names and signatures of the veterinarians in the documents: the city's chief veterinarian at that time, another man who was the meat factory's veterinarian and another who worked for the city SES. In response to Matthew's direct question, he says, "The documents are authentic because of the signatures of these specialists." So at least we have gotten that confirmed.

When Matthew offers to copy the documents for the SES archives, Krasnoperov dismisses the offer with a wave of his hand. "It is not important now," he says. He is more concerned about how his agency can get good vaccines now that the Tblisi factory, the old source in Georgia, is no longer part of Russia.

We then drive down past Chkalovskiy and take the highway south toward Chelyabinsk. After we pass miles of deep green forest, the landscape suddenly breaks open to field after field of sunflowers, their heads tilted up to the brilliant sky. Although they are an industrial crop, there is something wondrous about whizzing along through the high yellow blooms at their peak.

The village of Abramovo is no more than a hundred cottages in a small valley near a pond. Its dilapidated little brick church has grass growing on the roof. Geese waddle across the dirt roads. Except for a few parked cars and the many television antennas, it could be one of the villages described in Gogol's *Dead Souls*, "a string of huts, looking like old timber shacks, covered with gray roofs with carvings under them, that resembled embroidered towels" and from whose lower windows "a calf stared or a pig poked its small-eyed snout."[2] The garden plots are bursting with cabbages and tomatoes, and brilliant zinnias hang over wire fences.

In 1979, Abramovo had its own sovkhoz, or state farm, and local veterinarian, and the records for April show five households had anthrax-infected animals, the most and earliest cases verified by tests. As we walk the road in search of the documented addresses, a drunken man, his jovial face aglow with sweat, introduces himself as Mikhail and bares his broad hairless chest to show us the tattoo of a crow, the artwork of a fellow soldier. It should have been an eagle, he tells us cheerfully, but his army superiors interrupted the process, taking away the equipment, even the chair he'd been sitting on. He would like to talk more with us, but a harsh female voice from a cottage reins him in.

According to the documents from Dr. Burgasov, seven sheep and a cow died here between April 5 and April 10, 1979. In each case the diagnosis of anthrax was "confirmed by the examination of an expert." These animals, plus another sick sheep that went undiagnosed, were either burned in the local quarry, buried in the forest, or, it is implied, eaten by dogs. The veterinary documents also outline an aggressive program of animal vaccinations. On April 11, 1,019 cattle were vaccinated at the sovkhoz, along with 841 privately owned cattle, sheep, goats, pigs, and horses from the village area. From April 21 to 23, several hundred more animals were inoculated. The document relating to Abramovo states, "There were no complications among the vaccinated animals by April 25, 1979." The anthrax epizootic had ended.

The village is quiet. With low expectations of a response, Irina and I knock on the first door, the home of Alexander Lomovtsev. His wife answers and is willing to talk with us. Her cottage is like those on Lyapustina and Poldnevaya streets in Chkalovskiy, except that a small stable is appended to the back, with just a rudimentary door dividing a sheep stall from the kitchen. Behind the house is a large field for grazing. Lomovtseva straightforwardly recounts her story of the death of a single sheep in the beginning of April 1979. There was no snow on the ground, so the animals were let out to graze. The evening before, this sheep was fine, but the next morning, its belly was distended and it had blood coming from its anus.

Her first reaction was that it was her fault. The sheep had been healthy and strong, then it died. Had she done something wrong? She buried the carcass at the local dump and didn't inform the authorities until later in the day, after she learned that others in the village had also lost livestock and the local veterinarian was informing the villagers the disease could be anthrax. He made sure her sheep was dug up and burned.

The next day a public health crew descended on the village, dispensing tetracycline. To her mind, these strangers were rude and treated the villagers as if they had "committed a crime." Her yard was disinfected with chlorine. The floor of her shed was ripped up and the wooden boards over the mud in her yard were taken away. Veterinarians arrived from Sverdlovsk and stayed in a nearby hostel. No one was permitted to leave the village for two weeks, perhaps longer. She and her husband got paid leave from work for that time. Because of the quarantine some women, Lomovtseva adds, missed their planned abortions at a city clinic.

We knock next at the door of Yuriy Kostarov. His wife answers and agrees to talk with us. Kostarova lost a ram, after noticing it was sick and, on the advice of neighbors, calling in the local veterinarian. Her story is like her neighbor's: troops of outsiders appeared, the house and yard area were disinfected, the shed floorboards were torn up, a quarantine sign was put on the house. She thinks people from Moscow also came to the village. She remembers shearing her ram before it fell sick and storing its precious white wool in a can. That prize was confiscated and because she had handled the wool, strangers woke her one night "like a spy or criminal" and required her to be vaccinated on the hip. She is still furious at this indignity.

The Krutikovs, whose house we enter next, owned the first animal recorded to die of anthrax, a sheep that fell sick April 4 and was butchered April 5. They ate pies made from its meat. None of them fell ill, which is possible if the meat was well-cooked. Krutikov's father, a professional butcher, made them throw away the uncooked meat. The mother in this family indignantly recalls a Moscow investigator asking, "Who sent this bacteria to you? Where did you get it?" as if she and her husband were involved in a plot to kill livestock.

Their neighbors, the Kosterevs down the street, recall a "busful of Moscow veterinarians" arriving in the village and soon after arrogantly appearing at the doorstep to demand the ears of a calf that had died. Afterward, some women who lost animals were accused by their neighbors of not keeping the stalls clean, of being themselves dirty and slovenly. Among those interviewed, no one is sure if stray dogs ate the infected carcasses or whether dogs in the area were shot, although the rumor is that these things happened in other villages and towns and in Sverdlovsk city.

At the fifth and last door, there is no answer, but we have heard enough to believe that in April 1979 the little village of Abramovo was turned upside down by an epizootic.

We park the car on a pleasant rise overlooking the quiet village. The sky is brilliant blue, the air is warm, and the green landscape rolls for miles before us. The village is incredibly serene, as if it has fallen into a summer high-noon slumber. The geese and chickens have disappeared into the crawl spaces beneath the cottages and a yard dog, the kind Russians refer to as *sharik,* or little bull, is stretched out on a shady stair. We drink tea from a thermos and eat salted biscuits that taste like Ritz crackers, but this is not by any means a picnic. We have come to the outer limit of the 1979 outbreak, where a cloud of anthrax seems to have spent itself, diffusing the last of its lethal spores over this gentle valley. (See Map 3.)

Before our tea is finished, we begin checking the interviews against the Burgasov documents. Women are usually in charge of domestic livestock, so we were fortunate to talk with the ones in these four families. Until now, to be sure I would not ask leading questions, I have avoided reviewing the accounts about individual households. We find that the details of each family's narrative confirm what is reported in the veterinary documents. There is agreement on number and kind of animals that died in each household, when they died, how carcasses were disposed of, and the public health measures taken in each home. Even the seizing of Kosterova's tin of ram's wool was described by the veterinarians.

Other descriptions in the documents also corroborate the interviews. From April 16 to 20, "the floors in the suspected anthrax peasant homesteads were broken open. The soil from underneath the floors was removed for 20 cms, mixed with a 20 percent solution of chloride of lime, and taken away to the quarry for disposal. The boards from the broken floors were burned in the quarry." Manure "from the unfortunate and suspected anthrax peasant homesteads" was disposed of in the quarry, which is two miles from the village. In a measure that paralleled efforts undertaken in Sverdlovsk, though with more vigor, all the "peasant homesteads were disinfected five times with 10 percent solution of hot caustic sodium. The fifth disinfection, as recommended by the Moscow [veterinary] experts, was made with adding 1 percent chlorofos to the solution of caustic soda. . . . In the course of cleaning the premises and removing the floors and manure, the inventory of little value, items of maintenance and tools, were burned."

Unmentioned in the documents is the rough treatment the villagers received from officials: the forced vaccinations, the accusations of illegal activity, having parts of their homes ripped apart and equipment destroyed, the difficult quarantine, and the unreimbursed loss of livestock.

To vaccinate hundreds of animals within a month's time must have taken all the veterinary reserves in the area, which is what Dr. Romanenko remembered. To vaccinate villagers suggests there was a connection between the vaccination program Dr. Nikiforov ordered in the city and the busloads of Moscovites that descended on Abramovo. In short, the campaign going on in Sverdlovsk spilled over to the hinterlands, where SES and veterinarians took their marching orders from higher up, ultimately from Dr. Burgasov and the Extraordinary Commission. If we multiply the experience of Abramovo by that of the five other villages where animals died, we can conclude that havoc reigned here as well as in Sverdlovsk. Why Dr. Babich wanted to downplay the epizootic remains unclear. The veterinarians who refused to speak to our team last year, those in charge in 1979, surely participated in this frantic containment of the animal anthrax. But whether they could have told us anything conclusive about the source of the human anthrax outbreak is unlikely, since the animal cases did appear to precede the human ones.

The timing and interpretation of the animal cases is key to understanding the confusion. The first sheep died April 5, 1979, six days before laboratory tests confirmed that anthrax was the cause of the human deaths that hit the city starting about April 8. Hence Burgasov sees the veterinary reports as proof the outbreak originated from infected meat. The reports themselves are accurate, as we have just confirmed in a brief inquiry. But to presume a causal relationship, that infected meat killed people in Sverdlovsk, is to pursue a mirage. The animals were exposed soon after the people in Chkalovskiy, and like them sickened as early as

April 4. But because their symptoms were familiar to veterinarians, they were diagnosed more quickly than the human victims.

As we leave Abramovo, a flock of sheep, their thick wool clumped with dirt and briars, blocks our car. With no shepherd in sight, a ram with a bell around his neck confidently leads the rest across the road. We could be back in April 1979. On the highway, we pass a horse-drawn wagon that takes us even further back in time. On it rides an old woman in peasant's dress and kerchief who could easily be the proud witch Kubarikha in *Dr. Zhivago*, the one who advises the itinerant Red partisan wives on cures for animal sickness. After diagnosing anthrax on a cow's udder, she prescribes her special ointment and sings a magic chant: "Terror, terror, show your mettle, take the scab, throw it in the nettle." She also advises the women not to be fooled by "the red banner," which she tells them is the purple kerchief of the "Death Woman "who "nods and winks and lures young men to be killed, then she sends famine and plague."[3]

Unfortunately, Russian villages like Abramovo may be consulting their Kubarikhas in lieu of veterinary services. With the end of the Soviet Union, Chief Veterinarian Krasnoperov has told us, the number of privately owned sheep and cattle has skyrocketed, with no great assurance that they are being vaccinated against anthrax. The state is doing what it can, but it no longer has a ready supply of vaccine and cannot monitor private owners or the new private collectives that are springing up from the old communist models. In the old days, the 1920s to 1940s, livestock in anthrax-infected areas in Sverdlovsk oblast would be vaccinated twice a year. In more modern times, it was once a year. Now the vaccinations will be less frequent and the risks of epizootics will increase wherever old reservoirs of anthrax exist. In former soviet states like Kazakhstan and Izbekhistan, where anthrax has long been rampant, the rates of disease will be even higher.

What if diseases that affect humans take a parallel backward course here? The czarist empire was "a playground for epidemics," Henry Sigerist wrote in his 1937 apologia for Soviet health programs. Smallpox, typhus, tuberculosis, typhoid, and dysentery were endemic; cholera and plague broke out at regular intervals. "Health conditions there were so constant a menace to the West that Russia was looked upon with dread by the rest of Europe, as a permanent source of infections."[4] For all its failings, the Soviet Union expanded public health organizations, educated many professionals, and built many hospitals to provide citizens with medical care at several institutional levels. Factories played their part, providing clinics for workers, and health resorts and spas were opened to ordinary citizens. In the new Russia, citizens can no longer count on its health system, which is underfunded; and industry, already in bad shape, can barely support itself, let alone provide benefits for workers. AIDS is just beginning to appear here, along with a rise in other drug-related and sexually transmitted diseases. Since arriving, we have heard about serious increases in drug-resistant tuberculosis, in dysentery, ty-phus, and influenza, and in bronchial diseases related to pollution.

Safe in our car, we speed past the horse and carriage and head back through the fields of sunflowers to the city. No one wants to think about how much of Russia is rural and undeveloped or how it could, along with its Asian neighbors, regress to the level of a former century. Or how, as an industrial nation that began with the most utopian health-care in-tentions, it may founder in the proliferation of modern "man-made dis-eases," aggravated by the breakdown of social systems.[5]

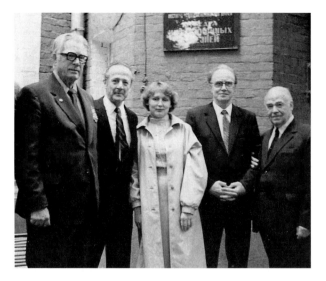

Deputy Minister Pyotr Burgasov, Matthew Meselson, Dr. Olga Yampolskaya,
Dr. Vladimir N. Nikiforov, Dr Ivan Bezdenezhnikh, Moscow, 1986.

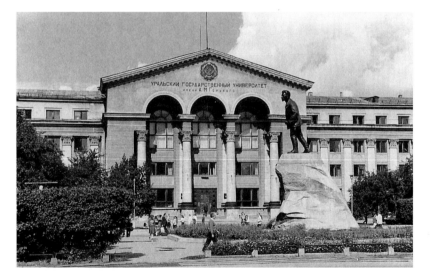

Ural State University, Yekaterinburg, with statue of Yakov Sverdlov, 1992.

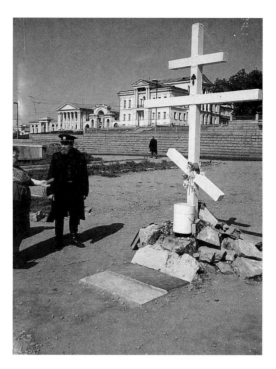

The shrine at the site of the now-destroyed Ipatiev House, where the family of the last Romanov czar was murdered. A donation is being offered by the woman at the left. Yekaterinburg, 1992.

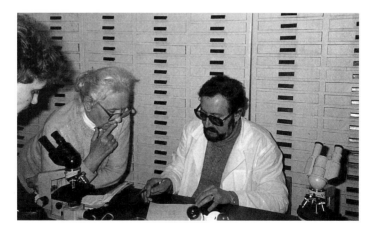

Dr. Faina Abramova and Dr. Lev Grinberg at the Tuberculosis and Pulmonary Diseases Unit, with Olga Yampolskaya at left. Yekaterinburg, 1992.

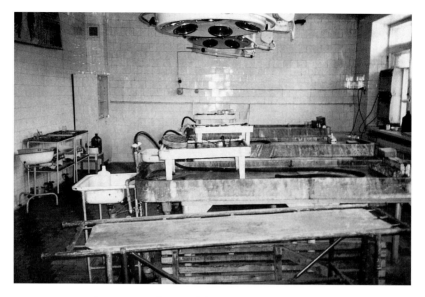

Autopsy room at Hospital 40, Chkalovskiy, Yekaterinburg, 1998.

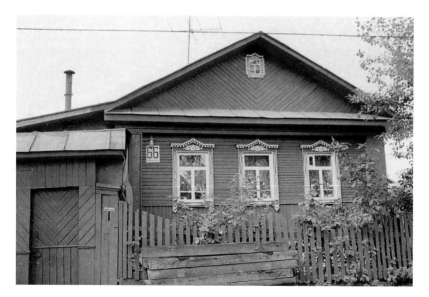

Cottage in Chkalovskiy rayon, 1992.

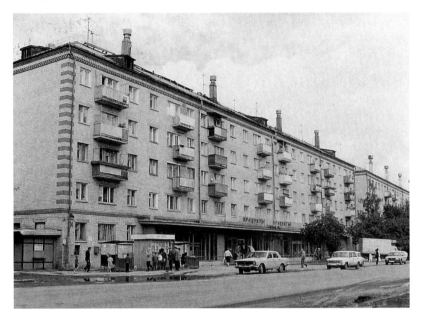

Apartment buildings on the boulevard bordering Chkalovskiy rayon, 1992. Two residents of these buildings died in the 1979 anthrax outbreak.

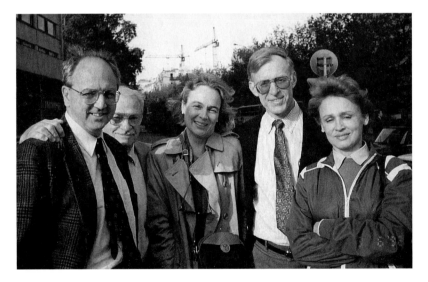

Martin Hugh-Jones, Alexis Shelokov, Jeanne Guillemin, David Walker, and Olga Yampolskaya, Moscow, 1992.

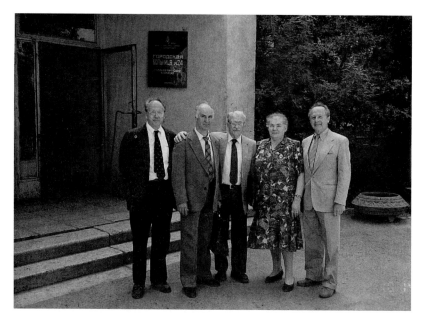

Martin Hugh-Jones, Professor Vladimir Shepetkin, Alexis Shelokov, Dr. Margarita Ilyenko, and Matthew Meselson, outside Hospital 24, 1992.

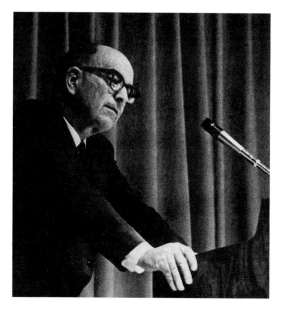

Alex Langmuir, lecturing at Johns Hopkins University in the 1980s.
(Photograph courtesy of the Johns Hopkins School of Public Health.)

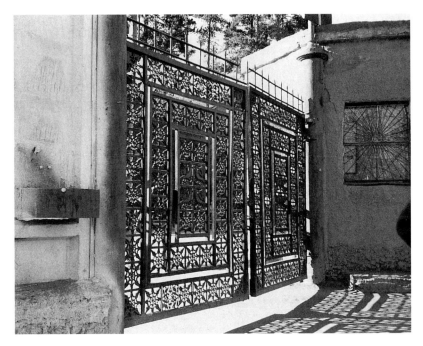

The gate at the entrance to Compound 19, 1998. The guard on duty uses an electric switch to control the coming and going of automobiles and trucks. Residents and workers enter through a nearby separate guardhouse. Notice the gate's elaborate ironwork, typical of Yekaterinburg architecture.

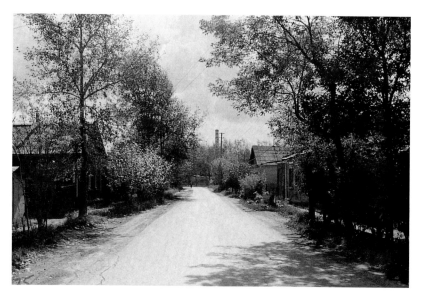

Looking south down Poldnevaya Street to the smokestack of the ceramic factory pipe shop, 1993.

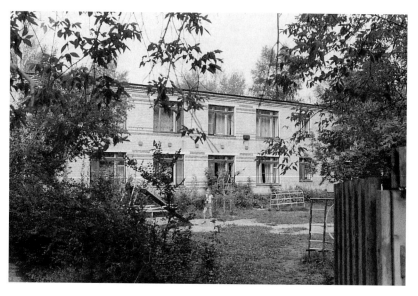

The ceramics factory kindergarten where, in 1979, twenty-four-year-old Tatyana Kosheleva was a teacher. Chkalovskiy rayon, 1993.

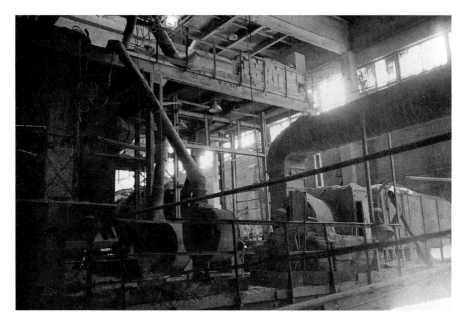

The interior of the pipe shop at the ceramics factory, 1993.

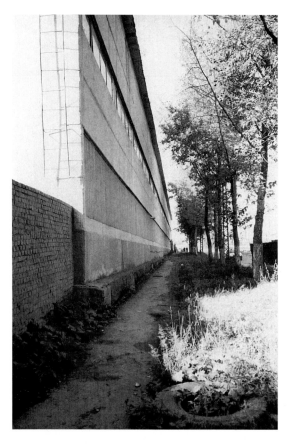

The exterior of the ceramics factory, 1998.

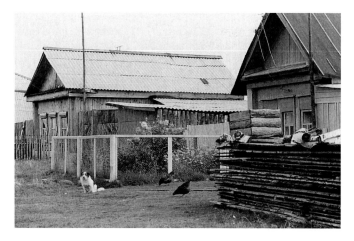

Typical cottage in Abramovo village, with the ever-present dog, 1993.

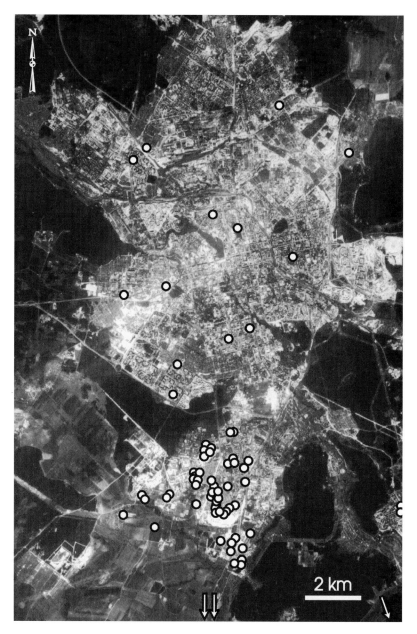

Map 1. Residences of 1979 anthrax victims from the KGB list acquired in 1992, plus four addresses added later that year. The city map used matched this 1988 SPOT satellite photograph of Sverdlovsk. A recently declassified U.S. satellite photo (Corona series) of the city in 1970 showed that little change had taken place over the intervening years. Arrows indicate addresses outside the city.

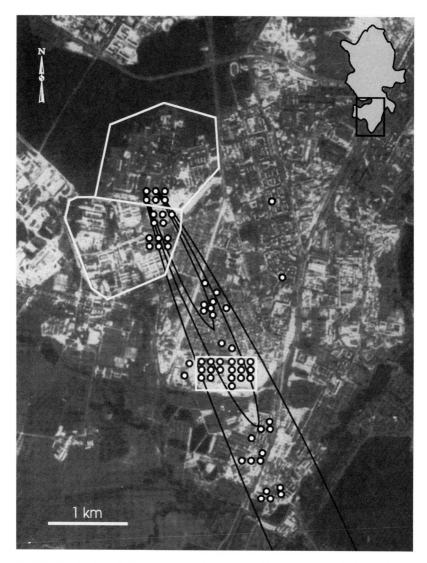

Map 2. Daytime locations of sixty-two anthrax victims in Chkalovskiy rayon on Monday, April 2, 1979. The insert at upper right shows Chkalovskiy's location in Sverdlovsk. Four outliers, in addition to the two that fall to the right of the plume here, lie outside this map's boundaries, in the north and west of Sverdlovsk. The irregular areas outlined in white indicate the perimeters of Compound 19, from which the emission emanated, and, to its south, Compound 32. The rectangle outlined in white indicates the location of and number of victims at the ceramics factory. The elliptical shapes (isopleths) indicate areas of decreasing concentration of dose, moving outward from the source.

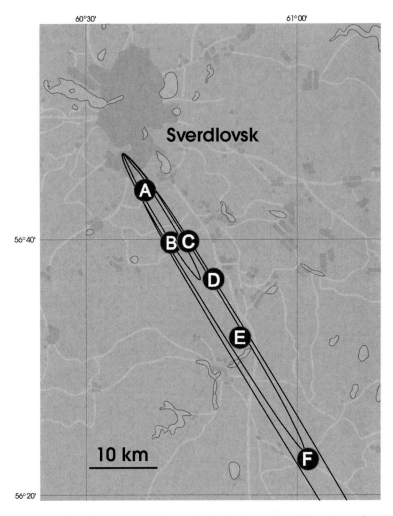

Map 3. Six villages that reported cases of animal anthrax in April, 1979, southeast of Yekaterinburg: A, Rudniy; B, Bolshoye Sedelnikov; C, Maloye Sedlnikovo; D, Pervomaiskiy; E, Kashino; and F, Abramovo. The elliptical shapes (isopleths) indicate areas of decreasing concentration of dose, moving outward from the source at Compound 19 in Sverdlovsk.

21

Chkalovskiy

THE FINAL PIECES

Back in Yekaterinburg, our efforts focus on the problem of the remaining outliers, the men who lived and worked outside Chkalovskiy. While we were in Abramovo, Ilona has confirmed by telephone that two of them were in Chkalovskiy at the beginning of April 1979, taking their required military reserve courses at Compound 32. The men's relatives are sure that Monday, April 2, was the first day of the week-long program. But what about the rest? Were they also military reservists at the same training course? There is only so far one can go to get precise data about events fourteen years in the past. Irina recently went to a military reserve office and was told that there is no way to ascertain the April 1979 dates for Compound 32 courses or who attended them.

Nonetheless, Ilona persevered with telephoning and soon has news. According to the widow of young Aleksandr Vyatkin, he was at Compound 32 for reserve training, but just for one day, either April 2 or 9, his wife isn't sure. A telephone call to Vyatkin's mother yields her assertion that he was at Compound 32 only on Monday, April 2, not later. By the end of our second day in Yekaterinburg, Ilona has contacted a second family and learned that on April 2, 1979, Valeriy Prokhorov was in Chkalovskiy for reserve classes at Compound 32. Just like the day shift at the ceramics factory, the reserve classes began at eight in the morning and ended at four in the afternoon, after which the reservists left the base.

Also by telephone, Ilona succeeds in reaching the family of Mikhail Lozhkin. His wife says that in early April he was taking a military reserve course at Compound 32. He had his meals there, except for sup-per, which he ate at home. Although she cannot say with certainty that the course started April 2, she gives Ilona the name of one of her late husband's friends who might know. Irina follows through on this con-tact and learns that Lozkhin's friend traveled with him every day to Com-pound 32. He is positive the course began April 2 and ended April 6.

Though we have made some progress tracking the outliers, the loca-tions of at least six will probably always elude us for lack of detailed in-formation. Three of them were mobile, with occupations that might have brought them to Chkalovskiy. Nikolay Vostrykhov was a driver in a pool and traveled the city. Mikhail Lavrov, who lived in a hostel and died in the ambulance before reaching Hospital 40, read meters in the Chkalov-skiy area. Ivan Makarov (not Pyotr who worked at Compound 19) was a pipe layer for a construction company. He, too, could have been in Chkalovskiy on a job. Along with Konstantin Chikalov, who was a welder at a factory outside Chkalovskiy, on SakkoVanzetti Street, these men have been confirmed by autopsy data as having died of anthrax. Nikolay Sha-tokin, who is on the KGB list, did maintenance for the telephone com-pany and might have passed through the district. In addition, some doubt exists that he died of anthrax. Since he died relatively early (April 10), he is not in Abramova and Grinberg's autopsy series. His death certificate, written at Hospital 20, indicates he died of "acute enteritis." Yet the de-cision was made by someone, probably a clinician, to list him as an an-thrax victim.

With the sixth of these outliers, a survivor, Aleksandr R., we have reached a complete impasse. We have documentation on his illness from Dr. Nikiforov's files, but he has moved away, and the new residents of his apartment cannot help us locate him. We have no information that places him beneath the plume. Like his home, the knitting factory where he worked as a welder is just east of Chkalovskiy, across a main boulevard.

Another mysterious outlier is Vitaliy Fyodosov, who lived north, near the university, on the street named for astronaut Yuriy Gagarin. We know almost nothing about him except for his photograph at the cemetery and that he died at age forty-three. But Professor Borisov, who has asked among friends about the 1979 outbreak, has discovered that Fyodosov was a computer programmer at the Institute Sofia Kavaleskaya, named for the famous mathematician. A friend and colleague of Fyodosov's wants to talk with us.

On our third afternoon in Yekaterinburg, Viktor D., a middle-aged, bearded academic, comes to our hotel. It is three in the afternoon and, after a rainy morning, the sun has come out. Irina and I sit across from our visitor at the table near the plate-glass windows overlooking the soaked, lush botanical garden.

Viktor begins his story in a soft voice. On April 10, he stopped by the apartment where Fyodosov lived with his mother. Viktor had heard from Fyodosov's mother that he had come down with the grippe and was suffering from a high fever and shortness of breath. At his best, her son was not the healthiest of men. Often suffering from influenza and colds, he was always trying to improve his health with herbal remedies and had, in fact, used his last vacation to collect medicinal herbs in the countryside. Nonetheless, Viktor stopped by to borrow a book; the two men had been at Compound 32 and were sharing the course material. When Viktor knocked on Fyodosov's door, he could hear the distant sound of his friend coughing on the other side. Then he heard Fyodosov, alone in the apartment, stumble to the door and try to open it, but instead he collapsed and fell heavily against it. Describing this moment, Viktor rubs his face, which has turned slightly gray. "There was nothing I could do," he says with grief in his eyes. "The door was locked."

He waited outside until, after five or ten minutes, Fyodosov's mother returned.

"We found Vitaliy unconscious on the floor and tried to revive him. Failing, we called for an emergency ambulance. The paramedics arrived quickly, but it was too late." Fyodosov died on the way to the hospital.

Everything else Viktor tells us about the outbreak is according to form: the apartment was disinfected, Fyodosov's body was never returned home, he was buried at Vostichniy Cemetery with a police escort. Barred from seeing her son's remains, Fyodosov's mother, in her early eighties, never really believed he was dead and feared that instead he had been taken away by the state. "What if it is only bricks in the coffin?" she wept. A few years later she died.

"The significance of all this," Viktor says, "only emerged later."

"And when did your military reserve course begin?" I ask, and hold my breath.

"On the first Monday of April," he answers, "April 2." He is sure of it.

Five of our outliers have now been placed at Compound 32 on the day of April 2, 1979, a coincidence that is beyond chance.

On our fourth day in Yekaterinburg, Irina, Matthew, and I take advantage of an opportunity to visit Compound 32. We are on the track of a rumor we heard in Abramovo that the postmistress there, named

Anna, knows a good deal about the outbreak, and we want to find any military victims we can.

Compound 32, with its broad streets and park benches under leafy trees, is a better maintained version of the 1960s garden apartments on Selkorovskaya. The military may be falling apart, but it is not yet evident here. The post office looks like any other briskly run depot for a small community. Anna, the postmistress, takes a break from her work and, across the counter, we talk about the outbreak. She believes her husband, Aleksis, was the first victim to die of anthrax, even though his medical diagnosis was kidney failure. He fell ill on April 2 and died on April 5. Another woman behind the counter joins in to affirm what Anna says, but they both realize the government doesn't recognize the claim and there is no hope for one of the pensions promised by Yeltsin.

We show them our list, pointing out the five names of victims who resided here at MSD34: Pavel Retnev, whose cemetery photo showed his many medals; Lilia Fokina, the Turgenev countess; Rosa Margamova; Aleksandra Chernyaeva; and Vladimir Sannikov. The two women shake their heads. Those families have all moved away, they say, except for one, Sannikov's widow. As for other military cases here or in Compound 19, they don't know of any. They point the way to the Sannikov apartment near the front entrance to the base. In a few minutes, while Matthew waits outside, we are talking with Sannikov's wife about the thirty-one-year-old husband she lost in 1979. She is herself still a young woman, and her pretty face fills with the same anxious grief as other relatives who have narrated their loss to us.

Her husband's case involves the confusion of a reaction to anthrax vaccination with actual onset of the disease. Sannikov fell ill with a fever on Tuesday, April 22, just after being vaccinated. When his wife called the Compound 32 clinic, she was told the fever was only a temporary reaction and that she should not disturb the doctors. On Wednesday her husband felt worse, and she arranged for him to be taken to a large military hospital just north of Chkalovskiy, in Leninskiy rayon. He died Friday, April 25, with a diagnosis of sepsis, and was buried in Sector 13 in Vostochniy Cemetery. As with Pyotr Makarov, who died at Compound 19 and is buried with the other 1979 victims, the military appears to have respected the public health directives laid down by the city and by Moscow. Sannikov, a lower-ranked officer, worked as a senior maintenance man. His office was at the west end of the compound, but he frequently went by car to check on repairs around the base, and he lunched at the canteen across from the apartment, which would have put him closer to where the reservists were at their courses. No, his wife doesn't know of any other victims' families at the bases.

Leaving the compound, we find ourselves on the bluff that overlooks Chkalovskiy; thirteen meters down a gradient three kilometers long is the ceramics factory. From there, we begin walking southeast, on the straight line toward the ceramics factory. This is a solemn trek, worthy of a dirge. We are now sure that sometime during the day on April 2, a lethal anthrax aerosol was emitted from Compound 19 and blew in the direction we are walking, over Chkalovskiy and out into the countryside. It is about noon, cloudy, with a chill wind at our backs; the streets are muddy from another morning rain. As Irina and I walk arm-in-arm, Matthew photographs the path, upwind and downwind, trying to recapture the invisible in images of fences, gardens, cottages, schools, and streets.

I try to concentrate on the facts. Dr. Romanenko at SES has provided us with the 1992 block-by-block census figures for this area of Chkalovskiy, and in particular for the area between Compound 19 and the ceramics factory. As we also know, in 1979 around twenty-four hundred people inhabited this danger zone. Since last year, Ilona has spoken to some sixty residents along these streets who lived here then, people unrelated to the anthrax victims but of the same mix of age, gender, and social background. These "controls," along with SES data, confirm that the victims were fairly like other people in the area, factory workers and pensioners; only about 15 percent of the population was under fifteen years of age. Except for some retired people, the great majority of them, both men and women, were routinely off at work during the day, as they probably are now, with most employed at local industries just outside the plume, where no one died of anthrax.

As we walk this path, Irina and I find ourselves feeling increasingly skittish, almost ill. Turn back the clock fourteen years, and we are one with the victims of the 1979 outbreak, who trusted the air and never guessed that it could kill them, who knew nothing of the danger they were in. Should such an event ever happen again, how would anyone know? There would be no smell, no taste, no way to know if one were inside the plume or out, or if one's family or friends were in jeopardy or not. This cloud could pass by like a biblical plague, striking down the unfortunate, sparing others.

The people we meet along the path are very much in the present. We stop briefly at a kindergarten for the local rubber factory, where a teacher complains the school will probably close down because the factory is failing. Moving on to Eskadronaya, we pass a little market where a babushka is selling, along with tomatoes and cucumbers, the ubiquitous Snickers bars and Western brands of soap, noodles, and canned goods. Yet as we continue southeast, I keep seeing the past. To the left and right are the homes of people who died in the anthrax outbreak: Fagim Dayanov, who missed his son's childhood; the gentle pensioner Maria Moseykina, whose daughter resembles her; the old cleaning woman Sophia Bliumova; dignified Ivan Vershinin, who never got his shaving razor; Anna Komina, who worked nights and had Monday April 2 off, all to herself at home. I begin to feel emotionally spent. Irina has the same fretful reaction.

Soon we reach Poldnevaya Street, parallel to Lyapustina, the two streets that are like corridors between Compound 19 and the ceramics factory. We pass the ceramics factory kindergarten, where Tatyana Kosheleva (at age twenty-four, the youngest anthrax victim) was a teacher. Children at recess play in the yard. Turn back the clock, and Kosheleva is there by the door, clapping her hands to get the children's attention, never guessing her life will soon end.

When we reach the ceramics factory, where the anthrax outbreak hit the hardest, I feel chilled to the bone, colder than I did in Vostochniy Cemetery, though this day is much warmer. The factory yard looks the same as last year, as I remember it from my first visit to Chkalovskiy with Olga Yampolskaya. Now, though, I don't envision a truck full of anthrax-infected meat pulling up to the loading dock. I just feel the wind at my back. Eighteen workers here died of anthrax.

We carry with us a letter of introduction from Peoples Deputy Larissa Mishustina. The foyer level of the factory is empty. On the first floor, we approach a man in his shirtsleeves checking a loose doorknob. He is factory director Yuriy Gusev, on the watch the way model managers in the Soviet Union were supposed to be. Waving our letter aside, he leads us downstairs to the factory clinic to meet Dr. Tamara Chernich, the clinic's head, who was at her post during the 1979 outbreak. She has some business to attend to before she can meet with us. Meanwhile, we discuss with the director the theory we once entertained that anthrax-contaminated clay fired here might have spewed spores into the atmosphere and been the cause of the 1979 epidemic. The same idea had occurred to him, he admits. He explains that four different kinds of clay are used in this ceramics factory, some local, some imported from Kazakhstan, where anthrax is known to occur. Green clay is aged by microbial action, but nothing so bizarre as an anthrax outbreak had ever happened in this factory before. He leaves us, and we browse through the brochures in what we know now we can tell his sister she is right, but not for the reasons she thinks.

The next day, Irina and I return to Chkalovskiy to interview the two survivors who may have been away in early April. Although the sun is out, autumn is in the air. We start on Lyapustina, looking for Anatoliy S., who may have been in Leningrad the first week of April 1979. By chance, we find him walking with his wife and daughter near his house. The two women stop to talk to us, but Anatoliy S. keeps on a straight path toward his home. I lead an undignified charge after him, trying to catch up before he disappears behind his door. He has his hand on the doorknob as we ask him to please answer just one question.

"In the first week of April 1979, were you in Leningrad or here at home?"

"Here at home, of course," he answers in an irritated tone, as if this fact is common knowledge. "We came back from Leningrad at the end of March." He was right here building his bathhouse in early April. He disappears inside the door.

In my mind's eye, another red dot appears in the high-risk zone in Chkalovskiy rayon.

Crossing over to Poldnevaya, we knock at the door of the cottage of the other survivor, Nina T., whose daytime work as a baker in 1979 took her well outside center Chkalovskiy. In her tidy yard, a small white dog, the kind one might see in a circus, greets us with tail-wagging. Her four-room cottage is impeccably clean. While we are talking with her in her kitchen, two handsome fair-haired grandchildren tumble home from school and, after shyly enduring introductions, disappear outside.

Nina, now sixty-three, has deep-set eyes and high cheekbones and, though she sits down to talk with us, she gives the impression of being in perpetual motion. She recounts that she first felt ill on May 4, and on May 11 she was transported to Hospital 40. While in the ambulance, she had difficulty breathing and complained when one of the paramedics lit up a cigarette. His response, she tells us, was "What does it matter? You are going to die anyway." But she says she never felt she would die. Even when two patients on beds near hers passed away, she felt she would survive. In Dr. Nikiforov's records, hers is the classic anthrax case, with X-rays showing clear mediastinal widening, the chest expansion that should have predicted her death. Her work life, which began on a collective farm when she was twelve, has been long and hard. For many years, before she got the job as a baker, she worked in a Sverdlovsk machine factory, grinding and polishing metal parts. She says her outlook

the waiting room, on dental and prenatal care. In the next room, in curtained cubicles, workers are being massaged by husky physical therapists.

Feisty and bright-eyed, Dr. Chernich greets us with impatience, as if we should have come sooner to ask about the epidemic. She begins her story by telling us that at first she and others thought the anthrax had come from burning infected animal carcasses in pits. But Compound 19 was also suspected. In the middle of the panic, no one knew what to think.

"For one whole month," she says, "I didn't go home. I stayed here night and day." As she talks, she digs into her file cabinet and comes out with index cards and pieces of paper with names, addresses, job categories, and dates of death during April and May of 1979. Most she thinks were from anthrax.

"One Friday," she tells us, "a man in the pipe shop died. The next Monday I came to work and found out that two more people were at home, very sick."

The numbers of sick increased so quickly that she ran out of antibiotics. She went to ask the director for more, and when she returned to her office she found two people from the local SES, who announced that the problem was respiratory (i.e., from pneumonia or influenza) and that her people were showing up sick at Hospitals 24 and 20. Her plan then (never fully realized) was to get everyone in the factory on a five-day regimen of antibiotics.

Matthew and I have each brought our summaries of case data and are checking Dr. Chernich's cards and lists to see if they match what we have patched together from interviews, lists, and clinical sources. By her reckoning, the first victim among the ceramics workers was Speridon Zakharov, first on the KGB list, the forty-four-year-old pipe shop worker for whom his doomed friend and coworker Ignat Maslennikov helped dig a grave. We have no autopsy data for him; his wife said that, although he was sick on April 6, he went to work April 7, only to collapse and be taken to Hospital 20, where he died.

As Dr. Chernich goes over other names with us, she muses on the individual victims: Dimitriy Vinogradov, Anna Komina, Vera Kozlova, Pytor Gayda, Mikhail Burmistrov, Valeriy Poletaev, the pensioner Lazar Korsayev. Like Dr. Ilyenko, she knows Chkalovskiy. In 1979 she lived on nearby Energetnikov and had a next-door neighbor, Mikhail Krivstov, a worker at a felt factory who died in the outbreak. Later, after the epidemic, she moved to an apartment at Selkorovskaya 102, where several other victims had lived.

Ivan Vershinin, whose son Aleksandr we interviewed last year, is missing from her list, an oversight, Dr. Chernich admits; she knows his widow, who lives just across the street from the factory. Four names she has records for are not on the official list, although three were cited in Dr. Ilyenko's records as having fallen ill during the outbreak. Otherwise, we have no records of these cases. Some chronically ill workers died during the outbreak, but not from anthrax. One worked as a cashier in the canteen; maybe this was Aleksandra Chizhova, whose death certificate read Friedländer's pneumonia, which particularly affects those with compromised immune systems. In all, ten of the victims Chernich cites were autopsied by Abramova and Grinberg, and all were unambiguously confirmed as having died of anthrax.

Dr. Chernich confirms other details about the victims. Yes, Mikhail Markov drove an electric car inside the pipe shop. Maslennikov was a pipe fitter, whereas Mikhail Burmistrov was a pipe welder. Vinogradov was employed to mix clays. Komina was a machinist in charge of the steam generator. Chernich knew them all. She says she would like to give us more precise information about the antibiotics and about vaccinations, but in 1979 the KGB took away the workers' records. She presumed they were brought to Hospital 40 for review by a high-level committee.

Dr. Chernich was among the doctors called together by the "Moscow physician with the refined accent" (Dr. Nikiforov) for a lecture on anthrax, the same that Dr. Ilyenko attended. He didn't discuss tainted meat, she says, although she had heard of the outbreak of animal anthrax; instead he talked about systemic infection. Then there followed the huge vaccination program, including the shots given at this factory to many of the workers. Panic was widespread in the neighborhood, which was why people cooperated. Chernich recalls an old woman of eighty who came to the factory demanding her vaccination, shouting "I want to live!" to the doctors.

The director has arranged a tour of the factory for us. We thank Dr. Chernich and follow a guide outside to the block-long pipe shop on the northeast edge of the plant. It is deserted now except for small area where a special heat-resistant pipe is being made. The conglomerate that optimistically bought the building last year failed to convert it to new industry; the pipe shop is now in a commercial limbo. Its interior space is cavernous and filled with unused engines, kilns, and troughs. Every surface is covered in a heavy, gray residue of grime and cobweb-like trailings, like a Halloween scenario in a disco loft. Delicate iron catwalks three stories up, on the level of the row of high windows facing north-

east, look like theater staging. Leaving Irina and our guide below, Matthew and I climb a rickety ladder up to the windows and look down over the maze of machinery. It is easy to imagine what it must have been like here in April 1979. Workers, mostly men, must have been sweating over the kilns. Vinogradov (who later collapsed in the street) would have been mixing clay. Markov (who became so sick he couldn't help his sister-in-law hoist the pig into the car) would have been buzzing around on a transport car. Maslennikov (who, we just learned, had a history of tuberculosis) might have climbed up here on the catwalk to adjust a window while his friend Zakharov and Vera Kozlova checked the new pipes for faults. Warm air heated by the ovens below must have risen and rolled like a wave as it met the incoming spring wind, carrying the fatal spores. Today the windows are closed and the vault of air is cool and still. Matthew and I descend the creaky metal ladders and continue the tour of the rest of the factory.

In the nearby tile shop (west of the pipe shop) a conveyor belt carries rows of wet ceramic squares into a great gaping furnace. At the other end, a young woman in a kerchief, her cheeks flushed from the heat, checks the fired tiles for cracks. Behind the tile shop is the boiler room, where Anna Komina worked. Through another door is the factory store, where tea sets are for sale, along with mugs, pitchers, and bathroom and kitchen tiles decorated with banal decals of flowers and fruit. Yeltsin's order about the sale of individual tea pots has been forgotten. One buys the whole set—or bargains with the shopkeeper.

We leave the ceramics factory to complete our walk on a straight line southeast. On the boulevard beyond it, we locate MEX44, the construction company truck depot. There, in a cramped office, a frowning clerk listens to our inquiry about Zinatulla Abusagitov, a twenty-nine-year-old victim, a Tatar, who we believe worked here. Abramova and Grinberg's estimate, based on bacteriological tests and autopsy, is that Abusagitov's case was "classic anthrax." We are certain that Pyotr Pilyasov, so handsome in his cemetery photo, also worked here. Irritated, the clerk goes to a large file cabinet and jerks open a long drawer bursting with hundreds of old handwritten receipts and index cards, her records for 1979. What do we expect her to do, waste her time searching that mess! Never! But she clearly remembers a pair of Abusagitov brothers employed here in the 1970s. Maybe, she suggests with a shrug, the other one still lives in the city. Ilona has already spoken to Abusagitov's sister, who says that, at his death, he had a skull injury and bruises on his body. The sister suspects his death was caused by foul play. Wi[...]

on life is positive because she was born in western Siberia, where people are optimistic and out-going. Besides, she insists, nothing now is as bad as the famines and deprivations during the Great Patriotic War, in which she lost her father and her two brothers.

And what about her work schedule in April 1979? In 1979 Nina worked as a pastry cook at the forest-machinery factory canteen, with only Sundays off. She held the job ten years and is certain about her schedule. To make her point, she carefully describes the route she traveled each day to the factory bakery. After feeding her hens, she left every morning at 5 A.M. With her finger she traces the route on the table. She always walked north on Dieselnaya to Ferganskaya, passing by the train station there. The walk, about twenty minutes, took her out of the high-risk zone.

But here is the crucial information: her workday was eight hours. She returned home each day by 1:30. Her husband, who worked at another factory outside Chkalovskiy, came home in the late afternoon, around four.

As Nina speaks, I am thinking about my first interview more than a year ago, with Anna Komina's son. It was a lucky one, in that it gave me the earliest onset date, April 4. This last of my interviews, with Nina T., is also lucky. If on April 2, 1979, Nina T. arrived home by 1:30 P.M. and the five military reservists left Compound 32 at 4 P.M., give or take some latitude of time for each, then their common exposure to the lethal anthrax spores (and that of the other victims) had to have occurred within that brief period. Nina has just narrowed the time of the anthrax emission to within two to three hours.

While I am distracted by this revelation, she talks about her grandchildren. I lose the details, but later, back at the hotel, Irina explains why Nina really believes she survived her anthrax infection. Several years after the epidemic, her daughter died of leukemia, leaving two small children, the grandchildren we have just met. Their father was unable to take care of them. They needed Nina and she took them in. She believes that God saved her in 1979 so she could raise her grandchildren. What other reason could there be, but that He watched over the children? Irina and I, overwrought perhaps, certainly tired, with our shoes and stockings splattered with pale Chkalovskiy mud, have already spent some time talking about the woes and joys of family life, about children and the effort it takes to raise them, and whether a collective sense of responsibility exists anywhere or if individual interests have completely taken over. In these modern times, Irina has remarked, "No one cares." In Nina T.'s world, simple faith in goodness endures. We are moved to tears.

This evening, we have dinner with the Borisov and Belaev families. Professor Borisov's granddaughter Masha, a bow in her hair, is only five but she has the demeanor of a princess, a very energetic one. Irina's son Andrey, a lanky, bright-eyed university student, gets to try out his English on us. We say nothing about our grim research in front of these two beautiful children. I think of the 1979 anthrax outbreak as an obscenity, the deaths themselves brutal and unnecessary, the handling of them a ritual of degradation for the families and friends of the victims. I want to warn the children about this evil and reassure them that the purpose of our trips has been to drag it out into daylight, to strip away the veil, to exorcise it with proven facts. Maybe another time. For now, Masha loves to dance. Andrey enjoys studying economics. They cannot know it, but their youth is a relief from the morbid solemnity of this investigation. I lead a toast to the future. Will we learn from the past?

Do No Evil, See No Evil

Professor Vladimir Gubanov, the physicist who arranged our invitation from the Ural State University, was our first link to Yekaterinburg. On Saturday, August 29, the last morning of our second trip to Yekaterinburg, he drives us to Koltsovo airport for our flight to Moscow. While waiting for the plane, we drink coffee with him in the Intourist lobby, which is as spare as a bus station. We laugh again at the coincidence that when Matthew telephoned Donald Ellis at Northwestern University in the spring of 1992, Gubanov was sitting right there in the office. (He continues to make trips to the United States.) We were only private citizens trying to solve an old puzzle. With no help from government, what would we have done without the assistance that the university provided us? Now our work in Yekaterinburg is done. We have said goodbye to the Borisov family, to the Grinbergs, to Ilona and Irina. I have the feeling of a circle closing. But there will be no closure until we have attended to unfinished business in Moscow.

On Monday, in the capital, we have a meeting scheduled with Major-General Valentin Yevstigneyev, who has been outspoken in the press about the former Soviet CBW program and with whom Matthew met in January. Beforehand, we lunch at the McDonald's restaurant across from the Foreign Affairs Ministry, with our interpreter, Bela Kaplan. Bela has been for many years a distinguished interpreter for Russian and American scientists. She is also a survivor of the Siege of Leningrad, the two-year stand against Nazi troops during which thousands of citizens died of cold and hunger. Bela, who received a medal for packing artillery shells, seems ageless. Her hair is jet black, her skin is winter white, her nails are bright pink, and she dresses immaculately. McDonald's has a theme park atmosphere. The young women in red caps behind the counter take our orders with un-Russian smiles and laughter. The orange walls in the upstairs dining area are decorated with modernistic gold stars and other pleasantly abstract designs. The piped-in violin music plays a soft Russian melody. The only thing that seems real is the dark Russian tea.

Bela is just back from a visit to a friend in Germany, and though she assures us all is well with her job at a Moscow patent office, we sense her life is not easy. The night before, Matthew and I had dinner at the home of friends, a Jewish scientist and his wife. He told us that Moscow has turned openly antisemitic. The table was set for six, but the other couple, also Jewish, did not come. They have just made the decision to move to Australia and were too upset by the planned uprooting to dine with us. Our friends have a son, also a scientist, currently working in the United States. Should he stay? It isn't the economy, they say, but what you feel when people on the street look at you and say, "You Jew!" They describe the banners carried by right-wing groups that read "Kill Jews!" The scientist has recently been to Munich and seen the same banner at the exhibit on Nazism at the Neue Pinakotek. Will this hostility in Russia grow?

The antisemitism isn't all. Prejudice against people from the Caucasus, against anyone who isn't ethnic Russian, is rampant. And there is corruption. The television story of the moment is about a government official who has been siphoning money from business deals to his Swiss bank account. He denies everything. According to a poll, 56 percent of Russians don't know whether to believe he is innocent or guilty. Certainly some people are making money. The streets of Moscow are full of expensive automobiles: Rolls Royces, Mercedeses, Jaguars. A young boy, certainly no more than eighteen, nearly ran me over with his BMW as I was crossing a street. Bela Kaplan says inflation is so bad that she cannot keep up with the zeros. But as "a senior citizen," as she humorously refers to herself, she cannot even think of emigrating.

The small Foreign Ministry office where we meet General Yevstigneyev seems hardly big enough to contain him. He is well over six feet and built like a wrestler. His face is round and boyish, and he looks under forty, yet he is the superior of General Karechko at Compound 19. High-ranking officers this young are more common than they used to be in Russia. In the last seven years, older officers have been retired by the hundreds to downsize their inflated ranks. Not only the massive reformations of the Yeltsin era, but the earlier, equally large turnover in military personnel that Gorbachev began in 1986 has put younger men like Yevstigneyev in charge. By the end of 1988, 80 percent of the Soviet officer corps was under forty. Military expenditures increased by almost 5 percent in the next two years to pay off early retirees cut from the personnel roster or eased out under Gorbachev's unilateral force reductions.[1] It is not clear that the younger officers are politically more liberal or reformist than the older, but they have accepted the retreat from offensive policy and rhetoric that characterized the Soviet Union until the later years of Leonid Brezhnev. Officers like Yevstigneyev are invested in advancing technology, in improving soldiering skills, and in becoming more professional. These are the trade-offs for the slashing of the military budget and the halving of the number of troops.

Perhaps most difficult of all, the military is witnessing the erosion of its science and technology. As with many areas of Soviet government, military and civilian science organizations often had overlapping boundaries. The dozens of laboratories under Biopreparat now suffer from military budget reductions and are working fast to convert to post–Cold War industrial production. Chemical and biological defense research, as General Yevstigneyev has explained to the press, commands a fraction of the personnel and resources that it had before Gorbachev.

As for the Sverdlovsk facility, General Yevstigneyev became science director there in 1984 and presumably had access to the laboratory's records. In the mid-1980s he supervised dismantling the compound's BW capacity; there is nothing left to see. Like officials in Yekaterinburg, he bemoans the fact that the major vaccine production facilities are now located in the former Soviet republics—in Georgia and Moldavia, not Russia. Outbreaks of anthrax keep occurring throughout rural Russia, and there is not enough vaccine for preventive use. As for his interpretation of the way the Sverdlovsk outbreak was handled, he is already on record as blaming senior officials in Moscow. "They isolated the camp and put it into quarantine. They immediately decided that all the infection came from there, you see. The security organs and the sanitary services created such an atmosphere of secrecy and intimidation around the population that there was no longer any doubt about it."[2]

What interests him most about our visit, he tells us, is any opportunity it might foster for professional exchange, the chance to visit and study at an American research institute. Meanwhile, he is grateful for the medical articles and copies of the *Chemical Weapons Convention Bulletin* (edited by Matthew and Julian Robinson) and the copy of our draft article we sent in advance.[3]

Seated in a tight circle of four chairs, the general, Matthew, Bela, and I get down to the business of discussing the outbreak. Yet in no interview with a Russian official, and certainly not with a two-star general, does one expect a simple answer to the question, "What do you know?" We begin with the autopsy data. In addition to Abramova and Grinberg's article in the *Proceedings of the National Academy of Science*, their data are also published in a Russian journal.[4] Yestigneyev, an immunologist by training, well understands the findings.

"But one thing bothers me," he says. "It presents the data and proofs of just a single hypothesis [inhalation anthrax]. I feel that doubts are still valid. I am trying to be objective, but I feel a personal and patriotic bias." He also hasn't much regard for pathologists, believing anything can be proven, depending on which autopsy slide one chooses.

A particular criticism he has of the Abramova and Grinberg publications is that they failed to pay attention to the nine cases with infected mesentery lymph nodes or give full weight to the fact that thirty-nine of the forty-two cases had intestinal lesions. Yevstigneyev points out that case 26 (Andrey Komelskikh, the old janitor at the ceramics factory) had significant intestinal lesions. The general tells us he himself has worked as a pathologist and feels that this exception should have been emphasized. He questions what happened to the early cases not represented in the Abramova series, the ones who died before April 10. He suggests that Komelskikh (who fell ill April 9 and died on April 13) might be the end of a series of intestinal anthrax cases that occurred even earlier, only the others were never autopsied, perhaps because the public health officials did a poor job and missed them.

Matthew concedes that, given how little we know about the differences between inhalation and intestinal anthrax, there are ambiguities in some of the cases and that the pathologists might have expressed that better.

"A word is like a sparrow," the general says reprovingly. "Once set free, you cannot catch it again."

He then begins to suggest alternate scenarios for the anthrax outbreak. For example, the first victims might have expired from eating bad meat and the later cases from inhalation anthrax caused by the burning of infected carcasses. Echoes of the 1980 U.S. Interagency Working Group and of Dr. Ponomaryev begin to ring in my ears. They too speculated there were two sources of infection in 1979.

Why this hypothesis? The general notes that the graph of the epidemic, with cases occurring over six weeks, represents a protracted epidemic. He would expect an anthrax aerosol to produce a sharp high spike. He would also expect that people close to the facility would get higher doses and die quickly. The dozen or so individuals who worked at the laboratory were vaccinated, but some five thousand people lived at Compound 19 and ten thousand lived at Compound 32. Yet only six of them died at one base and five at the other.

To substantiate the epizootic, Yevstigneyev shows us file photographs from Sysertskiy rayon in April 1979, pictures of dumps where dead livestock are piled one on another, with legs and necks at awkward angles. Most of these photographs were taken at a village southeast of Sverdlovsk, Oktyabrskaya, which until now we hadn't heard was affected in April 1979. It is directly in line with the six other villages where animals died of anthrax. One picture shows large piles of dead dogs, including the body of a shepherd mix that looks disturbingly like our own pet.

When he was in Sverdlovsk, Yevstigneyev says, many witnesses were still around from 1979 and gave him firsthand accounts of the outbreak in the area. For example, waitresses at the military cafeteria said they found many dogs dying of anthrax. One story goes that old Fyodor Nikolaev, who worked at Compound 19, fed some *tachlik* (shish kabob) he had made to his own dog and to stray dogs he befriended. The dogs died. Then Nikolaev himself became ill and also died. That old Nikolaev and his dog eat meat provided by the military at a time when meat is scarce, and then pass from this world together adds pathos to the general's story. But Nikolaev is also on Abramova and Grinberg's autopsy list as having had all the signs of inhalation anthrax.

While dogs in villages may have died from feeding on infected carcasses, just where dogs in the city would have discovered large stores of such meat is a puzzle. Virtually no one interviewed in Chkalovskiy could attest to livestock dying there. Even supposing some infected meat from the April epizootic made it past the roadblock to the city, it could hardly account for "many dogs dying." Instead, people in Chkalovskiy told of stray dogs being shot by the hundreds, a slaughter that takes on a quirky symbolism reminiscent of "the Great Cat Massacre" in eighteenth-century France.[5] Omnipresent, nonproductive, and always ravenous, stray dogs are Russia's most miserable creatures. "We have the souls of slaves, and a wretched fate!" moans Sharik, the dog in Mikhail Bulgakov's classic *Heart of a Dog,* who is also a kind of Soviet Everyman.[6] Stray dogs might have been a public health threat in the countryside, but there was probably no reason to destroy them in the city.

Even so, General Yevstigneyev is right about the autopsy data. It cannot stand alone—and it doesn't. We show him a draft of our article, with its nearly perfected epidemiological map. But he still takes issue with our case for an aerosol release for Compound 19. If Compound 19 was the source, he argues, that would mean that people closest to it were exposed to a higher dose and should have died early, while those at a distance should have died later. No such trend exists, as the three of us know. Also, repeating the objection he made to Matthew in January, Yestigneyev says many cases should have been clustered close to Compound 19, but that was not the case.

Matthew points out that an aerosol emission from a roof-top ventilator would be carried away from the compound at that height; in fact, one would not expect many victims in the area adjacent to the laboratory. Instead, the distribution of cases that we have already plotted shows the most vulnerable area was along the center line of Chkalovskiy between Compound 19 and the ceramics factory, in the direction of the wind on the afternoon of April 2, 1979. Further, the widening of the plume as it moved downwind (like an expanding tunnel) would have increased the geographic distribution of cases. The general reflects on this but seems unpersuaded.

Instead, he proceeds to what he thinks he knows, that no Compound 19 vaccine research or production was in process in late March or April 1979. He has found no documentary evidence that anything went wrong there the first week of April. Before April 1, work was done with a small amount of virulent agent. Yes, aerosol challenges of monkeys took place at the facility. But not in March or April, as far as the records he has seen go. During that period, work was on cutaneous anthrax.

Yes, there was communication then between Compound 19 and Boris Yeltsin, the Sverdlovsk head of the Communist Party. An order was given at the base to stop all work on virulent anthrax material and destroy it. On April 15, the director of the compound reported to Yeltsin, to Deputy Minister Burgasov, and to the KGB that the work had stopped as directed.

When we press for further details, the general balks. There is no annual report from Compound 19, he tells us, no existing secret library that will tell us more. "We shall only be going again into the same marsh," he comments philosophically, "if we continue this debate. There's a fifty-

fifty chance you have solved this puzzle, even though [you] Americans think it is more."

Still, he is willing to talk about the specific technology of the aerosol challenges. He describes the aerosol chamber as two to three cubic meters in size, large enough for two monkeys. A typical experiment in this chamber would be done with a spray of five milliliters of an anthrax suspension containing a total of five billion spores. There were special filtered channels for venting the aerosols. Each filter (of an older Russian type called Petrionov) met regulations. Such experiments had to be carried out in hermetically sealed rooms with pressure gauges. Before being ventilated, the contaminated air from the chambers would go through two disinfecting processes, what the general calls "cascades" of hydrogen peroxide at 30 percent strength. Then it went through two filters, each ten centimeters thick. Each filter, he assures us, was checked for reliability by special detectors.

"It was practically impossible that the filters didn't work," he insists.

But I have about as much confidence in what he is saying as I do in Russian light bulbs and nuclear reactors. Soviet engineering has a far from stellar past.[7] Why should a filter designed fifty years ago be especially effective for a modern laboratory? And it isn't clear to me that two washes of hydrogen peroxide are sufficient to lay waste to anthrax spores.

Even the general, after he does a rough sketch of the chamber and filter system, looks hesitant. He tells us that in 1979 the military suspected sabotage and investigated a "deviant individual" not in the military, but nothing came of it. Maybe someone sabotaged the facility for money, he suggests. At one point, even Donald Ellis, the American physicist, was suspected, though he arrived in Sverdlovsk after the outbreak began. Maybe the probability of an accidental emission at that time was the same as the probability of accident in any technological system.

"This cannot be rejected," he says, "but there is no evidence." He claims that his office staff, too, reviewed the epidemiological data, but only came up with a 42 percent probability of an emission from the Compound 19 laboratory. He praises our work as "scientific and objective," but he doesn't really believe anything conclusive can be known about this event so far in the past and so classified.

We have a question about the strain being used at Compound 19 at the time of the outbreak. The tissue samples Abramova and Grinberg are sharing with David Walker's laboratory in Texas are being examined, but no news has yet come about the strain that killed the 1979

Sverdlovsk victims. Was it some new invention? Yevstigneyev's understanding is that it was not appreciably different from what was available
to nonmilitary vaccine production facilities. He is on public record as
saying that the Soviet Union was violating the Biological Weapons Convention with offensive weapons programs, but he doubts these included
artificially intensifying the lethality of anthrax. "Some [Soviet] enthusi-
asts," he remarks, "tried to find strain differences but failed. Anthrax is
conservative. There is no experiment I know for artificially increasing
virulence." The new cellular biology techniques, he points out, were not
available here fourteen years ago.

As for the future, he thinks the next best steps lie with finding common areas of cooperation between the United States and Russia. Disease
prevention is certainly one. In fact, he was recently invited to a meeting
in Washington, but his passport was not ready and he missed it. Maybe
another time. Despite a reputation for being overbearing in Russian-U.S.
meetings, Yevstigneyev has been more than cordial.

The next day, we are in former Counselor Alexey Yablokov's new
office in a building in central Moscow. He has left the Kremlin and his
government post, and works instead as head of a consulting group that
reports to President Yeltsin on the environment. He seems more pleased
to see us than he was last year. He is familiar with the autopsy articles
and has looked over our draft article and maps. What have we done, after all, he declares, but proved what he said was true: that the military
was responsible for the 1979 outbreak. He is proud of having gotten pensions for the victims' families, although no funds have yet been transmitted.

He reviews with us the communications that led to the presidential decree for pensions to the Sverdlovsk victims' families. Following Larissa
Mishustina's letter to Yeltsin urging recompense, Yablokov and his staff
investigated the files and found the empty KGB folder. But there was more
in the file than he told us about last year. Of course, they found the written conclusion of the government anti-epidemic commission (Burgasov's
group) that contaminated meat was the cause and the outbreak had nothing to do with Compound 19. But, in addition, a secret document dated
June 5, 1979, also surfaced. It was a statement from four high-ranking
officials of the Department of Public Health, the KGB, the Central Military Institute of Defense, and the Council of Ministers that "causative
agents" were "isolated from samples of soil, air, washings from a woolen
wall hanging, the outside part of a door (the exterior door and a mail box)."

So Yablokov concluded in a preliminary report to Yeltsin that air transmission had to be responsible for these results. The absence of group and family infections, he felt, supported his conclusion. He had also had direct word from the KGB that autopsy records (probably the ones taken from Abramova) and environmental records were destroyed in December 1990, resulting in the empty files he referred to last year.

Yablokov reported to Yeltsin on December 2, 1991, with regard to Supreme Soviet member Mishustina's request, that financial support to "families of the deceased" hinged on proof that the Sverdlovsk deaths took place as the result of "activities of the Ministry of Defense of the USSR." He offered as that proof the destruction of the KGB files, plus "a number of indirect facts." According to the Russian law on state pensions, he wrote, Yeltsin could raise the issue of "granting them a maximum pension as in the case of war traumas or diseases acquired during the military service." On December 3, 1991, Yeltsin hand-wrote instructions to Yablokov to "prepare an appeal to the Supreme Soviet," which Yablokov did. On March 4, 1992, Yeltsin submitted the appeal to the Supreme Soviet of the Russian Federation. The decree itself makes no reference to the military or its responsibility for the Sverdlovsk outbreak, only to rules set "by enterprises, agencies, and organizations for the damage caused to workers."

Perhaps the most important fact that Yablokov discovered was that in 1990 the military procurator of the USSR abrogated the criminal code associated with the fatal cases in the epidemic, so that those responsible for the outbreak could not be prosecuted in a civil court. Yablokov's recommendation was for Yeltsin to follow the lead of the United States and introduce a law criminalizing the development of BW. In this way, future offenses could be prosecuted. That law is now close to passage, he is proud to say.

Today Yablokov is more worried about the environment than about the cause of the Sverdlovsk outbreak. This is understandable, considering the pervasive health problems that result from industrial pollution in Russia. German sociologist Ulrich Beck argues that modern industrial technology, while it generates wealth, produces environmental risks at such ever-increasing levels that they can no longer be considered side effects.[8] Yablokov is definitely attuned to the problem.

But he should also heed the warning of the Sverdlovsk case. Military technology also imposes risks for the environment, in its manufacture, in its potential deployment, and above all in its technological development. Behind us lies a century devoted to using modern scientific achievements to develop weapons of mass destruction, the ultimate risks. Out of physics came nuclear weapons, which were produced in such quantity in the second half of the twentieth century that it will take centuries to rid the planet of their noxious products. Out of chemistry came nerve gases, cheaper to make and use than nuclear weapons, but hard to control. And then, out of biology, the science of life and healing, have come weapons that can turn the worst of nature's devices against humans. Advances in molecular and cellular biology threaten new products and techniques that may not simply kill or wound, but manipulate our bodies and our minds, including the way our species reproduces, who lives and dies, and all the life processes that govern our survival. The military development of new biotechnologies could recreate the nuclear threat, cubed. Biological weapons even at their most primitive—the case of the 1979 Sverdlovsk outbreak is an example—represent a hideous assault on life.

It is understandable that in 1990 the Sverdlovsk file was destroyed by the Soviet Council of Ministers. The Sverdlovsk outbreak was probably just one among many embarrassments and crimes that the Council, the KGB, and the Defense Ministry wanted expunged from history. In a peculiar way, the destruction of the documents signifies the old guard's fear of the inevitable power of glasnost to destroy censorship, to allow the freedom of the press, and to lay government bare to any inquirers, even foreigners, even Americans like us. They must have believed that, without documents, the real cause of the collective deaths of the 1979 anthrax outbreak would never be revealed, that involved citizens would remain resigned and silent. History and our investigation have proved them wrong. Still, Yeltsin's pension decree, lacking any reference to the military, now also looks like a move to rebury the events surrounding the 1979 Sverdlovsk outbreak, rather like reburying the bones of the Romanovs.

23

The Summing Up

The afternoon of our final day in Moscow, we visit former Deputy Minister Burgasov at his dacha in Barvikha. Though it is still August, autumn has arrived, wet and cold. Dr. Burgasov looks more gaunt than he did a year ago, and his manner and dress have become countrified, as if in this exclusive enclave that mimics a village, he is simulating a return to his peasant roots. We begin with a late lunch much like the one we had a year ago, with fish, blini, tomatoes, cucumbers, and multiple bottles of vodka. Once again, the house is filled with Burgasov's offspring, his daughter, his grandchildren. The center of attention is a newborn, a great-grandchild. The usual rabbits, chickens, and dogs abound, and an addition to the menagerie, a large green parrot, perched on a stand, adds to the commotion.

Despite that commotion, we get right to the subject of our research. Dr. Burgasov says he appreciates how deeply we have been studying the 1979 anthrax outbreak and reaffirms the point that he himself never had time to do that, having been preoccupied with all the people who were dying. He knows about the Abramova and Grinberg articles and feels the pathologists do not understand epidemiology. But journalists, he declares, are worse. He is still bridling about the way he has been represented in the Moscow press. As for the Nikiforov article, he claims it is now lost, for which he blames Nikiforov's son. At this point, at the end of the investigation, we are interested only in confronting him with our conclusions and in knowing if he can accept a radically different explanation of the outbreak's cause than infected bone meal, contaminated animal feed, and tainted meat.

After the table is cleared, we open a bottle of whisky we have brought and fill glasses. Matthew gives the former deputy minister a Russian translation of our draft, which is just ten pages long.

"Please read this and be a student," Matthew urges.

"I am glad to be young again, a student," Burgasov laughs. As he takes the article, he protests that nothing will change his mind about Sverdlovsk. "I will never publish any official statement myself," he insists. And he predicts that if secret research on biology is published, Third World countries like China, Iran, and Iraq, will use it. "There are more countries in the world than the United States and Russia," he declares.

"Give advice, then," Matthew tells him.

I hand Burgasov a red pen so he can make notations. For about ten minutes, while we wait in silence and children race around the house and the dogs bark and the parrot squawks, he concentrates on reading our paper and makes check marks as he goes along.

Finally he looks up and says, "I have no objections. But I would like to state that in the end the truth remains unclear."

To begin, he questions why no people in Compound 19 were infected if they were in the path of the wind. Certainly he is not up to date. Matthew shows the former deputy minister the KGB list, which indicates four victims there, at the address NII44. Burgasov counters that from April 6 to May 15, several people who worked at Compound 19 but lived in Chkalovskiy became ill, but none who were residents at the base. Matthew responds that General Yevstigneyev, whom Burgasov knows, has told us six people there became sick and at least one died. "I never saw them," Burgasov says emphatically, "I cannot answer any question about those cases."

The incubation period of the disease is also a mystery to him. If on April 2 an aerosol was released, why were people falling ill in mid-May? As he did with General Yevstigneyev, Matthew explains that the incubation period for anthrax was also difficult for him to understand. He refers to the experimental literature that indicates spores can remain dormant in the lungs for weeks, even months, depending on the individual.

"If so, this is a new discovery," Burgasov exclaims, but he appears unconvinced. "I have one request," he continues. "The houses were cleaned and the roads paved—bear in mind, for the May First holiday. That was a central event. Only now, over the last few years, have we stopped cleaning up. It was a Soviet tradition to clean up everything, not just in Chkalovskiy, but in all the cities." He pauses. "Besides that, I have no objections [to the article]. It is the opinion of the authors, who did a lot of research. It's a scientific paper."

Matthew, in reference to the document we have seen at Yablokov's office, asks Burgasov if he knew anything about a report citing samples positive for anthrax being found on doors and in air and water in Chkalovskiy. Burgasov dismisses the discovery of positive samples as just a false rumor, one of many, including his having been somehow in league with Boris Yeltsin to cover up the source of the epidemic. "Yeltsin asked me to come to his office and gave me a clock-radio to thank me [for handling the outbreak]. I met him only once, that time."

As for the timing of the animal outbreak, we present Burgasov with our proposition that livestock in the villages succumbed to anthrax starting April 5, about the same time as the first human victims, but that the animals were diagnosed earlier than the victims in Chkalovskiy. Burgasov counters that the veterinary documents he gave us are incomplete, that animal deaths caused by anthrax happened earlier among private owners and were not well recorded. Burgasov still wants to pin the blame on a faulty vaccination program. He complains that information from veterinarians is often erratic. We respond with information about our five outliers who were at military reserve courses, about the baker Nina T., about wind data, about dormant spores in monkey lungs. Burgasov, an administrator, not a scientist, retreats.

"The defense of this country is sacred to me," he says. "I will never reveal anything that would jeopardize it. If people want to disagree, that's all right. But I am a patriot."

Burgasov is completely of the old Soviet order, an anachronism, an old bear hiding in the woods. Whether or not he really knew what was going on in Compound 19, he did not break rank. Even to raise the question of an airborne source would have betrayed the military's mission to defend the country. When he went to the United States with Dr. Nikiforov in 1988 and presented the official Soviet explanation of the outbreak, he probably believed everything he said and never thought of saying anything else.

Gorbachev's glasnost, which allowed Burgasov to appear as its emissary to the U.S. in 1988, is as onerous to him as the free market economy his country has adopted. He sees it producing prostitutes, dirty streets, inflation, the degradation of life for everyone. If the new government wants to blame the military for the 1979 Sverdlovsk outbreak, that only proves its corruption. Were he alive, Dr. Nikiforov, who was of the same generation and also benefited from the old rule, might have felt the same, though he might also have welcomed in private, if not in public, the new medical research on anthrax. Dr. Bezdenezhnikh, the epidemiologist who pursued the tainted-meat explanation, also older and privileged, did not live to see the end of the Soviet Union. With his avid search for animal cases and his record of the hospital admission dates, he was probably the most influential articulator of the tainted-meat explanation, although here and there we have heard that higher officials disapproved of his on-site queries in Sverdlovsk and brought him back to Moscow quickly.

The common characteristic of each of these three men, though, is not what they thought but what they did not dare to think. As Hannah Arendt proposed in *The Origins of Totalitarianism*, everyone in the USSR, including professionals, was dependent on the good will of the state.[1] In 1979, this dependence required every level of medical personnel to proceed exactly as if the origin of the outbreak was irrelevant, its possible military source unthinkable. Or, if contemplated, then it was only a rumor, circulating among those "back porches" Dr. Arenskiy referred to, with no connection to action of wider significance.

The scientific enterprise (and I include medical science) relies, in contrast, on intellectual honesty, integrity, a sense of skepticism, disinterestedness, and impersonality, which cannot endure when state authority is imposed.[2] The scientific standards that should have been applied to understanding the Sverdlovsk outbreak when it occurred were not. We can continue to speculate about how political pressure was exerted. Conditions in 1979 were certainly better than when Trofim Lysenko, the fraudulent scientist touted by Stalin, nearly destroyed Soviet biological sciences.[3] None of the three Soviet physicians, Burgasov, Bezdenezhnikh, or Nikiforov, necessarily compartmentalized their moral and professional lives to the extent of, for instance, German doctors and geneticists in the Third Reich. But all three certainly bowed to the state. Their silence about Compound 19, whether overtly or tacitly demanded, reinforced the army's right to remain aloof, as if without responsibility to local citizens. The state that should have protected its citizens, the military bound by honor to defend them, and the medical professionals dedicated to serve them were instead united in silence against them.

The exception, of course, was Dr. Faina Abramova, whose private reaction to the KGB sweep of documents was to hide her autopsy data, merely because it was hers. She refused to let the state rob her of professional integrity. But until the end of the Soviet state Abramova, and Grinberg too, had little choice but to bow to its authority. For example, the paper they brought to Moscow in 1982 describes general lymph node infection and the example used to illustrate their findings was mesenteric—in keeping with the tainted-meat explanation—and not thoracic, which would have pointed to an anthrax aerosol. It was only after 1991 that the two pathologists were free to present their scientific analysis of the autopsy data. That earlier paper takes nothing away from the courage later required, even in 1991, to present publicly information so obviously critical of the military and the state, but only underscores the repression of Soviet medical science.

The alliance of Burgasov, Bezdenezhnikh, and Nikiforov with the state does not mean that all facts in the official Soviet explanation of the 1979 outbreak were erroneous. The general presentation of numbers of victims and case outcome was correct. According to the paper given by the Soviet government to the U.S. State Department in 1988, the total number of anthrax cases was ninety-six: eleven pure cutaneous, six cutaneous that became systemic, and seventy-nine gastrointestinal cases. Of the latter, sixty-four were said to be fatal, leaving fifteen survivors. The survival rate was therefore around 20 percent among these most difficult cases. In our study, the identification of sixty-six victims who died with authenticated anthrax and nine survivors (eleven minus two with cutaneous involvement) gives a survival rate of around 14 percent. This estimate is probably low since, without full records, we had no way to estimate or cross-check the number of survivors, the way we did for those who died. We found five survivors through Dr. Nikiforov's preserved clinical files, while other names came from hospital lists or by hearsay. These facts imply that, with aggressive clinical management, as many as one-fifth of patients with inhalation anthrax can be saved. (See Appendix B for a tabular summary of case information.)

Our visit to Dr. Burgasov ends with another expression of his respect for the scientific work we have done, but he says this as if we are on the other side of a substantial cognitive divide, which we are.

Afterward, we focus on what exactly we have learned to this point and what we will add to the draft of our epidemiology article. Our best work this trip has been with the outliers, especially those on military reserve duty on April 2, and with Nina T. Alex Langmuir's faith and Donald Henderson's optimism that the interviews would yield precision have been justified. We have now circumscribed the time of common exposure to anthrax. The number of red dots we can plot on our spot map places nearly all of the victims within a narrow plume that stretches southeast from Compound 19 to the neighborhood past the ceramics factory. With the excursion to Abramovo, we have clarified the relation of the timing of animal and human deaths and believe the exposure for both was nearly simultaneous. All the data—from interviews, documents, lists, autopsies, and wind reports—now fit, like pieces of a puzzle. What we know proves a lethal plume of anthrax came from Compound 19.

On Monday, April 2, probably between 1:30 and 4:00 P.M., human victims were exposed to a plume of aerosolized anthrax that traveled southeast over Chkalovskiy at an average rate of about fifteen kilometers an hour. That same plume proceeded out into the countryside, infecting livestock. In a few days, sheep and cows began to sicken and die, with the indications of anthrax familiar to veterinarians.

By April 4, in Sverdlovsk, the earliest anthrax victims, like Anna Komina and Vera Kozlova, suffering initial symptoms, were either being sent home by unknowing physicians, who mistook their illness for the flu or the grippe, or were braving their headaches, dizziness, chills and fevers without consulting doctors. On April 7–8, Dr. Klipnitzer was alerted by his staff to several unexplained rapid deaths. He telephoned Dr. Ilyenko at her hospital, where the critical cases were beginning to accumulate. The Extraordinary Commission chaired by Dr. Babich met and decided that Hospital 40 would be the centralized care facility. Around this time, Moscow was contacted. On April 10–11, Dr. Abramova made the diagnosis of anthrax, while in the villages animal carcasses were being burned under veterinary supervision.

On April 12, after the laboratory test confirmed the disease was anthrax, Dr. Nikiforov arrived in Sverdlovsk with his assistants, including Olga Yampolskaya and two other physicians, to manage the medical responses. Dr. Nikiforov must have planned for a vaccination program right away, to have it running just a few days after his arrival. On his heels came Dr. Burgasov and Dr. Bezdenezhnikh, as well as Dr. Burgasov's son. By then, the ongoing anthrax epizootic south of the city was being handled by tearing down sheds, vaccinating owners of livestock, and quarantining the villages.

Around mid-April, with dozens of patients being screened daily for anthrax and the vaccination campaign begun, Dr. Arenskiy traveled with Dr. Bezdenezhnikh to the villages southeast of the city, where other Moscow experts, along with SES veterinarians, were probably involved. Along the way, the March 28 report of a sick sheep was folded into the April 5–10 animal cases verified by laboratory tests as anthrax; so too was the Chkalovskiy court case against the two people from Rudniy village who sold bad meat. Infected meat may, in fact, have made its way into the city from Sysertskiy; Romanenko reported ten positive samples from meat taken from homes. But infected meat has no bearing on our map, where the daytime locations of victims markedly delineate the path of the anthrax plume.

We know that in the city the public health response to the epidemic extended from neighborhood to city to oblast offices, with volunteer brigades and ambulance drivers working vigorously and with Hospital 40 and the local hospitals and clinics screening patients on the basis of symptoms. Still, thirteen people died at home; at least four others were dead on arrival at the hospital. Dr. Burgasov and Dr. Nikiforov eventually controlled the management of the outbreak, but who directed the washing of buildings remains unclear. Some city officials claimed credit for it; Dr. Burgasov did not. The interior and exterior of the ceramics factory were disinfected in somewhat the same way as the stables in Abramovo and other villages, because, as one official put it, so many workers had died there and "we just had to do everything possible."

After the end of the epidemic in May, Bezdenezhnikh drew his graph of the hospital admissions that resembled the progression of the disease in Yaroslavl (see Figure 1). Because many victims died relatively quickly after hospitalization and because the hospitals were also registering home and sudden deaths, the graph generally represents how the Sverdlovsk epidemic erupted and continued. The addition of onset and death dates from our research gives new dimensions to our understanding of the onslaught (see Figure 3). The first two weeks were the most perilous: some two-thirds of the victims fell sick and died by April 16. The deaths of the remaining third were spread thinly over the next month.

Are we sure, though, that we accounted for all or nearly all of the anthrax fatalities? In the family and neighborhood interviews, the question "Do you know of other victims?" was always asked. Sometimes we thought we had found leads; in the end, we returned to the KGB list, and even there some deaths may not have been caused by anthrax. We heard no rumors of many deaths occurring at Compounds 19 or 32, and we know the military itself referred several patients to Hospital 40. More important, although military officials remained aloof from the 1979 outbreak, the flow of ordinary people back and forth through the compound gates continued. People who lived on the military bases worked in town; people who lived in town worked on the military bases. Even today, workers going in both directions crowd the compound gates during morning and evening rush hours. Keeping thousands of deaths secret from the local

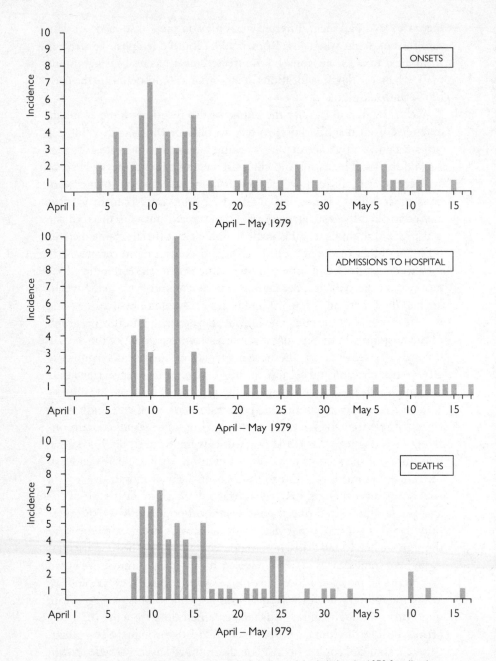

FIGURE 3. Dates of onset of symptoms, hospital admission, and death during the 1979 Sverdlovsk anthrax outbreak, from interview and medical record sources. Onset and admission data for survivors are included. The victims with the earliest onset, on April 4, were Anna Komina and Aleksandra Volkova.

population would have been difficult indeed. As for possible missing cases early in the outbreak, no proof exists that these were more than a few. In any event, the deaths of nearly seventy people is tragedy enough.

Still left out of these reckonings is the problem of individual susceptibility to anthrax. There was the super-chimpanzee who survived enormous doses of anthrax, and we know that many U.S. woolen-mill workers exposed to anthrax spores, even those new to the job, never became ill. Of the roughly seven thousand people who were within the boundaries of the plume on April 2, 1979, probably relatively few were susceptible. We know that some of the 1979 victims, like the computer programmer Vitaliy Fyodosov, had chronic problems with their immune systems. Some suffered from siderosis, asbestosis, or tuberculosis. A number of the men were heavy smokers. At the same time, fifteen victims had a spore or spores in their lungs for three or more weeks before falling ill. These include six survivors who felt symptoms thirty-four to forty-five days after exposure, for reasons that are unknown.

Age was certainly an important predictor of death in the 1979 outbreak. Of the victims for whom we have birth and death dates, fifty-two were over age thirty-seven; half were forty-five or older. Three-quarters of the fatalities were men, nearly all middle-aged; the median age was forty-two. The median age for women was fifty-five; the kindergarten teacher Kosheleva, age twenty-four, was the only woman in her twenties. The other women were thirty-two and older. Young people under twenty-four and children escaped being victims, perhaps because their immune systems were stronger or because their physiologic reactions to inhalatory infections are different than those of adults. We just do not know.[4] What is sure is that older men were more susceptible during the outbreak.

Instead of feeling jubilant about all we have learned, I am almost depressed. I cannot help envisioning the everyday lives of the 1979 anthrax victims as they were innocently trapped in the lethal swath of air. Officer Vladimir Sannikov was perhaps having a late lunch at the canteen. The military reservists were in class, trying to concentrate on some new fact about artillery. The sickly Fyodosov was about to get sicker. Maybe young Yuriy Kramskoy in his room at the hostel had plans for a date. One survivor, Anatoliy S., was hammering away on a new family bathhouse. Across the street, Anna Komina, on her day off, was washing lunch dishes, while around the corner, Nina T., the baker, had just returned from a day's work. Down the block, Tatyana Kosheleva might have been tying the shoe of a kindergarten child. Unaware of jeopardy, ten workers at the ceramics factory pipe shop, including the friends Maslennikov and Zakharov, were inhaling what would be for them lethal gusts of air through the windows. In other parts of the factory, without knowing it, eight more workers were also becoming mortally infected. Southeast of the factory, in the yard of MEX 44, Zinatulla Abusagitov could have been repairing an engine with Pyotr Pilyasov. Maybe the maintenance men who drove trucks were just crossing Selkorovskaya right into the invisible plume. Maybe Aleksandr R., the survivor we never located, decided to visit a friend in Chkalovskiy. Just ordinary people. All of them in the wrong place at the wrong time.

Our trip to Russia is done. On the last night, from our hotel window, we watch a magnificent fireworks display over Gorky Park. It seems to go on forever, a public diversion from Russia's economic and political woes, bouquets of flame simulating victory while the world around totters. The three interviews we have accomplished over the last few days, with General Yevstigneyev, the military scientist, with Dr. Yablokov, the government consultant, and with Dr. Burgasov, the retired public health official, give me little cause for celebration. The first, the general, hesitates to implicate Compound 19; he is skeptical and also has the military's interests at heart. The second, ex-Counselor Yablokov, downplays the importance of factual information about the outbreak; he wants us to look to the future, not the past. The third, retired Deputy Minister Burgasov, justifies the bad-meat explanation in the name of patriotism.

Each perspective is understandable. What disturbs me is that each is also an avoidance, a turning away from the strongest implication of our work: that the cover-up of the outbreak's source, no matter how or why it was perpetuated, was the real crime in this case. All five features of what the political scientist E. V. Walter calls "the process of terrorism" were present in the Sverdlovsk incident. The military was the structurally detached agent of violence against which no retaliation was possible. The victims were expendable people, but not the stigmatized types that might otherwise be punished by violence. The targeted population (call it those who lived and worked in Chkalovskiy) shared with the agents of violence the ideology that would let it survive terrorism. This population depended on the state and, in this city in particular, on the military itself, as its industrial mainstay in the Cold War economy. Further, local citizens, up and down the ranks, cooperated with measures to restore order, the submissive order which is the goal of organized terrorism and which it needs to maintain itself.[5] It mattered little that the anthrax emission was probably accidental. Its accidental nature was never communicated. Its lethal violence was. It mattered little that the violence was never repeated. It could have been, as far as the adjacent community knew. Chkalovskiy residents lived under that shadow for years.

All our efforts in this research have been to use science to capture the reality of the 1979 Sverdlovsk outbreak, to bring these deaths into a rational framework of analysis. I feel we have done that, as much as we could, and will be able to illustrate how the lethal plume traversed Chkalovskiy and reached the villages in Sysertskiy rayon. The revelation is incomplete, however, without some firsthand testimony about how this dread-provoking accident took place at Compound 19, although secondhand accounts of Compound 19's involvement have circulated from the beginning, and still do.[6] Did the death of General Mikhailov, the compound commander, really render an admission of culpability impossible? Were all the KGB files actually destroyed? Until there is accountability, the violence and the evil linger.

The fireworks in Gorky Park are over. We are packed and ready for an early flight to Amsterdam, where Julian Robinson will meet us. We have a lot to tell him. Before we leave, I write in my notebook, "In the end, it all seems so simple."

The Threat of Bioweapons

Once again back in Cambridge, we place the final dots on the map of daytime locations. The five men who were at reserve courses at Compound 32 are added. Survivors Nina T. and Nikolay S. are placed at their homes near the ceramics factory. All the daytime locations of the victims are then transposed to a satellite map of the city. After this, Matthew calculates the shape and direction of the April 2 plume. Three sets of curved lines (isopleths) illustrate the direction of the anthrax aerosol and its predictable diffusion; greater intensity of spores was likely in the center of the spreading cloud and diminished at the edges and as it diffused southeast (Map 2).[1] This illustration shows that Compound 32 and the ceramics factory, with relatively high population densities, bore the brunt of the aerosol. Our data, mapped with precision, are a stunning representation of the tragedy.

Our next step is to chart the locations of the six villages where animals died in the April epizootic (Map 3). All the villages lie along the extended axis of the plume that begins at Compound 19. The straight line from the military base right through to Abramovo that Matthew drew on our first trip to Yekaterinburg (and then showed to the dismayed Dr. Ponomaryev after his presentation) is confirmed. The compass bearing for the centerline of both the human and the animal cases is 330 degrees (plus or minus 10 degrees), from northwest to southeast.

Having gotten this far, we can return to the problem that has preoccupied Alex Langmuir and Matthew for some time: estimating what quantity of aerosolized anthrax spores could have caused the Sverdlovsk outbreak. The reckoning has two parts. The first is the calculation of how many spores a person would inhale, which would depend on that person's downwind and crosswind distance from the source, the number of spores released, and the prevailing meteorological conditions. Atmospheric diffusion theory can provide reasonably accurate estimates if the wind speed and the stability of the atmosphere are known. As has been mentioned, we have that information for Sverdlovsk's main airport in early April 1979 from the National Center for Atmospheric Research. Professor Borisov has also provided us with confirming data from two smaller airports reporting at the same time from Sverdlovsk.

The second and much less certain part of the calculation requires knowing the dose-response relation for the population that is at risk. Mercifully, no research has been done on this for humans. Instead, we have to assume that the dose-response for a human population will resemble what has been determined experimentally with nonhuman primates. Based on experiments with hundreds of monkeys done at Fort Detrick in the 1950s, the U.S. army standardized a value of eight thousand inhaled anthrax spores as the dosage lethal for 50 percent of a human population receiving it, the so-called LD50. But nowhere in Sverdlovsk was the fatality rate 50 percent. Even at the ceramics factory pipe shop, apparently right on the centerline of the passing spore cloud, only ten of about four hundred and fifty workers fell ill and died, a fatality rate of 2 percent. To estimate the dosage that would infect 2 percent of an exposed monkey (or human) population, one must extrapolate downward from data obtained from experiments with much higher dosages. Different mathematical models have been developed for doing this. The "log-normal" model used for years by U.S. army BW scientists to calculate anthrax munitions requirements and risk factors sensibly assumes that the exposed population is heterogeneous, that is, that some people are more susceptible to infection than others. In Sverdlovsk, for instance, adults certainly seemed more susceptible than children and teenagers; and it is not hard to believe that some adults were more resistant than others. Using the army's specific log-normal model for anthrax, one easily obtains the astonishing result that while the inhalation of eight thousand spores is required to infect half of an exposed population, a mere nine spores per individual would infect 2 percent of the population. Could a dosage of only nine spores have infected ten of the four hundred and fifty pipe shop workers? No one can say for sure. While the army's model was based on large-scale tests in Fort Detrick's one-million liter aerosol test chamber, other smaller experiments there and elsewhere (using various species of nonhuman primates, various anthrax strains, and various experimental conditions) have given LD50 values ranging from two thousand to fifty thousand spores.

In the face of all this uncertainty, Matthew follows the standard course of making a low estimate and a high estimate of the quantity of aerosolized anthrax spores that could have caused the 1979 outbreak. Using the old army model gives the smallest estimate of the quantity of spores that might have been released as aerosol at Compound 19—an almost unbelievable two to four milligrams, hardly enough to see, but containing billions of spores. For the upper estimate, using an LD50 of forty-five thousand spores and an extrapolation model (called a "one-hit" model) that gives higher values of the required dosage than the log-normal model, he gets an estimate of a release that is 150 times higher. But even that dosage is less than a gram, thousands of times less than the kilos estimated by the U.S. Defense Intelligence Agency.

These calculations have two important implications. First, the claim that the amount of anthrax released was so great that it exceeded any possible peaceful purpose is not supported by this information. Nonetheless, we know that after signing the 1972 Biological Weapons Convention, the Soviet Union violated it. Russia's own 1992 "Form F" declaration and statements by General Yevstigneyev have confirmed this fact and demonstrated the need for better mechanisms to ensure transparency, if biological weapons are to be effectively prohibited. But we cannot be sure that the Compound 19 facility in particular was in violation of the treaty. And until it is open to outsiders, we do not know its current status or the risks it poses to the city.

The second, more important, implication of Matthew's calculations is that while larger quantities of anthrax aerosol may be required to cause a very high casualty level, almost unimaginably small quantities might nevertheless pose a substantial threat if released in a densely populated area. The virulence of anthrax is patently clear.

Once infected with anthrax bacteria, what chances did the Sverdlovsk victims have of a cure? The aggressive clinical management of patients achieved a survival rate of at least 14 and possibly 20 percent. Dr. Nikiforov's interventions (which ran the gamut from penicillin, cephalosporin, chloramphenicol, anti-anthrax globulin, and corticosteroids to hydration and artificial respiration) saved perhaps fifteen lives. This is a clinical accomplishment to be proud of, as Dr. Nikiforov's colleagues and son understood. In ways we cannot reckon, the distribution of antibiotics at homes and workplaces may also have brought down the general attack rate, which looks to be about two to three percent, within the high-risk zone.

All these factors considered, the dose calculations and the outcome for victims underscore the dangerous nature of the research at the Sverdlovsk military facility. The laboratory obviously constituted a serious hazard for citizens in the adjacent community, as well as for soldiers and their families at the two military bases. In the end, the miasma surrounding the cause of the outbreak served the interests of the state, specifically the military, to the detriment of the people afflicted by death and illness and, we must not forget, by terror.

Three months after we return from our second expedition to Russia, in November 1993, Alex Langmuir, who has been in failing health, passes away. The following spring, *Science* (the journal of the American Association for the Advancement of Science), after customary peer review, accepts our article on the epidemiology of the Sverdlovsk outbreak.[2] The maps are perfected, with no compromises; the six outliers we could not account for, including those who were mobile and may have been in Chkalovskiy, remain outside the plume. The phrasing of the seven-page text is polished like a gem, thanks to Matthew's efforts. We dedicate the article to Alex and, when it is published in November 1994, we believe that anthrax and its controversies are over.

Not so. Like a bad genie, anthrax refuses to be contained. As fears of nuclear annihilation recede, chemical and biological weapons loom with increasing menace. The Sverdlovsk outbreak, instead of being consigned to the past, is like a tabletop model for future incidents against which we have to defend ourselves. Instead of being an account of an accidental emission, unlikely to be repeated, the scenario can be transposed to an intentional fatal assault on a vulnerable population that, like the victims in 1979, cannot feel or see the fatal spores.

But why are biological weapons, which have been around for decades, so important now? The answer lies in how national security issues are defined in the post–Cold War era. As the foremost world power, the United States must now reckon with the likelihood of dispersed hostilities and terrorist acts from a handful of economically disadvantaged non-Western countries. Dr. Burgasov was right when, in reference to biological weapons proliferation, he said there were more countries in the world than Russia and the United States. In recent years, the U.S. State Department has listed seven "rogue" nations that both support terrorism and have BW programs, in particular, Iraq, Iran, and North Korea.[3]

Foremost among these enemies is the recalcitrant Iraq, whose aggression is documented. The 1995 report of the United Nations Special Commission (UNSCOM), for example, delineated Iraq's active development of anthrax as a weapon. Mass production began in 1989, with strains imported from the United States and France, as well as with local varieties. By Iraq's own admission to UNSCOM, it had produced six thousand liters of anthrax slurry and had deployed fifty bombs and ten al Hussein missile warheads filled with it. In addition, one hundred bombs and still more warheads were filled with concentrated botulin toxin.[4] Despite the UN-supervised destruction of Iraq's major biological weapons facility at al-Hakam in 1991, the possibility that Iraq could reconstitute its BW program is being taken seriously.[5]

The potential threat of Iraq and other nations with offensive BW programs is only part of the picture. When a bomb exploded in February 1993 at New York's World Trade Center, killing six and injuring a thousand, American citizens realized their vulnerability to the free-floating political violence that ignores national boundaries. Other fanaticisms that cross borders trouble us. When in March 1995, the Aum Shinrikyo group released sarin nerve gas in Tokyo, a new model for terrorism was created. New York City officials immediately began exercises against the same potential terrorism in their city subways. At the federal level, American national security analysts were just as quickly called upon to explain why the Central Intelligence Agency had missed tracking the cult, whose activities included extensive anthrax production, until after the Tokyo attack. Eight months before, the world press had reported a sarin gas attack in a Japanese town that killed seven, which was also linked to the cult.

A month after the incident in Tokyo, when Timothy McVeigh blew up the Murrah Federal Building in Oklahoma City, killing 163 adults and children, the boundaries of terrorism were again expanded. This time the fanatic hostility against the U.S. government was home-grown, from within. McVeigh's inspiration came from the Patriot militia movement, one of many white male organizations that promote racism, antisemitism, and active protest against the federal government.[6] "Leaderless resistance" has emerged internationally as a strategy that appeals equally to a deracinated Gulf War veteran like Timothy McVeigh and to neofascists in Europe, Middle-Eastern suicide bombers, and fanatics in Northern Ireland. Sectarian fanaticism has surged in the past decade, analyst Walter Laqueur reminds us, and the means to the end of terrorism have expanded.

The power of terrorism lies in its threat of potential harm. To this coercion, the threat of biological weapons adds its own powerful symbolic implications of dissolution and despair. Disease has always had a special claim on our experience. "The body's integrity is the foundation of our sense of order and wholeness. When we sicken, so it seems does the world."[7] Nightmares of succumbing to terrible illness touch on our fears of losing our rationality to pain, our dignity to physical degradation and loss of control. On a collective level, a major epidemic can destroy social order. When it strikes, as Daniel Defoe described in *A Journal of the Plague Year*, civilization can fall apart: city dwellers flee in panic, the sick and dying are shunned.

Modern Western science, grounded in individual rationality, is supposed to protect us against the great plagues that afflicted our ancestors or that afflict the underprivileged in far-away countries. How can such random collective death assault us when we are so intelligent and our society is so advanced? But emerging diseases like AIDS and reemerging ones like tuberculosis and plague have invaded our modern world. Biological weapons evoke not just the fear of their violent assault on the individual body's life processes (Julian Robinson uses the term "biospecificity),[8] but also fears of attack on the body politic, on who we are as citizens of a particular nation.

During the autumn of 1997, the Department of Defense went full force to publicize bioterrorism as a top national security priority. The drumbeats began with a sequence of three reports that proclaimed biological weapons as the new, central threat to national security and laid the groundwork—reinforced by Congressional hearings and other public statements—for a whole new series of defensive programs against the threat of BW.[9] As in 1954, when the U.S. BW program had more money than it could spend,[10] anti-bioweapons programs soon became a well-funded top priority.

Some of the programs may result in discoveries that will have wider application. The Defense Advanced Research Projects Agency (DARPA) is investing hundreds of millions of dollars in contracts to commercial and university laboratories to investigate innovative measures to detect pathogens and combat infection. The Defense Department also funded ProMed, a free and highly interactive global reporting address for tracking and identifying disease outbreaks. Multiple organizations, from WHO to universities and even missionary societies, are participating; a network of networks for emerging and reemerging diseases is sure to evolve.[11] Of course, a major concern is how to differentiate natural outbreaks from BW attacks, no easy feat.[12]

Other programs are more strictly focused on reacting to the use of BW: technologies for detection of manufactured clouds potentially bearing biological weapons, Biological Integrated Detection Systems (BIDS), and another effort, Portashield, a network of sensors for air bases and seaports.[13] These are in addition to the usual programs for protective suits and masks.

One major program announced by the Defense Department in 1997 was the vaccination against anthrax of all 2.4 million members of the military, including reservists. The program of six inoculations over eighteen months will require at least sixty million dollars in vaccine orders and is justified, according to the Defense Department, by the deployment of American military around the world in more or less destabilized areas, as part of the nation's new role as "policeman to the world."[14] Resistance to the program by some U.S. soldiers and their families was immediate. Even the army is unsure the vaccinations are fully effective.

At the same time the Defense Department, in conjunction with the National Security Council, has established a program of nationwide BW civil defense exercises in 120 U.S. cities, virtually every large metropolis in the country. The idea is to fund each city's emergency preparedness program to deal with a Sverdlovsk or Aum Shinrikyo type of assault. New York and Washington were among the first to stage preliminary exercises and received several millions of dollars to develop programs to mobilize emergency forces, including police, firefighters, paramedics, ambulance corps, and medical and nursing staffs in hospitals with intensive treatment facilities.

Donald Henderson, the former Dean of Johns Hopkins School of Public Health and Alex Langmuir's protégé, worries especially about the lack of a public health infrastructure in the United States. He has focused attention on the problem of how contagion can extend the effect of a BW attack; that is, that human-to-human transmission of disease takes off where an aerosol stops and amplifies the weapon's power. Using the hypothetical example of smallpox (less hardy but far more contagious than anthrax), he argues that the United States lacks both the trained personnel and the hospital beds to respond to a large BW attack.[15] Our major health care investment has been instead in emergency and acute care, not in containing infectious diseases.

Compare this to the Sverdlovsk case. There, an extensive public health system made it possible to handle a relatively small outbreak. Residents relied on local clinics and hospitals, emergency transport, a central hospital, a special laboratory for disease identification, and a pediatric division at another hospital, as well as medical specialists, volunteer brigades from factories and hospitals, the police, and firemen. The government response rang in on every level, from the microrayons to Moscow. The stability of the Sverdlovsk social system extended to medical personnel and administrators who knew each other well and were in frequent communication, even before the outbreak, and who also knew their patients; in some instances, they were even neighbors. Despite these resources it took six days to discern the outbreak and nine days (until April 11) to confirm the diagnosis, by which time many victims were dead or dying.

An improved U.S. public health system might be able to better cope with infectious disease outbreaks, but could it reasonably contain the effects of a deployed biological weapon? A typical American city, large, impersonal, and culturally diverse, is a far cry from the Soviet city of Sverdlovsk. Most would need a complete civil defense–public health overhaul to deal with a full-scale biological weapons attack. Indeed, we have to ask if any public health response would be sufficient. An anonymous official from the Arms Control and Disarmament Agency has told the press, "Biological agents, both toxins and living organisms, can rival thermonuclear weapons—possibly producing hundreds of thousands to several millions of casualties in a single incident. Mortality levels from a biological attack could possibly exceed that of a large nuclear explosion."[16] This drastic level of threat implies the BW capacity of a state rather than an individual or cult, for which a public health response would be as futile as for a nuclear holocaust. Ultimately, we need to recognize, as we have done for nuclear and chemical weapons, that it is much more realistic to invest our resources in preventing weapons proliferation and use than to aim for damage control.

Another, perhaps inevitable, outcome of the new emphasis on bioweapons is greater surveillance by the FBI, the CIA, and Defense Intelligence. One 1998 committee report, with John Deutch, former Director of U.S. Central Intelligence, as cochair, recommends a federal consolidation of bioterrorism intelligence and the creation of decentralized Catastrophic Terrorism Response Offices (CTROS).[17] The report also outlines strategies for defense of electronic information systems against cyberwarfare and infoterrorism. Preparations may not be far behind for the kind of surveillance (strict immigration procedures, increased wire tapping and electronic media controls, photographing of license plates on highways, and generally greater government secrecy) that nations like Israel and the United Kingdom, targeted for terrorist attacks, long ago instituted.

Obviously government anti-bioterrorism programs raise a host of questions about increased centralization of authority, not because of actual aggression, but because of the potential use of biological weapons. As anthropologist Mary Douglas and political scientist Aaron Wildavsky warn us, "Risk aversion is a preoccupation with anticipating danger that leads to large-scale organization and centralization of power in order to mobilize massive resources against possible evils."[18] We may be facing the conversion of public health and hospital services to defensive units against biological weapons, at the same time that federal and local intelligence agencies increase surveillance. The conflict between such measures and democratic values is self-evident. The question turns on what kind of political socialization the American public is willing to support, if it is willing to submit to civil defense drills and routine invasions of privacy based on what is fundamentally military authority. Is the threat of bioterrorism sufficient to justify diminished civil liberties?[19]

The U.S. Department of Defense and the media have worked in synchrony to promote bioterrorism as a national security threat. Television coverage began in earnest in November 1997, with Secretary of Defense William Cohen hoisting a five-pound bag of sugar and claiming that the same amount of anthrax would lay waste to Washington, D.C. The media took off from there, with a frenzy of television and press stories about the horrors of possible anthrax, smallpox, or plague attacks.

In modern times, as sociologist Ulrich Beck cogently observes, the media profitably market the risks that confront society, whether or not those risks materialize.[20] In this regard, biological weapons offer almost unlimited potential for exploitation. They could be as diverse as the hundreds of illnesses that threaten human life (imagine them combined in "chimeras"), as earth-shaking as the fatal epidemics that have destroyed civilizations, as terrifying as the emerging diseases that leap environmental boundaries, and as awe-inspiring as the new microbiology. BW calls to mind Zymunt Bauman's observation that the "potential commercial value of risk-fright is infinite."[21] The media industry, which lives or dies by television ratings and print sales, must appeal to as broad an audience as possible, even if few or none of its consumers are at actual risk and even if the information presented is undocumented, false, or misleading. In one television program on bioterrorism, a commentator blew powdered cocoa off the palm of his hand to illustrate how easily anthrax could be disseminated in a crowd, conveying the erroneous impression that a puff was aerodynamically the same as a lethal aerosol.[22] An explanation of how difficult it has been to manufacture, weaponize, and use a bacterium or virus (most of which, anthrax excepted, degrade fairly quickly), of international negotiations to reduce biological and chemical weapons threats, and of the near zero statistical likelihood of any viewer's ever being in a BW attack would make for dull programming indeed, compared to the fright value of bioweapons.

For fifty years, whether in warfare or for terrorist purposes, the actual use of biological weapons has been highly unusual; Japanese aggression in Manchuria, for example, is historically an anomaly. The complex manufacture of an aerosol, the difficulties of calculating optimal wind direction and then waiting for it, of rigging spraying devices or bomblets, of having dissemination plans go awry and then risking one's own contamination and death from a painful disease seem to have deterred states and terrorists alike. In *Bioterrorism and Biocrimes*, a review of 128 alleged cases reported in the twentieth century up to 1997, the facts about actual incidents indicate that "few terrorists have demonstrated an interest in bioterrorism, and fewer still tried to acquire biological agents."[23] Publicized BW possession, threats, and alleged use, though, have been on the increase, with anthrax (no surprise) the preferred agent. Fifty-seven of the 128 reported BW hoaxes and plots occurred since 1984; forty-seven of these were in the 1990s. Most perpetrators of threats have been Americans: individual scientists or physicians with grudges against colleagues, former spouses, or employers, or white supremacists acting alone or in small groups.

What the media sows, the public often reaps. In the early 1990s, attempted or threatened HIV contamination of victims' food or blood accounted for six famous cases; publicity surrounding the case of the Florida dentist who infected his patients probably sparked the trend. More recently, anthrax hoaxes have become a fad, following directly on those Defense Department and media drumrolls. In late 1997 and continuing into 1998, they began to occur by the dozens (usually in the form of harmless powders sent in envelopes), at thirteen mid-Western abortion clinics, at schools, at a magazine publisher in Florida, in a court house, and among shoppers in California. These false alarms set off a variety of "civil defense" responses, usually involving firefighters, the police, and paramedics and emergency care physicians and staff, and including vigorous showers and antibiotics for all those threatened. Reports of anthrax hoaxes to the FBI reached two to three per day by the spring of 1999.

Since the recent anthrax incidents have been hoaxes, we might be tempted to dismiss them as expensive (the California responses cost tax payers four to five million dollars) but basically harmless. Yet their socializing effect, like the socializing effect of the Sverdlovsk outbreak or of any terroristic event, along with the media risk-fright exploitation of bioweapons, can only be to diminish trust in social interactions. It becomes inadvisable to go out in public, to risk the impersonal venue of the city, the mall, the office, the courthouse, the federal building. The public domain, already eroded in our times, becomes a landscape of fear from which we retreat even faster to more atomized private spheres.[24] This bioterrorism, a government-media simulacrum, is like other terrorisms in that it promotes the submission of the target population, which knows only the scare-mongering it has just seen on television or read in the newspapers.

As historian Gerald Holton pointed out, to keep the public ignorant of scientific facts is to cripple its ability to judge the politics of weapons technology.[25] We cannot assess the risks of bioweapons and government mobilization against them if our education consists solely of BW risk-fright. How many of us know, for example, whether we should be vaccinated against anthrax, participate in a CBW civil defense drill (which is much like a 1950s nuclear air-raid drill combined with disaster medicine), or support a build-up of CTROS and a paramilitary public health service? Are the anthrax hoaxes a passing fad or an antecedent?

Defensive measures aside, we should be asking whether U.S. leadership in world arms control is all it should be. Is there a firm insistence on global norms to promote transparency and compliance? The surge of international activity to control weapons proliferation and use (little reported in American media) finds the United States too often on the sidelines. The Chemical Weapons Convention, the strengthening of the Biological Weapons Convention, the international ban on land mines, and the establishment of an international criminal court are recent endeavors that have engaged nearly every nation on the globe. More often than not, the United States has been an apathetic or reluctant participant or, as in the case of the land mines ban and the international court, a dissenter siding with the very nations (like Libya and North Korea) it considers threats to its national security. We are proud of our legal system, yet how is it that we have been slow to develop an international law against those individuals, including heads of state, who dare to use and deploy biological or chemical weapons? Is the growth of a new "threat industry" the best we can do? Are landscapes of fear the American environments of the future? Or is there a middle ground, where reasonable tactics for legal restraints can be combined with reasonable tactics to identify real threats to national security?[26]

25

Return to Yekaterinburg

And what about the new Russia, where the story of the Sverdlovsk inquiry began?

During the 1990s the transformations in the former Soviet Union were almost beyond imagining, or imagining without anxiety. The economic "shock therapy" begun in 1991 was applied to an already debilitated post-Soviet economy. The Russian population, with its high literacy and educational levels, was required to forego the security of full employment and guaranteed pensions and throw itself into high-risk "byzniz" opportunities in a global world. Just as Russian workers were catapulted into twentieth-century industrialism by the inception of the Soviet system, so they were by its demise thrust into the high-risk arena of the global free market economy. In Moscow, the joke has been, "Everything they told us about communism was wrong. Everything they told us about capitalism was right."

In 1998, after five years of freedom, Russia is in financial crisis. Beset by millionaire entrepreneurs who channel their profits to Swiss banks, by domestic companies that circumvent taxation, by Western and Japanese corporations exploiting Russian natural resources, and by its failure to develop its own industries and legal and financial systems, it is approaching default on its enormous international debts. Russian rates of violent crime are now on a par with those of the United States and include assassinations of public figures—politicians and media personalities. The 1993 attempted coup against President Yeltsin was settled with more bloodshed and loss of life than anyone anticipated. The war in Chechnya became shockingly brutal. The vast Russian state, which gave the world Pushkin, Tolstoy, Dostoyevsky, Chekhov, Tchaikovskiy, the art of ballet, Metchnikoff and other Nobel laureates in science and medicine, as well as in literature, and produced some of the finest poets of the twentieth century, is the wild West and East.

But is Russia so different from the rest of the world? As sociologists Alex Inkeles and Raymond Bauer pointed out years ago, the similarities among large industrial nations may be greater than their differences, despite the divergence in Soviet and Western history.[1] Factories in cities like Sverdlovsk were based on the same assembly-line ideas of Henry Ford as those in Detroit or Gary, Indiana, and in Germany and Japan. The new Russia is a version, albeit a colossal one, of the transformations taking place in the rest of the post–Cold War world, as capitalism goes global and old industrial "fordism" becomes outmoded.

The Western uneasiness about Russian instability has quickly translated to media marketing of both past Soviet involvement in BW research and suspicions about present Russian investment. As the U.S. Department of Defense embarked on its biodefense campaign, the 1979 Sverdlovsk outbreak unexpectedly reemerged in the headlines, via a scientific article. Through Martin Hugh-Jones, the veterinarian on our 1992 trip, and his dean at Louisiana State University, David Huxsoll, tissue samples from eleven cases Dr. Grinberg brought to Galveston in 1993 were sent to the U. S. government laboratory at Los Alamos for PCR (polymerase chain reaction) analysis. Publishing in *PNAS* (where the summary of Abramova and Grinberg's work appeared), Paul Jackson and his Los Alamos colleagues reported finding four different strains of anthrax bacteria in some samples.[2] These multiple strains could mean that the 1979 aerosol was an invented concoction, meant as a new weapon. Or, as the paper cautioned, during autopsy and storage in Sverdlovsk, the samples could have become contaminated with multi-strain anthrax vaccine used in the April campaign. (One set of samples came from Pyotr Gayda, who had been vaccinated before dying.) Or the military strain may have mutated, as anthrax has been known to do in the soil.[3] The media fastened only on the first possibility, proclaiming that the Soviets had developed an anthrax weapon engineered to defeat existing vaccines.

Even more single-minded was the media reporting of a December 1997 article in the British journal *Vaccine* as evidence that now the new Russia's scientists were intent on developing ever more virulent anthrax weapons. The article reported the genetic modification of an anthrax strain that made it possible to infect hamsters which had been immunized with the standard Russian STI vaccine. It also described how to modify the vaccine so it could be highly effective, even against the genetically modified strain.[4] What got reported in the press was only the first part, the production of a more virulent anthrax. What was left out was the development of a vaccine to counter it—which is made clear in the article's title—and, significantly, the fact that scientists in the West had been kept informed of this work, which was done at the Obolensk facility outside Moscow. Two years before the press caught on, the research had been presented and discussed by the lead author of the article, Dr. Andrey Pomerantsev, at the Second International Workshop on Anthrax, held in Winchester, England.[5] The U.S. Army Medical Research Institute of Infectious Diseases (USAMRIID) at Fort Detrick was one of the sponsors of the workshop, the Pomerantsev research was reported in its program, and Pomerantsev himself kept his Western colleagues fully aware of it.

The American media still mine Russia for their own purposes, which are not simply commercial, but serve to contrast the perversity of the Soviet and now the Russian system with an uncritical estimate of our own.[6] So the Cold War lingers, and coverage of current international cooperation and increased transparency between former enemies lags behind events. Great contingents of Russian army generals, scientists, and administrators have been circulating through official Washington and other U.S. cities. Demilitarization programs like the one established by the Nunn-Lugar Cooperative Threat Reduction Act have been shoring up Russia's science facilities, where one major problem is keeping the underpaid and at times unpaid scientists from migrating to hostile nations. The result has been progress in converting laboratories to peace-time production and the increasing openness of Russian facilities, always the best political antidote to BW development.[7] This kind of positive news usually goes unreported.

In early September 1998, I fly to England to attend the Third International Workshop on Anthrax (they are held every three years). The papers presented vary from reports on subclinical infections in Canadian buffalo to sophisticated molecular biology from John Collier and Philip Hanna, pioneers in investigating the complex role of the macrophage in anthrax infection,[8] and from Robert Liddington, on the specific way lethal anthrax toxin penetrates cells.[9] Harry Smith, who discovered the three components of anthrax lethality, also attends; though he long ago moved on to other work, he is still considered the "father of anthrax research" within this small group of researchers.[10] Among molecular biologists,

B. anthracis, the first germ in germ theory, has become an important means for generally understanding inflammation and immune responses.

Just a handful of Russian scientists, fewer than expected, attend the Anthrax Workshop. Russia is in such a profound crisis that the West is predicting that any day Boris Yeltsin will fall from power. The phrase "the ailing President Yeltsin" has long been a media catchword for political destabilization, but this time it seems impossible that Yeltsin can endure. U.S. government scientists at the meeting, including Paul Jackson from Los Alamos and Arthur Friedlander from USAMRIID, receive last-minute instructions not to continue on to a planned meeting in Moscow with Russian colleagues. The political situation there appears too precarious.

Even so, after the Anthrax Workshop, I will head east for a third visit to Yekaterinburg. My colleagues at the Ural State University have invited me back to give a seminar to advanced sociology students. As I say good-bye to Matthew and to Julian Robinson at London's Heathrow Airport, that old dream about being trapped in Russia flashes through my mind. Is there hostility against Americans? How much dare I inquire about present politics, even from old friends? Once in the Urals, will I be indefinitely detained? The morning plane from London to Moscow has only seven other people on it, which adds to my anxiety. But I need this trip to achieve a sense of closure. I want to know how life in Yekaterinburg has gone on, if conditions have changed, if the families of victims ever received their pensions, if there is resignation or hope in the new Russia.

Olga Yampolskaya has agreed to meet me in Moscow, which is calm. Its mayor, Yuriy Luzkov, runs the city like a well-oiled machine, although now economic forces seem stacked against him. The Kremlin area is spotless and boasts a dramatic underground shopping mall. At this juncture in history, this mall and the nearby refurbished GUM building (supposedly the world's first shopping mall) house dozens of boutiques full of expensive European and American goods, but all are almost empty of customers. Many banks are ominously shut. In one day, the value of the ruble swings from nine to eighteen per dollar and then down to twelve. When I find an open bank, several of my worn twenty-dollar bills fail the counterfeit machine test, and I have to hand over the newer, crisper ones.

The immediate major disruption for Muscovites is the precipitous rise in prices for food and domestic necessities. A box of laundry soap that cost twelve rubles last week is now sixty rubles. Little now on the shelves is produced in Russia; as stocks run low and Russian credit is in the dumps, nothing will be left on the shelves to buy. Mars, Inc., which makes the widely popular Snickers bars, has announced it will pull out of Russia; maybe, Russian friends suggest, the better quality Russian chocolate will reappear. Meanwhile, the hoarding of sugar, flour, toilet paper, noodles, and canned goods has begun.

Worse still, a long winter lies ahead. The thousands of melons from the south for sale in depots along the highways will soon disappear. The potato and cabbage crops from country gardens that sustain many families will be used up before spring. Free market reforms, executed without the legal apparatus to control profiteering or ensure that taxes can be collected, without structures to control massive outflow of capital, without corollary investments in industry and marketing, have despoiled the new Russia. Why, I can only wonder, didn't Yeltsin look to Finland or Sweden for a model, instead of the United States?

But then Russians are curiously like Americans, impulsive risk-takers and ambivalent about authority. In one extreme case, a Russian pilot handed the controls of a passenger plane to his thirteen-year-old son, who crashed the aircraft, killing all on board. In America young boys, discovering their father's guns, have gone on homicidal rampages against their schoolmates. The reasons for defying authority in the two cultures, though, are different. Americans are individualists who create their social worlds de novo with each generation and largely reject political centrality. Russians find their identities in the social connectedness of family and friends, two institutions where the Soviet state had a great, but not completely destructive, impact. At the same time, they are cynical about authority, which they usually assume is corrupt.[11] Kin and friendship networks have provided important ways of resisting the law, for good and for bad. Trade, barter, and the black market (the same that was supposed to have figured in the Sverdlovsk outbreak) were the means by which most people coped with material shortages in Soviet times. In 1998, this underground economy is in full evidence around Moscow, near metro stations, among neighbors and friends, and between clients and anyone with a service to sell.

At Yampolskaya's, after I have slept off my jet lag, we watch the new film of *Lolita*. Vladimir Nabokov's X-rated rendering of American desires is now graphically depicted in dubbed-over Russian to an audience that just ten years ago held to an ideology that consistently deemphasized the sexual dimension of the individual.[12] Nothing then was worse than public mention of sex. Now here is Jeremy Irons groaning "pazhalista" ("please") atop the smiling nymphet, a symbol of American youth, spontaneity, and degeneration. With democracy, the Russians opened the

gates to a flood of erotic films and publications, with little government
or public outcry. Among some young Russian women, it is as if old restraints never existed. Prostitution and other activities that may involve
sexual barter (modeling, massage, and beauty contests) can be the means
to material benefits.[13] High rates of abortion continue, while venereal
diseases and AIDS have increased, along with teenage pregnancies.
Many Russians, reeling from social, political, and economic reforms, are
changing their expectations about the future, about sex and families.
"Bridal agencies" that export Russian women to the West are thriving.
Divorce rates among younger people, already high, have skyrocketed.
How to plan a family or a life has become a difficult question.[14]

The next figure on the television screen is an obviously debilitated Boris
Yeltsin. His by-pass operation in 1995, with American medical super-
star Michael De Bakey in attendance, has done his health no lasting good.
Staggering and pale, he ushers in his new prime minister, Yevgeniy Primakov, whose job it will be to get Russia out of its financial quagmire.
Meanwhile, the eighty-nine governmental subdivisons within Russia are
instituting their own price regulations, food rationing, the suspension of
taxes (including federal ones) on foodstuffs, and bans on exports.

Had I been a week earlier I could have seen Deputy Minister Burgasov
on television, still affirming the official tainted-meat explanation of the
Sverdlovsk outbreak and claiming he has more "proof." When I telephone him at his dacha, he is cordial but says there is no more documentary evidence than what I have already seen. His voice sounds old
and far away.

General Yevstigneyev has also been in the news, in March 1998, repeating his conjectures about the Sverdlovsk outbreak. "I did a computer
analysis using image recognition theory and mathematical modeling, and
I tried three versions: the institute [Compound 19] was responsible, a
natural epidemic, and a diversion with the aim of compromising the institute. Strangely enough, the latter version [sabotage] got the highest
score." He continues to admit that the testing of BW on an island in the
Aral Sea "was in direct violation of the anti-biological treaty."[15]

At the same time, articles in the sensational Russian press have re-
suscitated the 1980 dissidents' accounts of the Sverdlovsk outbreak,
protesting the killing of thousands by a secret military microbe. This ex-
aggeration justifies anger against the continued secrecy around Russian
military laboratories—as if sixty-six deaths were not enough. Western
disinformation about the outbreak also persists. In the 1997 Brassey series on modern military equipment, for example, the volume on nuclear,

chemical, and biological warfare states that it is "now understood that at least ten kg of anthrax were released in the accident," that the British estimate deaths in the hundreds, and that the American estimates are between one and two thousand.[16]

The morning after I arrive in Moscow, Yampolskaya and I take the two-and-a-half-hour flight to the Urals. She is glad for the break from her hospital work and the chance to see Lev Grinberg and Faina Abramova again. When we arrive, Yekaterinburg is enjoying languorous *babye leto*, a "woman's summer" of sunshine and 70-degree temperatures that briefly interrupts the chill of autumn. The city has just celebrated its 275th birthday. All the classic buildings in the center city overlooking the Iset River have been newly painted in gorgeous pink, blue, yellow, and green pastels; the streets and sidewalks are immaculate. The old Iron Works museum is newly refurbished and across the Iset embankment the Canon corporation has invested in a large art museum. On the street, young women are fashionably dressed in short skirts and oversized black shoes. The young men, with their close-cropped hair, jeans, and leather jackets, could be Europeans anywhere, East or West.

The struggle going on behind this facade, though, has been enormous. Like other Russians in industrial centers and like Americans as well, the people in Yekaterinburg have been adapting to the end of the "fordist" era of factory production. No less than Americans, and in a shorter time span, they have had to adjust to new "flexible" institutions of power where the risks (downsizing, the impermanence of markets, and the lack of protection for workers) are high, but the risks of not adjusting (poverty and starvation) are even higher. The end of the Cold War has meant serious retraction in the weapons industry. Though highly educated technicians and scientists still have an advantage in the job market, developing portable skills in trade, computers, management, or the service industries might bring greater advantage.[17] Like modern people all over the globe, each Russian must develop a "protean self," to use Robert Jay Lifton's term,[18] to adapt to change or sink into a poverty worse than anything the old system imposed.

Unlike Moscow, where Soviet statuary was torn down, Yekaterinburg city officials have left standing the colossal Lenin statue and, in front of the university, the larger-than-life figure of his protégé Sverdlov, for whom the oblast is still named. Yet the handful of communists demonstrating downtown at the foot of Lenin's statue are old, and their clothes are shabby. Their speakers blare the "International," but the bustling crowds ignore them. The Soviet hammer-and-sickle building is now a hotel.

The Ural State University, where we go on our first day, has dropped the name "Gorky"—all over Russia, the author's name has disappeared, even from Moscow's famous park. For the lecture I will give, I have rehearsed with Yampolskaya a concise overview of the 1979 Sverdlovsk outbreak, set in the context of Ulrich Beck's and Anthony Giddens's ideas on the social consequences of risk. Greeting us at the university is Professor Anatoliy Marenkov, who introduced me to Ilona in 1992, and Professor Yevgenia Baraznova, who has written a book on American sociology, an attempt to determine which founding father was more important, functionalist Talcott Parsons or knowledge systems analyst Robert Merton. Merton won.

Thirty students assemble in a classroom with big windows and high ceilings. As we planned, I speak four or five sentences in English and then Yampolskaya interprets. The faces of the students are intelligent and attentive, even when, as Yampolskaya warms to the subject, the translation is sometimes longer than the original statement. When we are done, the hands shoot up. The first question is, "Isn't it true that only young men died because the microbe was genetically engineered to kill soldiers?" The students' information is from recent newspaper stories and rumors; sometimes not much difference between the two is discernible. Reviewing the data about age and sex, I point out that the elderly had more to fear in the outbreak than young people.

The second question is one I like better: "How did you get your information?" I explain the interviews and the process of cross-checking sources. After that, we are all on the same wavelength. Though still undergraduates, they feel they are researchers, too, and have important problems to investigate—about the environment, about work, about the economy. Some have been exchange students in the West and have a global perspective on social change. Several students who have grown up in Yekaterinburg, infants at the time of the outbreak in 1979, want to investigate the local memories of the event. With students like these, I would never have nightmares of being trapped in Russia.

Still, looming like a shadow over this discussion is the continued secrecy that seems to surround Compound 19. The laboratory there may have converted to peacetime industry, but so far no confirmation of that exists. Moreover, the scientists involved in anthrax research there in 1979 have died or dispersed. With them went not only possible information on the outbreak but also the chance for understanding a social group that could develop weapons of mass destruction while at the same time holding to universal norms of science.

I spend several days catching up with Professor Borisov and his family, with my former co-researchers, Ilona Nikonova (now Popova) and Irina Belaeva, and with Lev Grinberg and Faina Abramova. In the five years since I have seen them, they have all in one way or another accommodated to Russia's enormous economic and social changes.

The Pulmonary Unit, where Yampolskaya and I meet with Grinberg and Abramova, looks unchanged. Grinberg spent seven months in America in 1993, at the Pathology Department at the University of Texas Medical Center in Galveston. (Yampolskaya also visited on a year-long fellowship.) During that time, he had expected to have all the Sverdlovsk samples analyzed with modern technology. Unfortunately, the researcher who was to have helped him hadn't enough time and, leaving samples from eleven cases with Hugh-Jones, he returned to Yekaterinburg with the analysis incomplete. Not until he received a final draft of the Jackson multi-strain article from Los Alamos, did he fully realize where the samples had gone and what the results were. In Russian press coverage of the article and its report of four anthrax strains, Grinberg and Abramova were accused of being CIA agents cooperating with the U.S. laboratory or, alternatively, of collaborating with the KGB in 1979. Personal recriminations came from colleagues, neighbors, and even close relatives reacting to the newspaper stories. Had the analysis of the samples been done together with Russian scientists, instead of having the United States take unilateral responsibility, more might have been learned about the various strains and whether they matched Soviet vaccines, and the two pathologists might have been spared some grief.[19] When, six years ago in this same center, Grinberg and Abramova raised the issue of intellectual property rights, they never imagined the peculiarly unpleasant risks of American contact.

Nonetheless, when I tell Abramova that I would like to see inside Hospital 40, something I never got to do on my last two trips, she immediately makes a telephone call to assure our entrance and, with a quick good-bye to Grinberg, Abramova, Yampolskaya, and I are on our way. Had I done nothing else in Yekaterinburg, seeing the autopsy area at the hospital justifies this trip, for this is where, in 1979, medical science wrestled with and, as Foucault would say, tried to exorcise the evil of those terrible deaths.

In the hall, metal gurneys, curved like cylinders to keep bodies from rolling off, are pushed against the wall. A cold-room on the left is where bodies are stored. Abramova leads me into the sparse, white-tiled room, not now in use, where she and Grinberg did the autopsies. It is dominated by three long soapstone tables on wooden legs, biers really, with a three-inch edge. A wide shallow groove has been carved on all four sides, surrounding where the body would lie, to channel the blood flow; a wooden block to support the neck is screwed into the soapstone. Each table has on top of it a tray of instruments on four legs and is lit by an adjustable round lamp. Each has a black hose for cleanup and a drain to the floor, the same ones Grinberg blocked in 1979 for sanitary reasons. Abramova and Yampolskaya know this place well. I can only imagine what it must have been like throughout the anthrax outbreak, with three bodies at a time ready for examination and more outside in the hall and in the storage area. And what poor, wretched bodies, infected by dreaded anthrax bacteria, devasted by toxic shock.

In the anteroom, Abramova shows me the cabinet where she hid the tissue samples. Only after we have had this glimpse into Abramova's world in 1979 does she tell the story about how Dr. Nikiforov earned her gratitude. Near the end of the outbreak, she went to him to ask what she should do with the autopsy materials. He implied he had to consult with some higher authority and would then get back to her. Shortly after, he told her she should save everything she wanted, but to proceed as if he didn't know about it; he would "just look the other way." Later, when Abramova was away from the hospital, men from the KGB came looking for the materials. But the area was locked, and the cleaning woman, named Maria, refused to let them in. She knew that Abramova had something special in the cabinet. She must have intimidated them, for they never came back. After that, Abramova took the samples in paraffin to her home.

"Every hospital has a Maria," she laughs.

Not every medical system, though, has an Abramova.

The next day Professor Sergei Borisov stops by the hotel for a late lunch. He has developed a second career, teaching general science to business students. Life is changing for everyone. Ilona, my first Yekaterinburg interpreter, now has two children. She has left the university to work for an adoption agency. Russia now has strict laws against international adoption, except of children with birth defects or other problems. The rise in illegitimate births, though, especially among teenagers, is crowding local orphanages.

There is more news. Dr. Klipnitzer and Dr. Arenskiy have both passed away. Dr. Ilyenko is retired from her spacious office at Hospital 24. Rector Suetin has also left his post. He is Professor Suetin again, an active physics researcher and teacher; several of his students have won coveted

Soros Foundation grants for science research. Vice Rector Tretyakov, whose office we borrowed in 1992, has become the new rector and seeks to develop the university's information technologies. General Kharechko still rules at Compound 19, but its activities remain uncertain. Its gates are guarded, but workers still pass through them.

Irina Belaeva, my interpreter in 1993, soon after went to work for the Yekaterinburg branch of a California company that offers commercial training to Russian entrepreneurs. When we meet for lunch, she tells me that she has just quit that job to return to the university; in the last six months, business had fallen off and other workers were let go. She decided she would rather be teaching than in a too-quiet office with just two other people. Irina's hair is fashionably cut, with blonde streaks; she is wearing a chic suit and scarf. Around us in the little cafe, all chrome and glass, are men in Italian jackets, their shoes polished, wearing expensive watches.

"The money has run out," Irina announces in her gentle, candid way. "We have had three good years, but it's over."

The two of us have an appointment with Dr. Romanenko at SES. The once shaggy-haired physician now occupies the spacious deputy director's office, which has a potted lime tree near the window. He wears a neat navy suit and his hair is trimmed short. I have had intermittent e-mail contact with him over the years, to keep up with changing health conditions in the city and the region. The old Soviet system bequeathed Russia massive industrial pollution that affects the water and air and literally makes people sick; the new system has brought extreme poverty (with its health consequences), drugs, and AIDS. The biggest health threat, Romanenko says, is drug abuse, which often involves AIDS as well. In 1993, he told us about the first handful of AIDS cases, among eight homosexual men who were segregated in Hospital 40. In 1997 there were ninety-six AIDS cases, not many given the size of the city, but still a shock, and nearly all drug-related. Hepatitis cases have also increased, along with tuberculosis, dysentery, and tick-borne encephalitis. More cars in the city in the past several boom years have meant more air pollution and respiratory problems; and the quality of the water could be better. On the bright side, he says, the oblast has been free of polio for five years, and in November, a World Health Organization panel will arrive to award a certificate to that effect.

As for anthrax, Dr. Romanenko proclaims that no cases have occurred on his watch, except for a diseased cow brought in from Kazakhstan. Around a thousand people in the oblast, including private owners of live-

stock, are vaccinated against anthrax each year. He believes that the vaccine, now made in Russia, at a facility in Stavropol, was developed at
Compound 19. But he isn't certain of that; he has had no contact with
the facility there.

His division continues to analyze soil samples from Chkalovskiy, but
after more than sixty-eight hundred tests over nearly twenty years, he
has found nothing. Asked for my explanation, I can only suggest that
the 1979 emission was small to begin with and that its impact, for example, on trees or the side of the ceramics factory, cannot be compared
with the burial of an infected carcass. Trillions of spores packed tightly
into the earth at one site may leave traces for a long time, but the same
number aerosolized over fifty kilometers might not. Still I understand
the question behind his question. He has long wondered if shorter-lived
bacteria, not spores, were emitted from Compound 19, or some combination of the two; perhaps the spores emitted were not strongly encap-
sulated. Any one of these suspicions might be true. But without definite
input from the military, we will never know. In the meanwhile, he routinely samples the area under the plume and into the countryside and
finds nothing, except where known reservoirs from infected animals still
exist. Some aspects of the Sverdlovsk mystery may never be solved.

26

"The World Is Global"

Irina has found a driver with a car, a young man named Kostya, who can take us down to Chkalovskiy rayon. Kostya is twenty-three years old, with startling blue eyes and straight, sandy hair. He knows Irina from the California company, where they both used to work when its business was better. He considers the two years he recently spent in the Russian navy a complete waste. After an idle time with the Black Sea fleet, he returned to a city he barely recognized. All his friends are entrepreneurs. He's been trained as a machinist; he's not sure what his future will be.

Kostya was born and raised in Chkalovskiy, not far from Compound 19. With no trouble, he drives us first to the ceramics factory. Dr. Chernich has retired, and in her place is a nurse, Nadia Krashchenko. In 1979, Krashchenko, as Dr. Chernich's assistant, worked in the clinic during the outbreak. Her recollection is that, although the official explanation was tainted meat, when the washing of buildings began, a general fear swept through the community, and people turned up in droves.

"Did the families ever receive their pensions?" I ask. It's been six years since Yeltsin's decree.

The nurse isn't sure about the pensions. No one talks about the outbreak any more. For the answer to the question, we will have to ask the families themselves.

Across from the ceramics factory are Poldnevaya and Lyapustina streets, the twin corridors down which the anthrax plume traveled in

1979. Once again, Irina and I are knocking on doors. The neighborhood looks the same as it did five years ago. The only difference is that a younger generation is growing up and taking it over. At the Komelskikh cottage, the grandson of Andrey (the hothouse builder) answers the door. He was a young child when his grandfather died in 1979. But about the pension, he is perfectly clear. Nothing has been done for the families.

His neighbors, the Vershinin family, have gone to pick mushrooms, not as a holiday jaunt but as a necessity, so I won't get to see Aleksandr. But over on Lyapustina, Anna Komina's son opens the gate; he has been working in the garden. There are heaps of small yellow potatoes by the shed behind him and an enormous vat of gooseberries by the stairs. Pushing aside a brown-and-black puppy, he invites us into the house, which is exactly as I remember it, sparsely furnished, with the little bedroom off the living room. His face is tan and without sorrow. Komin speaks with pleasure about his twenty-two-year-old son, who has just completed his army service and is living here with his girlfriend. Komin and his wife, who still both work at the ceramics factory, have moved into a nearby apartment, but he still tends the garden here. His wife remains in the same division as his mother was, and she has been promoted. Their daughter, age eighteen, has just graduated from technical school as an accountant.

"All she needs now is that important first job," he says good-naturedly.

About the ceramics factory, he remarks, "It is more dead than alive. But it is still kicking." Technology imported from Italy has helped. The pipe shop has been successfully converted to making bricks. New construction of apartments at the north end of Chkalovskiy improved business. At one point in the last year, though, the factory was broke and the workers were paid in sink bowls.

As for a pension, nothing has come through. He remembers that a few years back, some official put a notice in the newspaper about a meeting to discuss it; nothing ever came of it. But he is not waiting around. He has a life to live. "You are welcome any time," he says to us as we leave.

Around the corner, we knock on Nina T.'s gate. Before we can blink, she has us sitting at her table with two steaming cups of tea before us. She is as energetic as ever. On the kitchen counter is a huge casserole of scalloped potatoes, and other good things are cooking on the stove. On the windowsill are giant purple zinnias from her garden. Irina says it is like being at her grandmother's. As with everyone else, Nina's mind is on the next generation. Her grandson is in the army, in Leningrad, as she calls it. Her granddaughter, like Komin's daughter, has just graduated from technical school and is looking for a job.

We talk again about her time in Hospital 40. She reiterates her resolve that she would not die. Then she confesses that once she had passed the crisis, she never took the antibiotics that were given her. She hid them under her pillow and later threw them out. She didn't take any antibiotics when she first felt the flu-like symptoms of anthrax, either. Without saying so, I am thinking that if she had she might have saved herself some time in the hospital. But that's not absolutely certain. And why disturb her with such a thought? God protected her and the grandchildren.

In the last days I am in Yekaterinburg, I dash around wanting to do and see everything and feeling increasingly reluctant to leave. I run to the Military Museum, where on the top floor one of the curators, who politely introduces himself as Alfred, shows me the piece of Francis Gary Powers's U-2 plane, which was shot down near Sverdlovsk in 1960. I remember that being the only time Eisenhower, the war hero, was ever known to have lied. Alfred, who served in the tank corps during the Great Patriotic War, speaks glowingly of the American assistance program that helped support Soviet troops against the Nazi army. Yampolskaya and I revisit the hotel near the university where she and Nikiforov and two other physicians from Moscow stayed for two months in 1979. She remembers that one night, toward the end, Nikiforov bought them all tickets to a concert at the opera house. In the nearby square, for the equivalent of ten dollars, I buy a small oil painting of a garden. The bushy-bearded artist tells me his name can be found on the Yekaterinburg web-site.

Up on Ascension Avenue, I stop a minute to see the framework for the church being built for the Romanovs on the site of Ipatiev House. Their remains have been removed from Yekaterinburg and buried in a crypt in St. Petersburg. That historical episode is over, just as Yeltsin wanted. That his 1992 decree for pensions apparently hasn't been funded troubles me. Maybe it shouldn't. What does the gesture of a pension mean anyway? I have heard stories from Russians whose relatives were killed in Stalin's purges, after which a pension of a few hundred rubles a year was awarded to the surviving spouse to make up for the loss. What price can be put on a life? As one widow we interviewed cried out, what good is the money without my husband? And yet Yeltsin's 1992 decree was the only government acknowledgment that the families of 1979 anthrax victims had suffered a loss, and the KGB list is the only validation of the individuals who died.

On our last night in Yekaterinburg, the Borisov family, including the youngest member, nine-year-old Masha, and Irina and her son Andrey meet Yampolskaya and me for dinner in the new little café-bar at the Hotel Oktyabrskaya. The two children have grown since I last saw them in 1993, and I hardly recognize them. Masha, her honey-colored hair pulled back, is turning into a young lady; she no longer giggles and dances. Andrey, now twenty-two and robustly handsome, is a graduate student in economics and a computer whiz.

I raise a toast to Yampolskaya, for her work in 1979 and for her helping me to return on this trip. Still another toast is due, but just as five years ago, the presence of the younger generation restrains me. I feel tensely poised between my wish to honor the past and my desire to dispel the weight of the dreadful Sverdlovsk outbreak. Epidemics, even past ones, provoke both mourning and gaiety. The dichotomy is an old one. In Pushkin's *Feast in Time of Plague* the central figure defies evil with a blasphemous toast that celebrates life:

> And so, O Plague, we hail thy reign!
> We laugh at graves, at death and pain.
> We die no cowards in the night! We drink, carefree![1]

Yet even in Pushkin's little play, the revelers are admonished by a clergyman to cease their "indecent songs and revelry."[2]

The anthrax epidemic itself is an evil long past. The uneasiness that remains is not from its lethal threat (we are all safe here), but from the mystery still at its core. "A secret contains a tension that is dissolved in the moment of its revelation," the great sociologist Georg Simmel told us.[3] The revelation for me was when I first saw the plume manifest in victims' daytime locations on the map of Sverdlovsk. The *Science* article, coupled with Abramova and Grinberg's work, should have dissolved the tension. But the secret and the tension from 1979 are maintained by Russia's government, and the basis for the full revelation may have become irretrievable, lost as documents were destroyed, as principal actors have passed away, as surviving actors keep their silence in the belief that "certain insights must not penetrate to the masses."[4] Against the silence, the only redeeming noise is the sound of the names of the victims, a rich, musical murmur: Komina, Bliumova, Bubenshikov, Chikalov, Lavrov, Lyakhova, Nazarov, Nikolaev, Permyakov, Tarasenko, Tepikin, Tischenko, Zakharov, Zinatulin, and the rest. Beautiful names all.

The dinner goes on without toasts. We talk about Russia's future. Andrey says he thinks that General Aleksandr Lebed, the elite paratrooper who has challenged Yeltsin in the past, will lead the country. Sasha, Professor Borisov's son-in-law, disagrees. He and his wife, both trained as scientists, think Moscow's mayor Luzhkov will be president, because he has experience and policies, and "he gets things done." The rest, Yampolskaya, Sergei, and his wife Natalya, feel content for now with Yeltsin's new Prime Minister Primakov, who is stable and not a reactionary, and only hope he can pull together an effective coalition. I feel that we older people at the table can hardly imagine the future, with its new technologies, its new alliances and hostilities, though we are all engaged in it. Yampolskaya's daughter and son-in-law have moved to California to join the computer industry. Along with her teenaged son, Dimitriy, she is now preoccupied with two grandchildren who are American and Russian. The Borisovs, husband and wife alike, lead lives absorbed with new research, teaching, and travel in and out of Russia; their budget is small but their joy in life seems only to expand. I too have one foot in the future. Since last in Yekaterinburg, I have begun research investigating website programs on preventive health care and often inhabit the world of what is called "medical infomatics." Now, in this city of Stalinist industries, of World War II and Cold War weapons manufacture, we eat and converse in an atmosphere of blue and pink neon, with international rock music pulsing in the background. Yeltsin's retreat from government; Russia's economic crisis; disease, drugs, and prostitution; orphans and poverty; biological weapons, evil, and death—we banish them without blasphemy.

Throughout the adult arguments, Masha, who is seated between me and her grandmother, Natalya Borisov, is even more princess-like than she was five years ago. She watches us attentively and eats her food in small bites. Occasionally, as the night goes on, her invisible tiara slips, and she leans affectionately and with uncomplaining fatigue against her grandmother. I cannot help thinking that all our words are only for her, for her safety and well-being, for Andrey's, and for Yamploskaya's Dimitriy and for her grandchildren, that their world will be peaceful and free. And for Kostya, too, back from the navy, and for the other children in Chkalovskiy rayon, back from the army, finishing their schooling, trying to find their places in life.

I propose a final toast after all: "To the future!" It's the same toast I made five years ago, but it is the best I can offer.

I have little time to spend in Moscow, all of it on a weekend. One large chunk goes to waiting in line to see the Pushkin Museum's hundredth anniversary exhibit. My tenacity is such that once I take my place in the line, I cannot leave, even though two-and-one-half hours elapse before I reach the ticket booth inside. The nation is in crisis, yet Russians (I hear only Russian around me) of all ages are waiting obdurately like me to see the masterpieces on loan from the Louvre, the British Museum, the Prado, the Metropolitan Museum in New York, and other international "partners" in this celebration. The wait is festive, the exhibit even more so. It seems inconceivable that we ever planned to use weapons of mass destruction against this city and its people.

On a quiet, cloudy Sunday afternoon, I visit with former Peoples Deputy Larissa Mishustina, who now works in another branch of the national government on communications. She has recently become a grandmother, but like Yampolskaya, she defies the babushka image. For lunch, she lays out pickled fish, salad, then pastries, fruit juice, tea, a cof-fee-flavored aperitif, and a box of chocolates. She herself has a tiny waist and cannot weigh more than a hundred pounds.

"Have the pensions ever been paid?" I ask her.

"It was impossible," she answers. She tells again how in 1991 agents from the KGB brought to her office the list of the sixty-four Sverdlovsk victims. The KGB had been advised that she and Counselor Yablokov were petitioning President Yeltsin for recompense to the families. After the decree was signed in April 1992, she was optimistic that the pensions would be paid. It was only a matter of getting the list to the right office and having it pass through the usual bureaucratic channels. When she gave us a copy of the KGB list of victims in June 1992, she meant what she said, that it was no longer a secret. She herself had been on televi-sion talking about it.

A year later, though, she received word from Yekaterinburg that the list was not acceptable; it lacked an official seal or validation. Fair enough, Mishustina thought. But when she contacted the KGB, their response was negative: no such list of victims existed. When she countered that two agents had personally delivered it to her office, the response was again denial: that visit, that delivery had never happened. No pension would be paid because the list did not exist.

"Without your papers, you are an insect," Yampolskaya comments dryly. "With papers, you are a human being."

The other saying from Stalinist times is "no person, no problem."

But these are not Stalinist times. Russian politics are simply going through identifiable and sometimes disagreeable changes. The Boris Yeltsin who stood on the tank in front of the White House in 1991 be-came the Yeltsin who ordered the army to attack the White House in

1993, when the antireformists were against him. The repercussions within the Russian government have made it more conservative, so that democracy appears dispensable.[5] Old forces reasserted themselves, Mishustina explains. The window of time in which we researched the Sverdlovsk outbreak, between June 1992 and August 1993, was the most open the society has ever been.

"And you weren't able to seek redress for the victims?" I ask.

"More important things absorbed our attention," Mishustina replies. "The war in Chechnya, for one. The environment for another. We have so many problems right now that we cannot keeping looking back at the past."

That night I am unable to sleep, although I have to get up at five to make my flight out of Sheremetyevo 2. How does a government leader decree compensation for a past wrong and then let it become a sham? It seems bad enough that the decree in no way held the military accountable. The only mention Yeltsin has given the role of Compound 19 in the outbreak was his brief newspaper interview in 1992.

To claim that present problems blot out the past does not satisfy me. That argument measures other wrongs—the Chechnyan war, radiation, AIDS and drug problems—against the one perpetuated in Sverdlovsk and finds the deaths of nineteen years ago less significant than more recent ones. This logic is false. The wars, the pollution, the diseases, and the anthrax outbreak are connected by a common disregard for the value of human life. Who can ignore the faces of Komina, Vershinin, Kozlova, Fyodosov, and the rest? What state has the right to deny them?

Obviously, I have a personal stake in the KGB retraction of the list. To dismiss the names of the victims dismisses all our research, all the hours and days that I and Matthew and everyone involved have spent to resurrect those individuals by name, to give memory and meaning to their deaths. Anna Akhmatova's "Requiem" uncannily expresses the dilemma:

> I want to call everyone by name
> But they have taken the list, and
> There's nowhere to find out.[6]

Except that I still have those names; no one can take them back. And such a trite gesture by the KGB, as if the denial of the list could erase the event! I have to put it in the same category with the destruction of file documents in December 1990 that Yablokov told us about: the suppression of information out of fear of new norms of disclosure. "How much evil is averted by openness!" Dostoyevsky wrote.[7] Meanwhile, even with an empty decree and no pensions, Chkalovskiy rayon and its working-class families continue with their lives, probably less in jeopardy than they were from, say, 1970 to 1979. Yekaterinburg is restructuring itself. Russia lumbers on, bearing no current resemblance to an enemy,[8] except to itself. If we can keep talking to General Yevstigneyev, if the discussion can take the high road of science, maybe we can eventually persuade the Russian military of what we proved. On our side, the older generation like Alex Langmuir, is gone, but the dialogue must continue, somehow.

I remember a conversation I had with Irina Belaeva in Yekaterinburg, as we walked through the so-called "gangster" cemetery on the west side of town. In recent years, large lifelike statues have been erected to men killed in shoot-outs. The figures sport leather jackets and jewelry on their necks, and the monuments use all the rich minerals of the Urals, especially polished green malachite, but also other stones in shades of mauve and pink. Unlike modest little Vostochniy, this cemetery is huge, and these newer monuments are only the smallest part of it, near the entrance. The tall pines growing amid the graves give it the atmosphere of a cathedral.

As we walk, I am stuck on the subject of Russia's woes and begin to recite a litany of disasters. Corruption is rampant from top to bottom. I have heard of an entire village north of Yekaterinburg that is entirely under Mafia control, with residents employed at slave wages. The economy is about to collapse. Terrible things could happen in the government. The environment is killingly polluted, a threat to the nation's health.[9] Russia has huge underdeveloped areas whose natural resources are being exploited by more powerful economies. What about the leasing of Siberian timber rights to the Japanese? The environment not ruined by industrialism will be consumed by rich nations. Educated Russians have deserted their country for better jobs. Its weapons scientists may be lured away to build nightmare arsenals of biological weapons, if they have not already sold themselves on that market. I can hear myself going on and on about these problems while a wedding party assembles for photographs at the eternal flame for the War Dead next to the cemetery, just as their parents and grandparents did. The bride is dressed in the traditional froth of white tulle, the groom in his best suit. A bottle of champagne is being passed around, and the little crowd of young people is laughing. Their photos done, they pile into an assortment of cars to go to the wedding feast. The married couple takes the Toyota Corolla.

"Yes, it's all the way you say," Irina agrees. "But there is no turning back. The world is global."

She is right. Russia is moving forward. The old repressions are fast dissolving as communication flows through multiple channels. But social systems do not change overnight. The czarist epoch shaped the Soviet epoch, which will certainly, despite its repudiation, shape this democratic epoch. The institutions that the Russians, as agents of their own destiny, selectively retain or discard or invent are as hard to predict as the impact of outside influences on this once closed society.

Meanwhile, our globalizing world shows little sign of becoming more egalitarian or of promoting justice. Instead, the risks of poverty and repression fall hardest on those already deprived, while wealthier nations try to barricade themselves against instabilities generated by the ebb and flow of world capital. As U.S. national security centers on defense against potential bioterrorism, the real biological terror of preventable epidemics lands blow after blow on the economically undeveloped parts of the world. Our dread of becoming like the other four-fifths of the world, where most poverty and disease are located, subconsciously fuels our fear of terrorism. Those other places—Zimbabwe, India, Malaysia, Brazil, Honduras—are where nature runs amok and lays waste whole communities in tin-roofed shacks. Not in America, we say, which has wealth and rationality and medical science.

But how do we remain within the barricades? We cannot. We are joined to the world by communication, by travel, by trade, by common values, and by conflicts. We are increasingly interconnected by the mix of immigrants, displaced by war, fleeing poverty, seeking freedom, that settle at the edges of Western prosperity. Our fates, though we may not want it so, are increasingly linked with other nations and events in the rest of the world; the fall of the Japanese economy, the rise of the Chinese economy, Russia's unpaid debts, and Latin American currency crises have already rocked our insularity, as have political instability in the Middle East and ethnic cleansing in the Balkans. Wealth and violence, musical styles and disease, information and excess capital swirl around the globe in patterns we are just beginning to decipher. Young people, like Andrey and Masha, like the newly married couple in the Toyota, probably have a better grasp of what is coming than their parents. Irina's intuition, though, is right. There is no turning back.

Appendix A

LIST OF 1979 SVERDLOVSK
ANTHRAX FATALITIES

The list given to Larissa Mishustina in 1991 by KGB agents contained sixty-four names of people recorded as dying of anthrax in Sverdlovsk in 1979; the names were numbered and listed approximately in order of hospital registration, as far as we know. Four names were added to the list in 1992. An alphabetized list of all sixty-eight names is also included here for the reader's convenience.

The KGB List

Patronymics not included on the KGB list are given in brackets. In the case of Ignat Maslennikov, an alternate patronymic was reported by his wife.

1. Zakharov, Speridon Viktorovich
2. Markov, Mikhail Fyodorovich
3. Kozlova, Vera Ivanovna
4. Komina, Anna Petrovna
5. Nikolaev, Fyodor Dmitryevich
6. Romanov, Boris Georgevich
7. Fokina, Lilia Mikhaylovna
8. Tarasenko, Yekaterina Yakolevna
9. Loginova, Pavla Nesterovna
10. Syskov, Alexey Nikolayvich
11. Vyatkin, Aleksandr Ivanovich
12. Poletaev, Valeriy Fyodorovich
13. Kosheleva, Tatyana Fyodorovna

14. Maslennikov, Ignat Alekseyevich [Aleksandrovich]
15. Margamova, Rosa Timirovna
16. Retnev, Pavel Yakovlevich
17. Bliumova, Sophia Fyodorovna
18. Zheleznyak, Boris Andreyevich
19. Myasnikova, Anastasia Ivanovna
20. Shatokin, Nikolay Afanasyevich
21. Ivanov, Vasiliy Dorofeyevich
22. Borisov, Valentin Petrovich
23. Fyodosov, Vitaliy Konstantinovich
24. Volkova, Aleksandra Mikhaylovna
25. Chikalov, Konstantin Mikhaylovich
26. Komelskikh, Andrey Andreyevich
27. Korsayev, Lazar Nikolayvich
28. Vershinin, Ivan Andreyevich
29. Krivstov, Mikhail Andreyevich
30. Burmistrov, Mikhail Yegorovich
31. Nazarov, Vasiliy Mikhaylovich
32. Tepikin, Gennadiy Vasileyvich
33. Lyzlov, Vladimir Pavlovich
34. Bubenshikov, Viktor Ivanovich
35. Tretnikov, Vasiliy Ivanovich
36. Mochalova, Taisa Pavlovna
37. Buchelnikov, Vitaliy Aleksandrovich
38. Moseykina, Maria Semyonovna
39. Permyakov, Vasiliy Matveyevich
40. Makarov, Pyotr Vasilyevich
41. Markova, Valentina Davidovna
42. Bliznyakov, Georgiy Grigoryevich
43. Geptin, Pyotr Fyodorovich
44. Khudyakov, Nikolay Alekseyevich
45. Mukhametshin, Mukhametalin [Mukhametshinovich]
46. Pilyasov, Pyotr Yevstafyevich
47. Vostrykov, Nikolay Ivanovich
48. Lyakhova, Natalya Ignatievna
49. Vinogradov, Dmitriy Yegorovich
50. Chernyaeva, Aleksandra Andreyevna
51. Zinatulin, Kinzhabay [Khuskutdinovich]
52. Lavrov, Mikhail Fyodorovich
53. Makarov, Ivan Vasilyevich

54. Yasinskaya, Nina Fyodorovna
55. Sannikov, Vladimir Mikhaylovich
56. Spirina, Klaudia Maksimovna
57. Prokhorov, Valeriy Petrovich
58. Gayda, Pyotr Leonidovich
59. Klyestov, Ivan Yevgenyevich
60. Lozhkin, Mikhail Mikhaylovich
61. Dayanov, Fagim Zigantovich
62. Abusagitov, Zinatulla Chaikulovich
63. Sysikov, Yuriy Anatolyvich
64. Kramskoy, Yuriy Vladimirovich

Names Added in 1992

65. Dyedov, Filipp Mikhaylovich
66. Sergeyeva, Galina Pavlovna
67. Zhelnin, Aleksandr Mikhaylovich
68. Tischenko, Valentina Ivanovna

Alphabetized List of Names, with Numbers

Abusagitov, Zinatulla Chaikulovich 62
Bliumova, Sophia Fyodorovna 17
Bliznyakov, Georgiy Grigoryevich 42
Borisov, Valentin Petrovich 22
Bubenshikov, Viktor Ivanovich 34
Buchelnikov, Vitaliy Aleksandrovich 37
Burmistrov, Mikhail Yegorovich 30
Chernyaeva, Aleksandra Andreyevna 50
Chikalov, Konstantin Mikhaylovich 25
Dayanov, Fagim Zigantovich 61
Dyedov, Filipp Mikhaylovich 65
Fokina, Lilia Mikhaylovna 7
Fyodosov, Vitaliy Konstantinovich 23
Gayda, Pyotr Leonidovich 58
Geptin, Pyotr Fyodorovich 43
Ivanov, Vasiliy Dorofeyevich 21
Khudyakov, Nikolay Alekseyevich 44
Klyestov, Ivan Yevgenyevich 59
Komelskikh, Andrey Andreyevich 26
Komina, Anna Petrovna 4

Korsayev, Lazar Nikolayvich 27
Kosheleva, Tatyana Fyodorovna 13
Kozlova, Vera Ivanovna 3
Kramskoy, Yuriy Vladimirovich 64
Krivstov, Mikhail Andreyevich 29
Lavrov, Mikhail Fyodorovich 52
Loginova, Pavla Nesterovna 9
Lozhkin, Mikhail Mikhaylovich 60
Lyakhova, Natalya Ignatievna 48
Lyzlov, Vladimir Pavlovich 33
Makarov, Ivan Vasilyevich 53
Makarov, Pyotr Vasilyevich 40
Margamova, Rosa Timirovna 15
Markov, Mikhail Fyodorovich 2
Markova, Valentina Davidovna 41
Maslennikov, Ignat Alekseyevich [Aleksandrovich] 14
Mochalova, Taisa Pavlovna 36
Moseykina, Maria Semyonovna 38
Mukhametshin, Mukhametalin [Mukhametshinovich] 45
Myasnikova, Anastasia Ivanovna 19
Nazarov, Vasiliy Mikhaylovich 31
Nikolaev, Fyodor Dmitryevich 5
Permyakov, Vasiliy Matveyevich 39
Pilyasov, Pyotr Yevstafyevich 46
Poletaev, Valeriy Fyodorovich 12
Prokhorov, Valeriy Petrovich 57
Retnev, Pavel Yakovlevich 16
Romanov, Boris Georgevich 6
Sannikov, Vladimir Mikhaylovich 55
Sergeyeva, Galina Pavlovna 66
Shatokin, Nikolay Afanasyevich 20
Spirina, Klaudia Maksimovna 56
Sysikov, Yuriy Anatolyvich 63
Syskov, Alexey Nikolayvich 10
Tarasenko, Yekaterina Yakolevna 8
Tepikin, Gennadiy Vasileyvich 32
Tischenko, Valentina Ivanovna 68
Tretnikov, Vasiliy Ivanovich 35
Vershinin, Ivan Andreyevich 28
Vinogradov, Dmitriy Yegorovich 49

Volkova, Aleksandra Mikhaylovna 24
Vostrykov, Nikolay Ivanovich 47
Vyatkin, Aleksandr Ivanovich 11
Yasinskaya, Nina Fyodorovna 54
Zakharov, Speridon Viktorovich 1
Zheleznyak, Boris Andreyevich 18
Zhelnin, Aleksandr Mikhailovich 67
Zinatulin, Kinzhabay [Khuskutdinovich] 51

Appendix B

SUMMARY OF CASE DATA FOR KNOWN VICTIMS, INCLUDING SURVIVORS, OF THE SVERDLOVSK ANTHRAX OUTBREAK OF 1979

Case No.[a]	Age/Sex	Days of Onset/Death[b]	Residence/ Workplace
[c]	?/m	?/?	?/?
32	40/m	?/?	-/?
67	26/m	?/?	+/+
68	32/f	?/?	+/+
8	60/f	?/8	+/+
18	38/m	6/8	-/?
16	40/m	?/9	+/+
66	55/f	?/9	-/?
1	44/m	6/9	+/+
2	46/m	6/9	+/+
5	66/m	7/9	-/+
49	51/m	8/9	+/+
21	49/m	?/10	-/?
4	54/f	4/10	+/+
6	40/m	7/10	-/?
20	39/m	7/10	-/-
17	67/f	8/10	+/+
9	72/f	9/10	+/p
7	52/f	?/11	+/+
19	64/f	?/11	-/?
22	27/m	?/11	+/+
23	43/m	9/11	-/r
3	48/f	4/11	-/+
10	27/m	9/11	+/-
65	72/m	9/11	+/p
15	48/f	6/12	+/+
25	46/m	10/12	-/-
12	38/m	11/12	-/+
11	27/m	10/12	-/r
26	67/m	9/13	+/p
13	24/f	10/13	+/+
24	65/f	10/13	+/p
28	47/m	11/13	+/+
14	49/m	12/13	-/+
27	64/m	10/14	+/+
31	42/m	11/14	-/r
30	52/m	12/14	+/+
29	45/m	13/14	+/+
50	72/f	?/15	+/p

Case No.[a]	Age/Sex	Days of Onset/Death[b]	Residence/ Workplace
51	31/m	10/15	-/?
40	37/m	12/15	+/+
36	68/f	12/16	a/p
35	52/m	13/16	+/+
34	43/m	14/16	-/+
38	69/f	14/16	+/p
39	49/m	14/16	+/+
41	41/f	?/17	+/p
42	43/m	15/18	-/+
43	39/m	15/19	+/u
44	47/m	15/21	-/?
45	45/m	?/22	+/+
46	39/m	20/23	-/+
47	41/m	21/24	-/-
52	42/m	21/24	-/-
53	47/m	22/24	-/-
48	57/f	15/25	+/-
54	50/f	17/25	-/?
55	31/m	23/25	+/+
57	31/m	27/28	-/r
58	32/m	29/30	-/+
59	55/m	27/31	-/+
60	33/m	25/33	-/r
61	42/m	34/40	-/+
62	29/m	39/40	+/+
63	25/m	37/42	-/+
64	28/m	42/46	-/?
90	28/m	?/s	-/+
82	68/f	13/s	+/+
80	49/m	14/c	+/-
84	55/f	10/c	-/+
85	40/f	15/s	+/+
89	50/f	34/s	+/-
86	28/m	37/s	-/-
81	29/m	38/s	+/+
83	45/m	41/s	+/+
87	41/m	42/s	+/–
88	37/m	45/s	+/+

NOTE: Symbols and abbreviations used: ?, not known; -, outside high-risk zone; +, in high-risk zone; s, survivor; c, cutaneous survivor; a, had two residences, one in Compound 32; p, pensioner; r, daytime military reservist at Compound 32; u, unemployed. Patients 25, 29, 48, and 87 were home on vacation during the first week of April.

[a] Case numbers for fatalities are as they appear on the KGB list (see Appendix A; numbers 33, 37, and 56, whose status as anthrax cases is doubtful, are not included). Case numbers for survivors are arbitrary.

[b] Days of onset and death are counted from April 1, 1979.

[c] Unidentified man.

Notes

Chapter 1

1. Seeley et al. 1984; Robinson, Guillemin, and Meselson 1987.
2. Meselson's personal correspondence file, 1983–92, contains many such exchanges. One typical response by a Soviet official in 1986 was communicated via Dr. Martin Kaplan, Secretary-General of the Pugwash Conferences on Science and World Affairs: "I do not consider it expedient to organize this trip because of a lack of questions for discussion" (A. V. Fokin to M. M. Kaplan, February 26, 1986).
3. Fitzgerald 1974, 13.
4. Fairclough 1967, 195.
5. Abdullin 1976, 47–48.
6. Below about 10 degrees centigrade and above about 40 degrees, and without sufficient oxygen and the requisite complex nutrition, anthrax spores will fail to form. See Mims et al. 1999, 57, and the classic essay on anthrax, M. Sterne 1959, 19–21.
7. M. Sterne 1959, 21.
8. Manchee et al. 1981; Manchee et al. 1994.
9. World Health Organization 1991, 1993.
10. Herman Gold, 1955; see also Armitage 1992. Gold notes that he cannot account for the scarcity of inhalation anthrax "in the presence of virulent anthrax bacilli in the dust and air which is being inhaled by the workers of this plant." Nor can he explain the relatively very few cutaneous cases, except by apparent individual immunity. Length of employment or exposure seems to have nothing to do with immunity. He saw cutaneous anthrax in long-term employees as well as new ones.
11. Albrink et al. 1960.
12. Brachman, Pagano, and Albrink 1961.

13. See Gorbunova 1968 and Cowdery 1947. Cowdery cites a series of 340 cases occurring in Great Britain, of which 24 are described as both pulmonary and intestinal.

14. Carter 1988 offers a review of the Koch-Pasteur competition. Perhaps no other bacterium was as thoroughly researched as anthrax in the early days of germ theory and the science of disease.

15. Dubos 1950, 338–40; Geison 1995, 146–76. Geison presents evidence suggesting that the vaccine used at this trial was not made according to Pasteur's own formula, which he later perfected for manufacture.

16. See Williams and Wallace 1989; S. H. Harris 1994; Hal Gold 1996. Evidence points to a U.S. postwar arrangement to suppress information on Japanese biological warfare (BW) activities, while actively debriefing those Japanese scientists involved in BW research. In 1949 the Soviets put the Japanese military involved with BW on trial and sentenced the offenders to labor camps. See Williams and Wallace 1989, 220–32.

17. For background, see Robinson 1973. See also Harris and Paxman 1982; Bryden 1989.

18. A War Department document (U.S. War Department 1945) contains an exhaustive debriefing of German scientists involved in Nazi BW activities, which appear to have been curtailed as Soviet troops advanced toward Berlin in winter 1945.

19. R. Nixon, letter to *New York Times,* February 19, 1970.

20. *Posev* 1980. A similar article from the Paris publication *Russkaya Mysl* (Russian thought) was translated in 1980 by Freedom House Information Service in New York; it included a firsthand account claiming an explosion at the military facility and the deaths of at minimum one thousand people. Months after the epidemic, it claimed, women gave birth to infants with "cancer-like swellings."

21. As reported in Gelb 1981, 31–33, 59–69.

22. The definitive account of the Sverdlovsk and other CBW incidents for this era can be found in Robinson 1982 and 1985. See also E. Harris 1987; Leitenberg 1991.

23. See the summary of these presentations in Meselson 1988. Defense Intelligence Agency 1986 summarizes the U.S. position that twenty-two pounds of anthrax were emitted and a thousand or more people died.

24. See U.S. Senate 1990, 210: "The next step, it seems to me, in clarifying this issue, is to visit that facility"; see also 498ff. In a March 8, 1991, radio interview regarding the 1979 outbreak in Sverdlovsk, Meselson said, "In the late 1960s, the U.S. government had reason to believe that [Compound 19] was developing biological weapons, and to this day the Soviets have not let us go look. This is up to them to do, the ball is in their court" (Meselson 1991a, 3). Further corroboration of this scientific skepticism and efforts to effect an inquiry are found in U.S. State Department cables summarizing Meselson debriefings (Washington, August 26, 1986, 267418; Moscow, August 29, 1986, 14971; Washington, September 17, 1986, 267418; Washington, January 21, 1988 18151; Moscow, February 1, 1988, 01894). See also Meselson 1991b, 11.

25. Meselson, Kaplan, and Mokulsky 1990. Dr. Martin Kaplan at Pugwash was at every step a positive force in promoting the Sverdlovsk expedition. In 1996, the Pugwash Conferences on Science and World Affairs received a Nobel Peace Prize.

Chapter 2

1. See Taubman and Taubman 1989 for the atmosphere of hope that prevailed as the Soviet Union began dissolving.
2. MacMahon and Pugh 1970, 157.
3. Abdullin 1976, 56.
4. Bezdeneznikh and Nikiforov 1980, 111.
5. Pashkov 1991b.
6. Burgasov et al. 1970. See also Burgasov and Rozhkov 1974 on STI vaccine.
7. Mims et al. 1999, 97. See Weismann 1998 for the cultural history of "the battle of inflammation."
8. Meselson trip notes, 1988.
9. Burgasov et al., 1970, 36, 34.
10. In addition to Burgasov et al. 1970 (Russian title *Siberskaya Yazva*), another major Russian source on anthrax, Akulov 1976, would have pointed Nikiforov in the direction of the lymph nodes. It suggests that "bronchial" lymph nodes may be afflicted and that hemorrhagic lymphadenitis of varying degrees may develop in them.
11. For the textile worker, see Herman Gold 1955, 12; the rug salesman case is presented in Cowdery 1947.
12. See Sontag 1977, 156.

Chapter 3

1. This description appears in the late story "My Life"; Chekhov 1993, 467.
2. Barykin, Vygodchikov, and Sazhina 1929, 26.
3. Ibid., 27.
4. See Nelkin and Gilman 1988.
5. See H. Smith 1984, 708–11. Smith also describes pervasive organized crime that should have made the post-Soviet mafia and "robber barons" predictable to economic reformers.
6. Balayev 1980. This article is an interview with Ivan Pavlovich Balayev, jurist and representative of the Chkalovskiy Municipal People's Court of Sverdlovsk.
7. Bezdenezhnikh, Burgasov, and Nikiforov 1988, 10–12.
8. See Lilienfeld and Lilienfeld 1980, 50–57.
9. See the descriptions in Averyanov 1940 and Benenson 1990, 18. The latter claims that illness in "most cases occurs within 48 hours after exposure."
10. Snow 1855.
11. Pashkov 1991b, 4.
12. Pashkov 1991a.

13. Burgasov et al. 1970, 80.

14. Smith, Keppie, and Stanley 1955; Turnbull 1991, 535.

15. Pasternak 1961, 115.

16. See Tuan 1984.

17. Burgasov et al. 1970, 3–4.

18. Turnbull 1991, 534. The United States and the United Kingdom use cell-free filtrates of anthrax cultures. See also Cherkasskiy 1979, 3, which notes considerable increase in animal vaccination in the Soviet Union from 1960 to 1979.

19. World Health Organization 1991, 1993.

20. Cherkasskiy 1979, 3.

21. Gogol 1923, 264.

Chapter 4

1. Chekhov 1947, 141.

2. Radzinsky 1992, 327–31.

3. Duval 1976, 230.

4. See the discussion of Russian renaming and displacement in Stapanian-Apkarian 1994.

5. Kotkin 1995.

6. Service 1998, 260.

7. Bonet 1995, 3.

8. These exchanges are in Meselson's personal correspondence: Meselson to A. V. Yablokov, January 22, 1992; Yablokov to Meselson, February 5, 1992; Meselson to Yablokov, March 3, 1992; e-mail from E. D. Sverdlov to Meselson, March 17, 1992; and Yablokov to Meselson, March 23, 1992. Other exchanges cited in this chapter are also from this personal correspondence.

9. Gelb 1981, 34.

10. For a cogent explanation of the Soviet health system divisions, which survive in present-day Russia, see Field 1967.

11. Boym 1994, 223–24.

12. Pfohl 1994, 289.

Chapter 5

1. Nothing in this 1982 manuscript, which we obtained a copy of from Dr. V. V. Nikiforov, alludes to infection of the thoracic lymph nodes. The only illustration shows mesentery lesions. Close comparison between this manuscript and the 1988 official Soviet statement given to the U.S. State Department by the Soviet Foreign Office reveals striking similarities of wording between the description of infected lymph nodes in both. The Abramova and Grinberg paper offers a general description of three stages of lymph node infection without differentiating between thoracic or mesentery. The Soviet report is written at the same level of description, but refers specifically to gastrointestinal anthrax.

2. See Foucault 1994, 138.

3. Hughes 1984, 87–97. Hughes's general point is that marginal figures can

be employed for tasks the majority do not want to be associated with. He makes no connecting reference to the medical profession in this essay, although he writes extensively about status in medicine in other essays in this volume and elsewhere. Hughes was on my dissertation committee (while he was at Brandeis University) and later we co-taught a course on sociobiology at Boston College. In our conversations, he asked the question, "What do we know about dirty work? Who washes down the operating room when the doctors and nurses have left?"

4. Shipler 1983, 21.

5. Hingley 1977, 120.

6. The Irish under British rule invented multiple forms of word play—jokes, witticisms, blarney, teasing, and even poetry that distanced and confused outsiders (Scheper-Hughes 1979, 82–83). Black English as it developed in African-American ghettos has these same facets of double-talk, scam, and "jiving" to circumvent the power of "the Man" (Abrahams 1976).

7. Goodenough and Thomas 1987, 3–14. See also Goodenough 1996.

8. Balmer 1998, 3, documents "Project Harness."

9. Foucault 1994, 196–97.

10. In Roueché 1967, xvii.

Chapter 6

1. Sontag 1977, 16. See also Avery Gordon's (1997, 108–11) discourse on the photographs of the "disappeared" in Argentina.

2. See Hokanson 1998.

Chapter 7

1. Metchnikoff 1884. In this article Metchnikoff refers to anthrax as the most researched of all bacteria.

2. Barnes 1947; Ross 1957. See also Young, Zelle, and Lincoln 1946.

3. Albrink et al. 1959.

4. Brachman, Pagano, and Albrink 1961.

5. S. H. Harris 1994, 48–69.

6. Pashkov 1991c.

7. See *Veterinaria* 1980, which mentions specific villages and animal deaths.

8. Glassman 1966.

Chapter 8

1. See Tuan 1974, 63.

2. Baidukov 1991.

3. Benjamin 1986, 98–99.

4. Filtzer 1986, 209.

5. Giddens 1991, 113.

6. Tuan 1979, 71.

7. Guillemin and Holmstrom 1986.

Chapter 9

1. Meselson to K. M. Dyumayev, July 14, 1983; Dyumayev to Meselson, October 10, 1983; this and letters cited in notes 2 and 3 are in Meselson's personal correspondence file.

2. Meselson to P. N. Burgasov, September 30, 1986.

3. Meselson to Y. Chazov, September 30, 1988; Meselson to E. V. Kosenko, November 4, 1988; J. Federov to Meselson, December 30, 1988; Meselson to Federov, March 9, 1989.

4. Mandelstam 1983, 83.

Chapter 10

1. Yeltsin (1992a, 81) describes this with regret.

2. Zhenova 1990, 12.

3. Miller 1952 (declassified 1978); Cochrane 1947 (declassified 1975).

4. Covert 1993, 40–41. At Ft. Detrick, Boyles Street and Willard Place are named in honor of these victims; Nickel Place is named in honor of an animal caretaker who died of Machupo virus. The fourth case, that of a young Army lieutenant, was "handled quietly," and Covert could obtain no information about the incident.

5. Averyanov 1940, 10. Averyanov summarizes major outbreaks from 1854 to 1936 and describes his own cases as well.

Chapter 11

1. Gomes 1911, 66–67. Sea Dyaks is the old name for one of the modern Iban tribes in Borneo. Gomes writes: "Other punishments are soon forgotten, but this remains as a testimony to a man's untruthfulness for succeeding generations to witness, and is a standing disgrace to his children's children."

2. See Couto 1986; Brown and Mikkelsen 1990.

3. Coser 1956, 127. See Covert 1993, 43–48, for guarded but still interesting accounts of local community protest against air and well-water contamination from Fort Detrick.

4. Cochrane 1947; Miller 1952, 77ff.; Manchee et al. 1981, 294; Manchee et al. 1994.

5. Vaughan 1996.

6. Agee and Evans 1941, 156.

7. Dostoevsky 1917, 171.

8. See Keller 1968; Gans 1982; and see Tuan's discussion of neighborhood and community, 1974, 210–24.

Chapter 12

1. Hochschild 1994, 199.

2. Grandin 1994.

3. Zisk 1993, 109–10.

4. See Covert 1993, 51: "There was considerable gloom and doom in Frederick and Fort Detrick in 1969 when the decision to stop offensive biological research was made by President Richard M. Nixon. It meant a loss of jobs and struck hard at both the employees and the community." The "ghost of Building 470" is described on pp. 48–49.

5. Pashkov 1991a, 8.

6. See Field's (1967, 103–4) description of the Red Cross and, in Moslem areas, the Red Crescent in Soviet medicine providing relief funds for victims of natural catastrophes, usually outside the USSR. It remains uncertain how many Sverdlovsk families actually received their Red Cross allotments.

7. Russian Federation 1992.

8. Wolff 1976.

Chapter 13

1. See Sacks 1976, 110–34.

2. Parfenov 1990.

3. See Goffman 1967, 5–45.

4. Khubova, Ivankiev, and Sharova 1992, 89. See also Sherbakova 1992.

5. Wallace 1956.

6. Erikson 1994.

7. MacNeill 1977 offers a sweeping overview of epidemics through history destroying poor or marginal populations; Watts 1997 writes on epidemics and imperialism.

8. See Wolfenstein 1957; although her discussion of victims' feelings of abandonment is brilliant, she ignores political contexts. See in contrast Fanning's 1995 account of socialist East European immigrants in Norwood, Massachusetts, victimized by the 1918 influenza epidemic even as they are politically stigmatized by local elites.

9. Erikson 1994, 230.

10. Coser 1956, 129–30.

Chapter 14

1. Chekhov 1930, 181–82.

Chapter 15

1. Zhenova 1990a and 1990b.

2. Zhenova 1991a; and see Meselson 1988. Zhenova mistakenly refers to Meselson supporting the Soviet explanation in 1980, with the implication that he supported it to the present.

3. Zhenova 1991b.

4. Pashkov 1992.

5. Carr and Renfrew 1957.

6. Giddens 1991.

Chapter 16

1. Kuran 1995; see pp. 105–56 and 261–88 on communism.
2. Taylor 1977, xix.
3. Quoted in Colton 1982, 162.
4. Muratov, Sorokin, and Fronin 1992.
5. Barylski 1998, 80.
6. Remnick 1994, 372–422.
7. Ibid., 467.
8. Barylski 1998, 139–43.

Chapter 17

1. Miller 1952, 9–10.
2. President's Air Policy Commission 1948, 12; this is cited in Miller 1952, 13.
3. The panels included, in Washington, Wilhelm Albrink, Philip Brachman, Joshua Lederberg, James Steele, John Steinbruner, and Fred Murphy, dean of the School of Public Health at University of California, Davis; and in Cambridge, Lederberg, Alexander Rich, and Leon Kass and Mary Wilson from Harvard, experts in infectious disease.
4. This survivor died of asphyxiation due to "larynx occlusion" in March 1992. Ilona Nikonova interviewed his widow.
5. Pashkov 1991c.
6. Gusterson 1996, 108.
7. Covert 1993, 57–58.
8. Rothschild 1964, 81. See CBS News 1969, 5–6, in which Rothschild, in an interview with Mike Wallace, argues that biological and chemical weapons are more "humane" than others.
9. U.S. Army 1954, 10–11.
10. See Keegan 1977, 322.
11. See Kaldor, Albrecht, and Schméder 1998, 1–8; see also Kaldor 1998 for a comprehensive analysis of global militarism.

Chapter 18

1. E. Harris 1987.
2. E. Harris 1992. The account of the meeting is taken from this document as well as from personal notes by Meselson and the author.
3. Davidovsky 1956, 384–88.
4. Meselson meeting notes.
5. Bok 1982, 177.
6. See Hirsch 1951 for the World War II debriefings of a Soviet prisoner-of-war and a deserter that include specific descriptions of BW agents, munitions, and targets being developed at various institutes.
7. Robinson 1973, 128–31.
8. Gerz 1992, 4. See also Alibek 1999, 226–40.

9. R. J. Smith 1992.

10. Litovkin and Eggert 1992.

11. Golts 1992, 3.

12. Interview with the author, July 23, 1998.

13. Uralmashzarod Production Association 1993.

Chapter 19

1. Henderson, Peacock, and Belton 1956.

2. Glassman 1966 draws on the unpublished work of J. Jemski.

3. Friedlander et al. 1993.

4. For example, cases were scattered over a general area in the Q fever epidemic originating from a rendering plant that affected the San Francisco Bay Area in 1953 (Wellock and Parker 1959; Wellock 1960); a long plume pattern was reported from the U.S. BW "St. Jo" experiments (U.S. Army 1954, 10–11). The Q fever epidemic may have been caused by multiple emissions from the factory, which varied depending on wind directions. The U.S. experiments were based on single-source scenarios.

5. Frolov 1992.

6. Urban 1996, 131.

7. Ibid., 227.

8. U.S. Senate 1995, 41–44.

9. U. S. Senate 1996, 273–76.

10. See Nicholas de B. Katzenbach's perennially ignored article against the support of covert groups (1973) and Sissela Bok's discussion of military secrecy (1982, 191–209) for philosophical arguments concerning military secrecy and covert action.

11. Kelly 1998, 28.

12. See the case summary in Carus 1998, 133–35.

13. Meselson trip notes, Moscow, January 18, 1993.

14. This notation is undated, but was probably made during the summer of 1992.

15. E. Harris 1992, 24.

16. Lévi-Strauss 1982.

Chapter 20

1. Guillemin 1998, 13–14.

2. Gogol 1923, 31.

3. Pasternak 1958, 365–66.

4. Sigerist 1937, 208. See Field 1967, x–xi, on Sigerist's sympathetic account of the Soviet Union.

5. See Watts 1997, 269–79, for a discussion of the "epidemiologic transition" from natural epidemics to man-made diseases; Watts enlarges on the work of Abdel Omran.

Chapter 22

1. Herspring 1990, 218; Zisk 1993, 173–75. See also Jones 1989, 92–98.
2. Pashkov 1992.
3. The journal's present title is *The CBW Conventions Bulletin*.
4. F. A. Abramova, L. M. Grinberg, O. V. Yampolskaya, and D. H. Walker, 1993, "Pathology of Inhalational Anthrax in 42 Cases from the Sverdlovsk Outbreak in 1979," *Proceedings of the National Academy of Science* 90, 2291–93; F. A. Abramova and L. M. Grinberg, 1993, "Pathology of Anthracic Sepsis According to the Materials of the Infectious Outburst in Sverdlosk, 1979," *Arkhiv Patologii* 55, no. 1, 12–14. The *Arkhiv Patologii* article is a more detailed version of the *PNAS* article; Abramova and Grinberg had submitted it for publication before we arrived in Yekaterinburg in 1992.
5. Darnton 1984, 5–104.
6. Bulgakov 1968, 6.
7. See Loren Graham's 1993 book on engineer Pyotr Palchinsky as the symbol of the engineering with human values that the Soviets rejected in favor of short-term efficiency and mass production.
8. Beck 1992.

Chapter 23

1. Arendt 1958, 431.
2. Merton (1938, 327) noted that the institutionalized norms of science are "dismissed by the totalitarian state as 'liberalistic' or 'cosmopolitan' or 'bourgeois' prejudices, inasmuch as they cannot be readily integrated with the campaign for an unquestioned political creed."
3. Soyfer 1994.
4. A 1976 article on epizootics contains a passing reference that veterinarians often find young lambs relatively immune to anthrax, whether or not the ewes have been vaccinated, and that in wild animals like reindeer the young seem to have a similar immunity (Abdullin 1976, 45). Perhaps nature is kind, and some feature of their lungs or general immune system protects young mammals, including humans, from this particular hazard.
5. Walter 1969, 335–43.
6. Ken Alibek in his autobiographical account of the Soviet BW program (1999, 74–75) attempts a secondhand reconstruction of the Sverdlovsk outbreak. He stipulates the cause as an accidental failure to replace a filter in an area of Compound 19 where anthrax spores were being dried in preparation for weaponization. However, Alibek also confidently promotes important factual errors about the event—that the emission occurred on Friday, March 30 (contrary to wind data; see Chapter 19 and Figure 2); that it occurred at night; that nearly all the night-shift workers at the ceramics factory were killed; and that army employee Nikolayev was the first victim and died April 2—which undermine the credibility of his other assertions.

Chapter 24

1. See Meselson 1995 for the specifics on these calculations.

2. Meselson et al., 1994, "The Sverdlovsk Anthrax Outbreak of 1979," *Science* 226, no. 5188:1202–8.

3. Carus 1998, 42, compiled from data from three U.S. government reports.

4. UN Security Council 1995a, 1995b.

5. Zilinskas 1997, 421–23.

6. Levin 1998, 117–19.

7. Tuan 1979, 87; in the same passage Tuan writes, "Sickness forcefully directs a people's attention to the world's hostility."

8. Robinson 1973, 131–32.

9. The first of these reports, *DoD Responses to Transnational Threats*, was a study by a panel of experts, issued in October 1997, describing a panoply of defense programs in the making. In November came the *CB 2010 Study*, which assessed future chemical and biological threats, calling them "innumerable." In December, the third, *Transforming Defense: National Security in the 21st Century,* restated the threat of biological weapons to U.S. security. In January 1998, Defense Intelligence Agency and CIA officials at a U.S. Senate hearing also spoke to what they believed was a growing terrorist interest in acquiring biological weapons. See Carus (1998, 5–8) for a summary of this "evolving perception."

10. Miller 1952, 54.

11. Heymann and Rodier 1998. Today (as opposed to 1979), hardly a significant epidemic occurs in the world that is not immediately broadcast electronically—the only surveillance fast enough for BW response. Electronic discussion sites such as ProMed and TravelMed are global and free. Health Canada has developed the Global Public Health Information Network with search engines that scan the World Wide Web for reports of communicable diseases.

12. Franz et al. 1997.

13. Beal 1998, 2.

14. Hersch (1998, 88) reports that this campaign was influenced by new though slender evidence that Iraqi soldiers had been inoculated against anthrax. Even before the American program began, nongovernment physicians raised questions about the efficacy and safety of the vaccination—that it may not protect against various strains of anthrax or against inhalation anthrax, the main BW threat, and that it may pose unknown health risks—as well as about the use of a medical program to address international political stability. See Sidel, Nass, and Ensign 1998 and Istock 1998. In the United Kingdom and Canada, anthrax vaccinations for the military are voluntary.

15. Henderson 1998, 490–91: "Even if only 100 persons were infected and required hospitalization, a group of patients many times larger would become ill with fever and rash and receive an uncertain diagnosis. Some would be reported from other cities and other states. Where would all these patients be admitted? In the Washington, D.C., metropolitan area, no more than 100 hospital beds provide adequate hospitalization [for such patients]. Who would care for the patients? Few hospital staff [today] have any smallpox immunity."

16. Quoted in Hasenauer 1998, 16.

17. Carter, Deutch, and Zelikow 1998.

18. Douglas and Wildavsky 1982, 195.

19. See Horowitz 1989, 408–9.

20. Beck 1992; 56: "Demands, and thus markets, of a completely new type can be *created* by varying the definition of risk, especially demand for the avoidance of risk—open to interpretation, casually designable and infinitely reproducible" (italics in original).

21. Bauman 1993, 204.

22. Pringle 1998.

23. Carus 1998, 9. Only one terrorist incident with a real pathogen has ever been recorded in the United States. In 1984 members of the Rajneeshee religious cult contaminated restaurant salad bars with *Salmonella typhimurium* to cause food poisoning among their neighbors in Wasco County, Oregon. Their goal was to decrease the number of negative votes on a zoning issue concerning their commune. Around 750 people fell ill, and 45 were hospitalized; no one died. At the time the event was blamed on restaurant workers' poor sanitary habits. Only when the cult group was disbanding a year or so later did the Federal Bureau of Investigation and the Centers for Disease Control gain access to the inside story of the plot (Carus 1998, 9ff).

24. See Sennett 1974, 259–340, on the modern transmutation of political categories to psychological categories and the retreat from public life.

25. Holton 1986, 301–3.

26. See Falkenrath, Newman, and Thayer 1998, 261–336.

Chapter 25

1. Inkeles and Bauer 1961, 383.

2. Jackson et al. 1997.

3. Cherkasskiy 1979, 4.

4. Pomerantsev et al. 1997.

5. Pomerantsev et al. 1995.

6. See Mannoff 1995, 26–27. Journalists under the influence of American Sovietology presumed the Soviet Union to be a static monolith and were late to report on the reform process. The more current strategy, according to Mannoff, is to normalize Russian adaptation to capitalism and the free market, that is, to be satisfied when Russians appear "like us" and critical when they seem reluctant to accept reforms.

7. In 1998, for example, following a nine-day oversight mission to Russia and Ukraine, Senator Richard Lugar spoke publicly on the "complete access" he had to the Obolensk facility, which is the Soviet Union's "premier biological weapons research and development institute for the bacterial pathogens plague, tularemia, and glanders, as well as the world's leading anthrax research institute" (*CBW Conventions Bulletin* 42 [December 1998]:45–46).

8. See Hanna, Accosta, and Collier 1993 for the beginning of this inquiry, which shows the role of macrophages in the spread of anthrax toxins; and Hanna 1998 and Collier 1998 for reports on recent research.

9. Liddington 1998.

10. See Merton 1957 on eponymy and "fathers" in the sciences, which means more to the specific professional group than to science itself.

11. See Boym 1994. On the cultural level we can wonder how Russian citizens will unlearn the lessons of seventy years of totalitarianism. Boym (1994, 288–89) recounts the story of two people leaving a political demonstration against the Gulf War, one American, the other a visiting Russian. The American, placard still in hand, stops at a crosswalk because the light is red. His protest is lawful; he respects the law. The Russian, ready to jaywalk, is amazed. He is accustomed to routine violations of an official order he does not respect or trust. Almost anything illegal could be done in Soviet Russia through networks of family and friends. Getting the law to work for you was harder.

12. Boym 1993.

13. Stishova 1996, 191; see also Bridges, Kay, and Pinnick 1996, 165–92.

14. Randolph 1996, 86–97, 185–236.

15. Felgenhauer 1998a, 1998b.

16. Norris and Fowler 1997, 30.

17. See Sennett 1998, 46–63.

18. Lifton 1993; see also Martin 1994.

19. General Yevstigneyev made the suggestion that Soviet anthrax strains from Sverdlovsk should be identified as one means of solving the puzzle, remarking that all it would take is money; see Pashkov 1992.

Chapter 26

1. Pushkin 1965, 92–93. See poet Marina Tsvetaeva's analysis of this toast (1992, 151).

2. Albert Camus, in his novel *The Plague* (1948, 120–21), presents the same tension among citizens in the quarantined city of Oran.

3. Simmel 1950, 333.

4. Ibid., 355; Simmel was writing about secret societies but could have been describing agencies within totalitarian governments.

5. See Goldman 1992, 246, on Yeltsin, dispensable democracy, and presidential decrees in 1991.

6. Akhmatova 1993, 201.

7. Dostoyevsky 1955, 173.

8. Remnick 1998, 367: "Russia is no longer an enemy or anything resembling one."

9. See Feshbach and Friendly 1991.

References

Abdullin, K. K.
  1976.   "Epizootology." In Kolesov 1976.
Abrahams, R. D.
  1976.   *Talking Black*. Rowley, Mass.: Newbury House Publishers.
Abramova, F. A., and L. M. Grinberg.
  1993.   "Pathology of Anthracic Sepsis According to the Materials of
              the Infectious Outburst in Sverdlovsk, 1979 (Some Problems of
              Morpho-, Patho-, and Thanatogenesis." *Arkhiv Patologii* 55, no.
              1:12–14.
Abramova, F. A., L. M. Grinberg, O. V. Yampolskaya, and D. H. Walker.
  1993.   "Pathology of Inhalational Anthrax in 42 Cases from the Sverd-
              lovsk Outbreak in 1979." *Proceedings of the National Academy
              of Science* 90:2291–93.
Agee, J., and W. Evans.
  1941.   *Let Us Now Praise Famous Men: Three Tenant Families*. Boston:
              Houghton Mifflin.
Akhmatova, A.
  1993.   "Requiem: Epilogue II." Trans. P. Perkins. In *The Burden of Suf-
              ferance: Women Poets of Russia*, ed. P. Perkins and A. Cook. New
              York: Garland Publishing.
Akulov, A. V.
  1976.   "Pathomorphology and Pathomorphological Diagnosis." In Ko-
              lesov 1981.
Albrink, W. S., S. M. Brooks, R. E. Biron, and M. Kopel.
  1960.   "Human Inhalation Anthrax: A Report of Three Fatal Cases."
              American Journal of Pathology 36:457–71.
Albrink, W. S., and R. J. Goodlow.
  1959.   "Experimental Inhalation Anthrax in the Chimpanzee." *Ameri-
              can Journal of Pathology* 35:1055–65.

Alibek, K., with S. Handelman.
    1999.   *Biohazard: The Chilling True Story of the Largest Covert Bio-logical Weapons Program in the World, Told from Inside by the Man Who Ran It.* New York: Random House.

Arendt, H.
    1958.   *The Origins of Totalitarianism.* 2d ed. New York: World Publishing.

Armitage, H. V.
    1992.   "Anthrax in Delaware County: A Historical Perspective." *Delaware Medical Journal* 64, no. 5:331–32.

Averyanov, K. K.
    1940.   "Epidemiological Outbreaks of Anthrax." *Journal of Microbiology, Epidemiology, and Immunobiology* 8: 35–44.

Baidukov, G.
    1991.   *Russian Lindbergh: The Life of Valery Chkalov.* Trans. P. Belov. Washington, D.C.: Smithsonian Institution Press.

Balayev, I. P.
    1980.   "Strict Observance of Veterinary Regulations." *Chelovek i Zakon (Man and the Law).* Interview, September 9, 9:70–72.

Balmer, B.
    1998.   "Using the Population Body to Protect the National Body: Germ Warfare Tests in the UK after WWII." "Using Bodies" Conference, Wellcome Institute for History of Medicine, London, September 3–4.

Barnes, J. M.
    1947.   "The Development of Anthrax Following the Administration of Spores by Inhalation." *British Journal of Experimental Pathology* 28: 385–94.

Barykin, V., G. Vygodchikov, and Y. Sazhina.
    1929.   "Outbreak of Intestinal Anthrax in Yaroslavl." *Zhurnal Gigiyena I Epidemiologiya (Journal of Hygiene and Epidemiology)* 1:25–30. U.S. Department of State translation.

Barylski, R.
    1998.   *The Soldier in Russian Politics. Duty, Dictatorship, and Democracy under Gorbachev and Yeltsin.* New Brunswick, N.J.: Transaction Books.

Bauman, Z.
    1993.   *Postmodern Ethics.* Oxford: Blackwell.
Beal, C.
    1998.   "Facing the Invisible Enemy." *Jane's Defence Weekly* 30, no. 18 (November 4):1–4.

Beck, U.
    1992.   *Risk Society: Towards a New Modernity.* Trans. M. Ritter. London: Sage.

Benenson, A. S., ed.
    1990.   *Control of Communicable Diseases in Man.* Washington, D.C.: American Public Health Association.

Benjamin, W.
    1986.   *Reflections: Essays, Aphorisms, Autobiographical Writings*. Ed.
             P. Demetz. New York: Schocken Books.
Bezdenezhnikh, I. S., P. N. Burgasov, and V. I. Nikiforov.
    1988.   *Soviet Response to U.S. Regarding Information on Sverdlovsk,
             1979*. 9 September. U.S. Department of State translation.
Bezdenezhnykh, I. S., and V. I. Nikiforov.
    1980.   "Epidemiological Analysis of Incidences of Anthrax in Sverdlovsk."
             *Zhurnal Mikrobiologiy, Epidemiologiy, i Immunobiologiy (Jour-
             nal of Microbiology, Epidemiology, and Immunobiology)* 5:111.
Bliss, C. I.
    1935.   "The Calculation of Dosage-Mortality Curve." *Annals of Applied
             Biology* 22:134–67.
Bok, S.
    1982.   *Secrets: On the Ethics of Concealment and Revelation*. New York:
             Pantheon Books.
Bonet, P.
    1995.   "Lord of the Manor: Boris Yeltsin in Sverdlovsk *Oblast*." *Oc-
             casional Paper #260*. Washington, D.C.: Kennan Institute for Ad-
             vanced Russian Studies.
Boym, S.
    1993.   "Loving in Bad Taste: Eroticism and Literary Excess in Marina
             Tsvetaeva's 'The Tale of Sonechka.'" In *Sexuality and the Body
             in Modern Culture*, ed. J. T. Costlow, S. Sandler, and J. Vowles.
             Stanford, Calif.: Stanford University Press.
    1994.   *Common Places: Mythologies of Everyday Life in Russia*. Cam-
             bridge, Mass.: Harvard University Press.
Brachman, P. S., H. Gold, S. A. Plotkin, F. R. Fekety, M. Werrin, and N. R.
Ingraham.
    1962.   "Field Evaluation of a Human Anthrax Vaccine." *American Jour-
             nal of Public Health* 56:632–45.
Brachman, P., J. Pagano, and W. S. Albrink.
    1961.   "Two Cases of Fatal Inhalation Anthrax, One Associated with
             Sarcoidosis." *New England Journal of Medicine* 265, no. 5 (Au-
             gust 3):203.
Bridges, S., R. Kay, and K. Pinnick.
    1996.   *No More Heroines: Russia, Women, and the Market*. New York:
             Routledge, 165–92.
Brown, P., and E. J. Mikkelsen.
    1990.   *No Safe Place*. Berkeley: University of California Press.
Bryden, J.
    1989.   *Deadly Allies: Canada's Secret War, 1937–1947*. Toronto: Mc-
             Clelland & Stewart.
Bulgakov, M.
    1968.   *Heart of a Dog*. New York: Grove Press.
Burgasov, P. N., B. L. Cherkasskiy, L. M. Marchuk, and Y. F. Shcherbak.
    1970.   *Anthrax (Sibirskaya Yazva)*. Moscow: Editions Medicine. Trans.

1981, Foreign Broadcast Information Service, Washington, D.C. (January 5).

Burgasov, P. N., and G. I. Rozhkov.
1972.   "Evaluation of Immunity to Anthrax from the Preventive Properties of Serum." *Zhurnal Mikrobiologiy, Epidemiologiy, i Immunobiologiy* 6:124–34.

Camus, A.
1948.   *The Plague.* Trans. S. Gilbert. New York: Knopf.

Carr, E. A., and R. R. Renfrew.
1957.   "Recovery of *Bacillus anthracis* from the Nose and Throat of Apparently Healthy Workers." *Journal of Infectious Diseases* 100:169–71.

Carter A., J. Deutsch, and P. Zelikow.
1998.   "Catastrophic Terrorism. Tackling New Danger." *Foreign Affairs,* November/December: 80–94.

Carter, K. C.
1988.   "The Koch-Pasteur Dispute on Establishing the Cause of Anthrax." *Bulletin of the History of Medicine* 62, no. 1:87–95.

Carus, W. S.
1998.   *Bioterrorism and Biocrimes: The Illicit Use of Biological Agents in the 20th Century.* Washington, D.C.: Center for Counter Proliferation Research, National Defense University.

CBS News.
1969.   "Sixty Minutes Highlights." July 8, transcript.

Chekov, A.
1930.   *The Plays of Anton Tchekov.* New York: Modern Library. Trans. C. Garnett.

1947.   *Letters of Anton Chekhov.* Ed. A. Yarmolinsky. New York: Viking Press.

1993 [1920]. "My Life." In *Longer Stories from the Last Decade.* Trans. C. Garnett. New York: Random House (Modern Library ed.).

Cherkasskiy, B. L.
1979.   "Current Problems in the Prophylaxis Against Anthrax." *Journal of Microbiology, Epidemiology, and Immunology* 8:3–6.

Cochrane, R. C.
1947.   *Biological Warfare Research in the United States.* EA-S-1089 (71). Ft. Detrick, Md.: Office of Chief, Chemical Corps, November.

Collier, J.
1998.   "Mechanisms of Membrane Translocation by Anthrax Toxin: Insertion and Pore Formation by Protective Antigen." Paper presented at the Third International Conference on Anthrax, University of Plymouth, U.K., September 9.

Colton, T.
1982.   *The Dilemma of Reform in the Soviet Union.* New York: Council on Foreign Relations.

Coser, L.
1956.   *The Functions of Social Conflict.* New York: Free Press.

Couto, R. A.
1986. "Failing Health and New Prescriptions: Community-Based Approaches to Environmental Risks." In *Current Health Policies and Alternatives: An Applied Social Science Perspective,* ed. C. E. Hill. Athens: University of Georgia Press.

Covert, N. M.
1993. *Cutting Edge: A History of Fort Detrick, Maryland, 1943–1993.* Fort Detrick, Md.: Public Affairs Office.

Cowdery, J. S.
1947. "Primary Pulmonary Anthrax with Septicemia." *Archives of Pathology* 43:396–99.

Darnton, R.
1984. *The Great Cat Massacre and Other Episodes in French Cultural History.* New York: Basic Books.

Davidovsky, I. V.
1956. *Pathological Anatomy and Pathogenesis of Human Diseases.* Moscow: Medgiz. Trans. 1993, Institute of Medicine (NIH).

Defense Intelligence Agency.
1986. *Soviet Biological Warfare Threat.* Washington, D.C.: Department of Defense. DST-1610F-057-86, 4.

Defoe, D.
1966 [1722]. *A Journal of the Plague Year.* London: Penguin.

Dostoyevsky, F.
1917. *The House of the Dead.* Trans. C. Garnett. New York: Macmillan.
1955. *The Insulted and the Injured.* Trans. C. Garnett. Westport, Conn.: Greenwood Press.

Douglas, M., and A. Wildavsky.
1982. *Risk and Culture: An Essay on the Selection of Technological and Environmental Dangers.* Berkeley: University of California Press.

Dubos, R.
1950. *Louis Pasteur: Free Lance of Science.* Boston: Little, Brown.

Duval, C.
1976. "Iakov Nikhailovich Sverdlov: Founder of the Bolshevik Party Machine." In *Reconsiderations on the Russian Revolution,* ed. R. C. Elwood. Cambridge, Mass.: Slavica Pubishers.

Erikson, K.
1994. *A New Species of Trouble: Explorations in Disaster, Trauma, and Community.* New York: W. W. Norton.

Fairclough, H. R., trans.
1967. "Georgics." *Virgil.* Vol. 1. Cambridge, Mass.: Harvard University Press.

Falkenrath, R. A., R. D. Newman, and B. A. Thayer.
1998. *America's Achilles' Heel: Nuclear, Biological, and Chemical Terrorism and Covert Attack.* Cambridge, Mass.: MIT Press.

Fanning, P. J.
1995. "Disease and the Politics of Community: Norwood and the Great

Flu Epidemic of 1918." Ph.D. diss., Dept. of Sociology, Boston College.

Felgenhauer, P.
1998a.   "Everything They Are Saying about Us Is a Myth." *Novye Izvestiya*. March 4, 4.
1998b.   "Biological Arms Bogeyman." *Moscow Times*. March 9, 3.

Feshbach, M.
1999.   "Dead Souls." *The Atlantic Monthly*, January: 26–27.

Feshbach, M., and A. Friendly.
1991.   *Ecocide in the USSR: Health and Nature Under Siege*. New York: Basic.

Field, M. G.
1967.   *Soviet Socialized Medicine. An Introduction*. New York: Free Press.

Filtzer, D.
1986.   *Soviet Workers and Stalinist Industrialization: The Formation of Modern Soviet Production Relations 1928–1941*. Armonk, N.Y.: M. E. Sharpe.

Fitzgerald, R., trans.
1974.   *The Iliad*. New York: Doubleday.

Fleck, Ludwig.
1979 [1934]. *Genesis and Development of a Scientific Fact*. Trans. F. Bradley and T. J. Trenn. Chicago: University of Chicago Press.

Foucault, M.
1994.   *The Birth of the Clinic: An Archaeology of Medical Perception*. Trans. A. M. Sheridan Smith. New York: Vintage Books.

Franz, D. R., P. B. Jarhling, A. M. Friedlander, D. J. McClain, D. L. Hoover, W. R. Bryne, J. A. Pavlin, G. W. Christopher, and E. M. Eitzen.
1997.   "Clinical Recognition and Management of Patients Exposed to Biological Warfare Agents." *Journal of the American Medical Association* 278, no. 5:399–411.

Freedom House Information Service.
1980.   "Eyewitness Confirms 1,000 Deaths from Germ-Warfare Explosion in USSR; Clifford Case Expresses Concern at the Soviets' Breach of Agreement." New York, July 11.

Friedlander, A. D., S. L. Welkos, M. L. M. Pitt, J. W. Ezzell, P. L. Worsham, K. J. Rose, B. E. Ivins, J. R. Lowe, G. B. Howe, P. Mikesell, and W. B. Lawrence.
1993.   "Postexposure Prophylaxis against Experimental Inhalation Anthrax." *Journal of Infectious Diseases* 167:1239–42.

Frolov, D.
1992.   "Russia Promises to Discontinue Production of Bacteriological Weapons: Military Maintains That Americans Confused Them with Veterinary Scientists." *Nezavisimaya Gazieta* 2 (December):6.

Gans, H.
1982.   *The Urban Villagers*. New York: Free Press.

Geison, G. L.
　1995.　　　*The Private Science of Louis Pasteur*. Princeton, N.J.: Princeton
　　　　　　　University Press.
Gelb, L.
　1981.　　　"Keeping an Eye on Russia: A Mysterious Event Has Raised Se-
　　　　　　　rious Doubts about Arms-Treaty Surveillance." *New York Times
　　　　　　　Magazine*, November 29, 31–33, 59–69.
Gerz, Bill.
　1992.　　　"Defecting Russian Scientist Revealed Biological Arms Efforts."
　　　　　　　Washington Times, July 4, A4.
Giddens, A.
　1991.　　　*Modernity and Self-Identity: Self and Society in the Late Mod-
　　　　　　　ern Age*. Stanford, Calif.: Stanford University Press.
Glassman, H. N.
　1966.　　　"Discussion." *Bacteriologic Review* 30:657–59.
Goffman, I.
　1967.　　　*Interaction Ritual: Essays in Face-to-Face Behavior.* Chicago: Aldine.
Gogol, N.
　1923.　　　*Dead Souls*. Trans. C. Garnett. New York: Modern Library.
Gold, Hal.
　1996.　　　*Unit 731 Testimony*. Tokyo: Yenbooks
Gold, Herman.
　1955.　　　"Anthrax: A Report of 117 Cases." *Archives of Internal Medi-
　　　　　　　cine* 96:387–96.
Goldman, M.
　1992.　　　*What Went Wrong with Perestroika*. New York: W. W. Norton.
Golts, A.
　1992.　　　"Military Biology: Hardly Any Secrets Remain. But How to Get
　　　　　　　Rid of Suspicions?" *Kraznaya Zvezda*, September 29, 3.
Gomes, E. H.
　1911.　　　*Seventeen Years Among the Sea Dyaks of Borneo*. Philadelphia:
　　　　　　　J. B. Lippincott.
Goodenough, W. H.
　1996.　　　"Navigation in the Western Carolines: A Traditional Science."
　　　　　　　In *Naked Science: Anthropological Inquiry into Boundaries,
　　　　　　　Power, and Knowledge*. ed. L. Nader. New York: Routledge.
Goodenough, W. H., and S. D. Thomas.
　1987.　　　"Traditional Navigation in the Western Pacific." *Expedition* 29,
　　　　　　　no. 3:3–14.
Gorbunova, M. M.
　1968.　　　"A Case of Recovery from Intestinal Anthrax." *Zhurnal Mikro-
　　　　　　　biologiy, Epidemiologiy, i Immunobiologiy* 45, no. 3:150.
Gordin, M. D.
　1997.　　　"The Anthrax Solution: The Sverdlovsk Incident and the Reso-
　　　　　　　lution of a Biological Weapons Controversy." *Journal of the His-
　　　　　　　tory of Biology* 30:441–80.

Gordon, A.
    1997.   *Ghostly Matters: Haunting and the Sociological Imagination.*
                 Minneapolis, University of Minnesota Press.
Graham, L.
    1993.   *The Ghost of the Executed Engineer: Technology and the Fall of
                 the Soviet Union.* Cambridge, Mass.: Harvard University Press.
Grandin, T.
    1994.   *Thinking in Pictures and Other Reports from My Life with
                 Autism.* Boston: Beacon Press.
Gray, F. du P.
    1989.   *Soviet Women: Walking the Tightrope.* New York: Doubleday.
Guillemin, J.
    1998.   "Detecting Anthrax: What We Learned from the 1979 Sverdlovsk
                 Outbreak." NATO Advanced Research Workshop, Prague, Czech
                 Republic, October 15.
Guillemin, J. H., and L. L. Holmstrom.
    1986.   *Mixed Blessings: Intensive Care for Newborns.* New York: Ox-
                 ford University Press.
Gusterson, H.
    1996.   *Nuclear Rites: An Anthropologist Among Weapons Scientists.*
                 Berkeley: University of California Press.
Hanna, P.
    1998.   "Lethal Toxin Activities and Their Consequences." Paper pre-
                 sented at the Third International Conference on Anthrax, Uni-
                 versity of Plymouth, U.K., September 9.
Hanna, P. C., D. Acosta, and R. J. Collier.
    1993.   "On the Role of Macrophages in Anthrax." *Proceedings of the
                 National Academy of Science* 90, no. 10 (November):198–201.
Harris, E.
    1987.   "Sverdlovsk and Yellow Rain: Two Cases of Soviet Noncompli-
                 ance." *International Security* 11, no. 4:41–95.
    1992.   "Preliminary Transcript of Brookings Meetings on Sverdlovsk."
                 Brookings Institute, Washington, D. C., July 2. Photocopy.
Harris, R., and J. Paxman.
    1982.   *A Higher Form of Killing: The Secret Story of Chemical and Bi-
                 ological Warfare.* New York: Hill and Wang.
Harris, S. H.
    1994.   *Factories of Death: Japanese Biological Warfare 1932–45 and the
                 American Cover-up.* London: Routledge.
Hasenauer, H.
    1998.   "Anthrax Update." *Soldier* 53, no. 9:16–17.
Henderson, D. A.
    1998.   "Bioterrorism as a Public Health Threat." *Emerging Infectious
                 Diseases* 4, no. 3 (July/September):488–92.
Henderson, D. W., S. Peacock, and F. C. Belton.
    1956.   "Observations on the Prophylaxis of Experimental Pulmonary
                 Anthrax in the Monkey." *Journal of Hygiene* 54:28–36.

Hersh, S.

1998.   *Against All Enemies: Gulf War Syndrome, The War Between America's Ailing Veterans and Their Government.* New York: Ballantine Books.

Herspring, D. R.

1990.   *The Soviet High Command 1967–1989.* Princeton, N.J.: Princeton University Press.

Heymann, D. L., and G. R. Rodier.

1998.   "Global Surveillance of Communicable Diseases." *Emerging Infectious Diseases* 4, no. 3:362–65.

Hingley, R.

1977.   *The Russian Mind.* New York: Scribner.

Hirsch, W.

1951.   *Soviet BW and CW Preparations and Capabilities.* Washington, D.C.: U.S. Department of Defense, May 15.

Hochschild, A.

1994.   *The Unquiet Ghost: Russians Remember Stalin.* New York: Viking.

Hokanson, K.

1998.   "Pushkin's Captive Crimea: Imperialism in *The Fountain of Bakhchisarai.*" In *Russian Subjects: Empire, Nation, and the Culture of the Golden Age,* ed. M. Greenleaf and S. Moeller-Sally. Evanston, Ill.: Northwestern University Press.

Holton, G.

1986.   *The Advancement of Science and Its Burdens.* Cambridge, Mass.: Harvard University Press.

Horowitz. I. L.

1989.   "The Texture of Terrorism: Socialization, Routinization, and Integration." In *Political Learning in Adulthood: A Sourcebook of Theory and Research,* ed. R. S. Sigel. Chicago: University of Chicago Press.

Hughes, E. C.

1984.   "Good People and Dirty Work." In *The Sociological Eye: Collected Papers of Everett Cherington Hughes.* New Brunswick, N.J.: Transaction.

Inkeles, A., and R. Bauer.

1961.   *The Soviet Citizen: Daily Life in a Totalitarian Society.* Cambridge, Mass.: Harvard University Press.

Istock, C. A.

1998.   "Bad Medicine." *Perspectives,* November/December, 21–23.

Jackson, P. J., M. Hugh-Jones, D. M. Adair, G. Green, K. K. Hill, C. R Kuske, L. M. Grinberg, F. A. Abramova, and P. Keim.

1997.   "PCR Analysis of Tissue Samples from the 1979 Sverdlovsk Anthrax Victims: The Presence of Multiple *Bacillus anthracis* Strains in Different Victims." *Proceedings of the National Academy of Sciences* 179:818–24.

Jones, E.
1989.   *Red Army and Society: A Sociology of the Soviet Military*. Boston:
           Allen & Unwin.

Kaldor, M.
1998.   *New and Old Wars*. Stanford, Calif.: Stanford University Press.

Kaldor, M., U. Albrecht, and G. Schméder, eds.
1998.   *Restructuring the Global Military Sector*. Vol. 2, *The End of Mil-
           itary Fordism*. London: Pinter.

Katzenbach, N. de B.
1973.   "Foreign Policy, Public Opinion, and Secrecy." *Foreign Affairs*
           52: 1–19.

Keegan, J.
1977.   *The Face of Battle*. New York: Viking.

Keller, E. F.
1985.   *Reflections on Science and Gender*. New Haven: Yale University
           Press.

Keller, S.
1968.   *The Urban Neighborhood*. New York: Random House.

Kelly, R. J.
1998.   "Armed Prophets and Extremists: Islamic Fundamentalism." In
           Kushner 1998.

Khubova, D., A. Ivankiev, and T. Sharova.
1992.   "After Glasnost: Oral History in the Soviet Union." In Passerini
           1992.

Kolesov, S. G., ed.
1976.   *Sibirskaya Yazva (Anthrax)*. Moscow: Editions Kolos. Trans.
           1981, Foreign Broadcast Information Service, December 5.

Kotkin, S.
1995.   *Magnetic Mountain: Stalinism as Civilization*. Berkeley: Univer-
           sity of California Press.

Kuran, T.
1995.   *Private Truths, Public Lies: The Social Consequences of Pref-
           erence Falsification*. Cambridge, Mass: Harvard University
           Press.

Kushner, H. W., ed.
1998.   *The Future of Terrorism: Violence in a New Millennium*. Thou-
           sand Oaks, Calif.: Sage Publications.

Langmuir, A. D.
1961.   "Epidemiology of Airborne Infection." *Bacteriology Reviews*
           25:173–81.

Laquer, W.
1996.   "Postmodern Terrorism." *Foreign Affairs*, September–October,
           24–36.

Leitenberg, M.
1991.   "A Return to Sverdlovsk: Allegations of Soviet Activities Related
           to Biological Weapons." *Arms Control* 12, no. 2:161–90.

Levin, B.
    1998.   "The Patriot Movement: Past, Present and Future." In Kushner 1998.

Lévi-Strauss, C.
    1982.   "Science—Forever Incomplete." In *Anthropological Realities. Readings in the Science of Culture*, ed. J. Guillemin. New Brunswick, N. J.: Transaction Books.

Liddington, R.
    1998.   "Crystallographic Studies of Anthrax Lethal Toxin." Paper presented at the Third International Conference on Anthrax, University of Plymouth, U.K., September 9.

Lifton, R. J.
    1993.   *The Protean Self: Human Resilience in an Age of Fragmentation.* New York: Basic Books.

Lilienfeld, A. M., and D. E. Lilienfield.
    1980.   *Foundations of Epidemiology.* New York: Oxford University Press.

Litovkin, V., and K. Eggert.
    1992.   "Biological Research Is of Course a Secret, But Not a Military One." *Izvestiya,* September 1, 2–3.

MacMahon, B., and T. Pugh.
    1970.   *Epidemiology: Principles and Methods.* Boston: Little, Brown and Company.

Manchee, R. J., M. G. Broster, J. Melling, R. M. Henstridge, and A. J. Stagg.
    1981.   "*Bacillus anthracis* on Gruinard Island." *Nature* 294: 254–55.

Manchee, R. J., M. G. Broster, A. J. Stagg, and S. E. Hibbs.
    1994.   "Formaldehyde Solution Effectively Inactivates Spores of Bacillus-Anthracis on the Scottish Island of Gruinard." *Applied and Environmental Microbiology* 60, no. 11:4167–71.

Mandelstam, O.
    1983.   *Selected Poems.* Trans. C. Brown and W. S. Merwin. New York: Atheneum.

Manoff, R.
    1995.   "Understanding the Soviet Other: Speculations on the End of History, the End of the Cold War, and the End of Journalism." In *The Conditions of Reciprocal Understanding,* ed. J. W. Fernandez and M. B. Singer. Chicago: The Center for International Studies, University of Chicago.

Martin, E.
    1994.   *Flexible Bodies. Tracking Immunity in American Culture from the Days of Polio to the Age of AIDS.* Boston: Beacon.

McNeill, W. H.
    1977.   *Plagues and People.* New York: Doubleday.

Merton, R.
    1938.   "Science and the Social Order." *Philosophy of Science* 5:321–27.

1957.   "Priorities in Scientific Discovery: A Chapter in the Sociology of
               Science." *American Sociological Review* 22, no. 6:635–59.

Meselson, M.
1988.   "F.A.S. Public Interest Report." *Journal of the Federation of
               American Scientists* 41, no. 7:1–6.

1991a.   "Interview Regarding the 1979 Outbreak in Sverdlovsk." UPI Ra-
               dio Network series "Harvard Newsmakers." *Harvard University
               Gazette* 86 (March 8):5–6.

1991b.   "Implementing the Biological Weapons Convention of 1972."
               *UNIDIR (United Nations Institute for Disarmament Studies)
               Newsletter.* June 4, 2: 10–13.

1995.   "Note Regarding Source Strength." *ASA (Applied Science and
               Analysis) Newsletter* 48:1, 20–21.

1998.   "Distinguishing Disease Outbreaks That Are Natural from Those
               That Are Not: Some Elementary Principles of Atmospheric Dif-
               fusion Theory." Paper presented at NATO Advanced Research
               Workshop, Prague, Czech Republic, October 15.

Meselson, M., J. Guillemin, M. Hugh-Jones, A. Langmuir, I. Popova, A. Shelokov,
and O. Yampolskaya.
1994.   "The Sverdlovsk Anthrax Outbreak of 1979." *Science* 266, no.
               5188:1202–8.

Meselson, M., M. M. Kaplan, and M. A. Mokulsky.
1990.   "Verification of Biological and Toxin Weapons Disarmament."
               In *Verification: Monitoring Disarmament,* ed. F. Calogero, M. L.
               Goldberger, and S. Kapitza. Boulder, Colo. and London: West-
               view Press.

Metchnikoff, E.
1884.   "Concerning the Relationship between Phagocytes and Anthrax
               Bacilli." English trans. 1984. *Reviews of Infectious Diseases* 6:
               761–70.

Miller, D. L.
1952.   *History of Air Force Participation in Biological Warfare Program
               1944–1951.* Wright Patterson Air Force Base, Dayton, Ohio: His-
               torical Office of the Executive Air Material Command, Histori-
               cal Study No. 194, September.

Mims, C. A., N. J. Dimmock, A. Nash, and J. Stephen.
1999.   *Mims' Pathogenesis of Infectious Disease,* 4th ed. London: Aca-
               demic Press.

Muratov, D., Y. Sorokin, and V. Fronin.
1992.   "Boris Yeltsin: I Am Not Hiding the Difficulties and I Want the
               People to Understand This." *Komsomolskaya Pravda.* May 27, 2.

Nelkin, D., and S. L. Gilman.
1988.   "Placing Blame for Devastating Disease." *Social Research* 55, no.
               3:361–78.

Nikiforov, V. I.
1973.   *Koznaya Forma Sibirskaye Yazva Cheloveka (Cutaneous Anthrax
               in Humans).* Moscow: Medicinia.

Norris, J., and W. Fowler.

1997.   *NBC: Nuclear, Biological, and Chemical Weapons on the Modern Battlefield*. Cambridge, Eng.: Cambridge University Press.

Parfenov, S.

1990.   "The Secret of the 'Sarcophagus.'" *Rodina* 5 (October 24):31–40.

Pashkov, A.

1991a.   "How We Got 'Inoculated' for Anthrax: Military People in White Coats Still Are Potentially Dangerous for the Society." *Izvestiya*, November 11, 8.

1991b.   "'I Know Where the Anthrax in Sverdlovsk Came From,' A Former Counterintelligence General Informed the Editorial Office." *Izvestiya*, November 25, 4.

1991c.   "The End of the Urals Anthrax Legend." *Izvestiya*, December 11, 8.

1992.   "Military Deny Involvement in Mysterious Illness." *Izvestiya*, April 17, 7.

Passerini, L., ed.

1992.   *Memory and Totalitarianism: International Yearbook of Oral History and Life Stories*. Vol. 1. New York: Oxford University Press.

Pasternak, B.

1958.   *Dr. Zhivago*. Trans. M. Hayward, M. Harari, and B. G. Guerney. New York: Pantheon.

1961.   "On First Seeing the Urals." In *The Three Worlds of Boris Pasternak*, ed. R. Payne. New York: Coward-MCann Inc.

Pfohl, S.

1991.   *Images of Deviance and Social Control: A Sociological History*, 2nd ed. New York: McGraw-Hill.

Pomerantsev, A. P., N. A. Staritsin, L. I. Marinin, N. P. Kuzmin, T. B. Kravchenko, and A. N. Noskov.

1995.   "Immunomodulating Effect of Phospholipase C and Sphingomyelinase of *Bacillus cereus* in Protection against Anthrax." International Workshop on Anthrax, Winchester, England, September 19–21.

Pomerantsev, A. P., N. A. Staritsin, Y. V. Mockov, and L. I. Marinin.

1997.   "Expression of Cereolysine AB Genes in *Bacillus anthracis* Vaccine Strain Ensures Protection against Experimental Hemolytic Anthrax Infection." *Vaccine* 15 (December): 1846–50.

Posev.

1980.   36, no. 1 (January):7–8.

President's Air Policy Commission.

1948.   *Survival in the Air Age*. Historical Office, Office of the Executive Air Material Command files, January 1.

Preston, R.

1998.   "Annals of Warfare: The Bioweaponeers." *The New Yorker*, March 9, 2–65.

Pringle, P.
    1998.   "Bioterrorism: America's Newest War Game." *The Nation*, Oc-
                 tober 26, 1–6.
Pushkin A.
    1965.   *Little Tragedies*. Trans. E. M. Kayden. Yellow Springs, Ohio: An-
                 tioch Press.
Radzinsky, E.
    1992.   *The Last Czar: The Life and Death of Nicholas II*. Trans. M.
                 Schwartz. New York: Anchor/Doubleday.
Randolph, E.
    1996.   *Walking the Tempest: Ordinary Life in the New Russia*. New
                 York: Simon & Schuster.
Reed, J.
    1977 [1919]. *Ten Days That Shook the World*. London: Penguin.
Remnick, D.
    1994.   *Lenin's Tomb: The Last Days of the Soviet Empire*. New York:
                 Vintage.
    1998.   *Resurrection: Struggle for a New Russia*. New York: Vintage.
Robinson, J. P. P.
    1973.   *The Problem of Chemical and Biological Warfare*. Vol. 2, *CB
                 Weapons Today*. New York: Humanities Press.
    1982.   "'The Soviet Union and the Biological Weapons Convention' and
                 a Guide to Sources on the Sverdlovsk Incident." *Arms Control*
                 3:41–56.
    1985.   "Chemical and Biological Warfare: Developments in 1984." In
                 World Armaments and Disarmament, SIPRI (Stockholm Inter-
                 national Peace Research Institute) Yearbook. London: Taylor and
                 Francis.
Robinson, J. P. P., J. Guillemin, and M. Meselson.
    1987.   "Yellow Rain: The Story Collapses." *Foreign Policy* 68 (Fall):
                 100–117.
Ross, J. M.
    1957.   "The Pathogenesis of Anthrax Following the Administration of
                 Spores by the Respiratory Route." *Journal of Pathology and Bac-
                 teriology* 73:485–95.
Rothschild, J. J.
    1964.   *Tomorrow's Weapons, Chemical and Biological*. New York: Mc-
                 Graw-Hill.
Roueché, B.
    1967.   *Annals of Epidemiology*. Boston: Little, Brown and Company.
Russian Federation.
    1992.   "Law on the Improvement of the Pensioner Support to Families
                 of Citizens Deceased after Contracting Siberian Ulcer in the City
                 of Sverdlovsk in 1979." *Rossiykaya Gazieta*, April 27.
Sacks, M. P.
    1976.   *Women's Work in Soviet Russia*. New York: Praeger.

Scheper-Hughes, N.
  1979.   *Saints, Scholars, and Schizophrenics: Mental Illness in Rural Ireland*. Berkeley: University of California Press.
Schiebinger, L. L.
  1989.   *The Mind Has No Sex? Women in the Origins of Modern Science*. Cambridge, Mass.: Harvard University Press.
Seeley, T., J. Nowicke, M. Meselson, J. Guillemin, and P. Akratanakul.
  1986.   "Yellow Rain." *Scientific American* 253, no. 3:128–37.
Sennett, R.
  1974.   *The Fall of Public Man*. New York: W. W. Norton.
  1998.   *The Corrosion of Character: The Personal Consequences of Work in the New Capitalism*. New York: W. W. Norton.
Service, R.
  1998.   *A History of Twentieth-Century Russia*. Cambridge, Mass.: Harvard University Press.
Sherbakova, I.
  1992.   "The Gulag in Memory." In Passerini 1992.
Shipler, D.
  1983.   *Broken Idols, Solemn Dreams*. New York: Times Books.
Sidel, V. S., M. Nass, and T. Ensign.
  1998.   "The Anthrax Dilemma." *Medicine and Global Security* 2, no. 5 (October):97–104.
Sigerist, H. E.
  1937.   *Socialized Medicine in the Soviet Union*. New York: W. W. Norton.
Simmel, G.
  1950.   *The Sociology of Georg Simmel*. Trans. and ed. K. H. Wolff. New York: Free Press.
Smith, H.
 1984 rev. ed.   *The Russians*. New York: Ballantine Books.
Smith, H., J. Keppie, and J. L. Stanley.
  1955.   "The Chemical Basis of the Virulence of *Bacillus anthracis*." *British Journal of Experimental Pathology* 36:460–72.
Smith, R. J., with L. Shackelford.
  1992.   "Russia Fails to Detail Germ Arms: US and Britain Fear Program Continues in Violation of Treaty." *Washington Post*, August 31, A1, A15.
Snow, J.
  1855.   *On the Mode of Communication of Cholera*. London: John Churchill.
Sontag, S.
  1977.   *On Photography*. New York: Farrar, Straus, & Giroux.
Soyfer, V. S.
  1994.   *Lysenko and the Tragedy of Soviet Science*. Trans. L. Gruliow and R. Gruliow. New Brunswick, N.J.: Rutgers University Press.
Stapanian-Apkarian, J. R.
  1994.   "Ironic Vision in M. Bulgakov's *Master and Margarita*." In *Rus-*

sian Narrative and Visual Art, ed. R. Anderson and P. De-
breczeny. Gainesville: University Press of Florida.

Sterne, J.
   1999.   *The Ultimate Terrorists.* Cambridge, Mass.: Harvard University
                 Press.

Sterne, M.
   1959.   "Anthrax." In *Infectious Diseases of Animals.* Vol. 1, *Diseases
                 Due to Bacteria,* ed. A. W. Stableforth and J. A. Galloway. New
                 York: AP.

Stishova, E.
   1996.   "'Full Frontal': Perestroika and Sexual Policy." In *Women in Rus-
                 sia and the Ukraine,* ed. R. Marsh. Cambridge, Eng.: Cambridge
                 University Press.

Taylor, A. J. P.
   1977.   "Introduction." In Reed 1977.
Taubman, W., and J. Taubman.
   1989.   *Moscow Spring.* New York: Summit Books.
Tolstoy, L.
   1935.   "The Death of Ivan Ilych." In *Ivan Ilych and Hadje Murad and
                 Other Stories.* Trans. L. Maude and A. Maude. London: Oxford
                 University Press.

Tsvetaeva, M.
   1992.   *Art in the Light of Conscience: Eight Essays on Poetry by Ma-
                 rina Tsvetaeva.* Trans. A. Livingstone. Cambridge, Mass.: Har-
                 vard University Press.

Tuan, Y.
   1974.   *Topophilia: A Study of Environmental Perception, Attitudes, and
                 Values.* Englewood Cliffs, N.J.: Prentice-Hall.

   1979.   *Landscapes of Fear.* New York: Pantheon.
   1984.   *Dominance and Affection.* New Haven, Conn.: Yale University
                 Press.

Turnbull, P. C. B.
   1991.   "Anthrax Vaccines: Past, Present and Future." *Vaccine* 9 (Au-
                 gust):533–39.
UN Security Council.
   1995a.   Report of the Secretary-General on the Status of the Implemen-
                 tation of the Special Commission's Plan for the On-going Mon-
                 itoring and Verification of Iraq's Compliance with the Relevant
                 Parts of Section C of Security Council Resolution 687 (1991).
                 S/1995/864. New York: United Nations.

   1995b.   Tenth Report of the Executive Chairman of the Special Com-
                 mission Established by the Secretary-General Pursuant to Para-
                 graph 9 (b) (I) of Security Council Resolution 687 (1991) and
                 Paragraph 3 of Resolution 699 (1991) on the Activities of the
                 Special Commission. S/1995/1038. New York: United Nations.
Uralmashzarod Production Association.
   1993.   "The Generals and Anthrax." Broadcast September 19.

Urban, M.
　1996.　　*UK Eyes Alpha: Inside British Intelligence*. London: Faber and
　　　　　Faber.
U.S. Army.
　1954.　　Munition Expenditure Panel, St. Jo Program. *Preliminary Dis-
　　　　　cussion of Methods for Calculating Munition Expenditures, with
　　　　　Special Reference to the St. Jo Program*. Camp Detrick, Md.
U.S. Senate.
　1995.　　*Hearings on the Global Proliferation of Weapons of Mass De-
　　　　　struction: A Case Study of the Aum Shinrikyo*. October 31.
　1996.　　Committee on Governmental Affairs. *Global Proliferation of
　　　　　Weapons of Mass Destruction*. Washington D.C.: Government
　　　　　Printing Office. Part I.
U.S. War Department.
　1945.　　*A Review of German Activities in the Field of Biological War-
　　　　　fare*. September 12. Washington, D.C.
Vaughan, D.
　1996.　　*The Challenger Launch Decision: Risky Technology, Culture, and
　　　　　Desire at NASA*. New York: Oxford University Press.
Veterinaria.
　1980.　　10:3.
Walker, D. L., L. Grinberg, and O. Yampolskaya.
　1993.　　"Death at Sverdlovsk: What Have We Learned?" *American Jour-
　　　　　nal of Pathology* 144, no. 6:1135–41.
Wallace, A. F. C.
　1956.　　*Tornado in Worcester: An Exploratory Study of Individual and
　　　　　Community Behavior in an Extreme Situation*. Disaster Study
　　　　　No. 3. Washington: National Research Council Committee on
　　　　　Disaster Studies, National Academy of Sciences.
Walter, E. V.
　1969.　　*Terror and Resistance: A Study of Political Violence*. New York:
　　　　　Oxford University Press.
Watts, S.
　1997.　　*Epidemics and History: Disease, Power, and Imperialism*. New
　　　　　Haven, Conn.: Yale University Press.
Weissmann, G.
　1998.　　"Inflammation as Cultural History." In *Darwin's Audubon: Sci-
　　　　　ence and the Liberal Imagination. New and Selected Essays*. New
　　　　　York: Plenum.
Wellock, C. E.
　1960.　　"Epidemiology of Q Fever in the Urban East Bay Area." *Cali-
　　　　　fornia's Health* 18, no. 10 (November 15):73–76.
Wellock, C. E., and M. F. Parker.
　1959.　　"An Urban Outbreak of Q Fever in Northern California." Mimeo.
Williams, P., and D. Wallace.
　1989.　　*Unit 731: Japan's Secret Biological Warfare in World War II*. New
　　　　　York: Free Press.

Wolfenstein, M.
   1957.   *Disaster: A Psychological Essay.* Glencoe, Ill.: Free Press.
Wolff, K.
   1976.   *Surrender and Catch: Experience and Inquiry Today.* Boston: D. Reidel.
World Health Organization.
   1991.   *Report of WHO Consultation Group on Anthrax Control and Research.* November 13–15. Geneva: World Health Organization.
   1993.   *Guidelines for Surveillance and Control of Anthrax in Humans and Animals.* Geneva: World Health Organization.
Yeltsin, B.
   1992a.   *Against the Grain: An Autobiography.* Trans. M. Glenny. New York: Summit Books.
   1992b.   Interview in *Komsomolskaya Pravda,* May 27.
Young, G. A., Jr., M. R. Zelle, and R. E. Lincoln.
   1946.   "Respiratory Pathogenicity of *Bacillus anthracis* Spores. I. Methods of Study and Observation on Pathogenesis." *Journal of Infectious Diseases* 79:233–46.
Zhenova, N.
   1990a.   "Military Secret: Reasons for the Tragedy in Sverdlovsk Must Be Investigated." *Literaturnaya Gazieta,* August 22, 12.
[Zenova]. 1990b. "The Deadly Cloud over Sverdlovsk." *Wall Street Journal,* November 28, A22.
   1991a.   "Military Secret. Part II. More on Alleged Sverdlovsk Bacteriological Accident." *Literaturnaya Gazieta,* October 2, 6.
   1991b.   "Continuing a Topic: Once Again on the 'Military Secrets.'" *Literaturnaya Gazieta,* November 13, 2.
Zilinskas, R. A.
   1997.   "Iraq's Biological Weapons: The Past as Future?" *Journal of the American Medical Association* 278, no. 5:418–24.
Zisk, K. M.
   1993.   *Engaging the Enemy: Organization Theory and Soviet Military Innovation, 1955–1991.* Princeton, N.J.: Princeton University Press.
   1997.   *Weapons, Culture, and Self-Interest: Soviet Defense Managers in the New Russia.* New York: Columbia University Press.

Index

Abramova, Faina, 20, 44, 50, 51, 52, 53, 54, 55, 196; author's dream about, 56, 97; autopsy notes of, 109, 140; collaboration and, 69, 76–77, 140; controversy between Burgasov and, 96; gathering of autopsy material and, 127; identification of disease by, 132; life of, 96; professional findings of, 20, 73–74, 130, 222, 284n1, 290n4; records and, 60; state authority and, 232–33; tissue samples and, 70–75, 130; victim addresses and, 108; visit to Hospital 40 and, 259–60

Abramovo (village), 22, 200, 201–5, 234

Abuladze, Tengiz, 124

Abusagitov, Zinatulla (victim), 215–16

age, as risk factor, 237. *See also* children

AIDS, 245, 261

airborne hypothesis: autopsy evidence for, 31; burning of carcasses and, 78, 111; ceramics factory workers and, 99; children and, 65; Compound 19 and, 111; criticisms of, 223; local beliefs and, 83, 88; Nikiforov, 17; path of anthrax aerosol and, 211–12; Russian views on, 46; Soviet public health response and, 14, 15; spore quantity and, 9, 79, 240–42; 1980 U.S. working group and, 9; vaccine research and, 107–8. *See also* inhalation anthrax

Akhmatova, Anna, 269

Albrink, Wilhelm, 19, 73, 79, 93, 288n3

Alfred (curator), 265

Alibek, Ken, 187, 192–93, 290n6

Alibekov, Kanatjan. *See* Alibek, Ken

American Embassy in Russia, debriefing at, 158

animal outbreak. *See* epizootic

anthrax hoaxes, 249–50

anthrax infection in animals, 2–3. *See also* epizootic

anthrax infection in humans: bacterial strains in Sverdlovsk outbreak, 197, 252–53; diagnostic characteristics of, 17, 18–19, 87–88; dose calculations and, 9, 240–42; forms of, 4–5; human response to, 17, 31; incubation period and, 26, 27–28, 189, 230; individual reactions and, 141–42, 143–44, 189, 237; international code for (022), 133; lethal components of, 32; primary lesion school, 72–73; risk calculation and, 156; survival rate and, 242; symptoms of, 14, 32. See also *Bacillus anthracis*

anthrax outbreaks, historic: in industrialized nations, 34; in Russia, 33–34, 261–62

anthrax research: aerosol challenges and, 224, 225; airborne hypothesis and, 111–12, 224–26; animal research process and, 107–8; for defensive purposes, 7; lack of, 19, 189; scientific interest and, 5–6; vaccine development in Russia and, 34, 107–8, 195–96, 252–53. *See also* biological weapons research

Antigua, British West Indies, 57

Text: 10/13 Sabon
Display: Grotesque
Composition: Integrated Composition Systems, Inc.
Printing and binding: Sheridan Books